W9-DCA-417

Double *the* Power

of Your

Immune System

⚡John Heinerman⚡

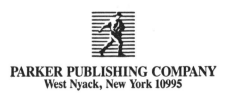

PARKER PUBLISHING COMPANY
West Nyack, New York 10995

© 1991 *by*

PARKER PUBLISHING COMPANY, INC.
West Nyack, New York

All rights reserved. No part of this book
may be reproduced in any form or by any means,
without permission in writing from the publisher.

10 9 8 7 6 5 4 3 2 1

This book is a reference work based on research by the author. The opinions expressed herein are not necessarily those of or endorsed by the publisher. The directions stated in this book are in no way to be considered as a substitute for consultation with a duly licensed doctor.

Library of Congress Cataloging-in-Publication Data

Heinerman, John.
    Double the power of your immune system / John Heinerman
      p. cm.
    Includes index.

    1. Natural immunity--Popular works. 2. Medicine, Popular.
3. Health. I. Title
QR185.2.H45 1991
613--dc20   91-15192
                                                      CIP

ISBN 0-13-218025-1

ISBN 0-13-218017-0 (pbk)

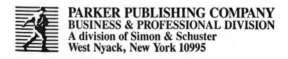

PARKER PUBLISHING COMPANY
BUSINESS & PROFESSIONAL DIVISION
A division of Simon & Schuster
West Nyack, New York 10995

Printed in the United States of America

Other Books by the Author

Heinerman's Encyclopedia of Fruits, Vegetables, and Herbs

Joseph Smith & Herbal Medicine

The Treatment of Cancer with Herbs (I)

East/West Cancer Remedies for Wellness & Recovery (II & III) (co-authored with Dr. Henry Yun)

The Complete Book of Spices

Herbal Research Manual for Professional Therapeutics

The Herbal Pharmacy

Herbal Dynamics

Spiritual Wisdom of the Native American

People in Space

Understanding Herbal Medicine & Natural Childbirth (co-authored with E. P Donatelle, M.D.)

Basic Natural Nutrition (Edited with co-authors: E. P. Donatelle, M.D., Lendon Smith, M.D., Vaughn Bryant, Ph.D.)

Bible Nutrition & Medicine

Folk Remedies from Around the World

Martyr's Glory The Life & Times of David W Patten

Health Secrets from Ancient Empires

(plus 17 other titles)

To

Matthew and Jason Fountaine

Love and peace, joy and truth,
Characterize their simple youth.
And I am privileged above all
Them as my *dearest* friends to call.
If we had more of their nobility,
This world would see far less hostility.
True Brotherhood, as I know it,
Are for both pair a perfect fit.
They are, as wise men and prophets might say,
Men for our time, and a hope for today.

Introduction

A FEW YEARS AGO a young woman wrote to me from Minneapolis, Minnesota. Part of her letter asked about where to obtain more information about the immune system. "Before you start recommending a whole bunch of titles for me to read up on about immunity," she wrote, "let me say that I'm looking for a book on *how to take care* of my immune system." She complained that almost all of the books she had previously consulted told how the immune system worked, but said virtually nothing about how to take care of it. "What we *really* need," she pleaded, "is something that tells you *what to do* about improving your resistance to disease."

That letter was the catalyst for this book—a volume you can use for reliable, up-to-date information on taking care of yourself better. This is information that you can work with and put into action—down-to-earth, practical, needed by all of us for one thing or another. This isn't just another book to read through once and then leave on a shelf. *Use* it; thumb through it, mark it up, turn the corners down, circle the subheads, make notes in the margins. Keep it with the books you use often—your favorite cookbook, your dictionary, or atlas, or almanac, or your Bible. Use this book as a manual for the maintenance of the health and welfare of your human body.

Here you'll find *natural* ways to build the power of your immune system to help your body fight diseases before they occur and to treat them in the event they do Here you'll find:

- the facts about candidiasis
- ten ways to cope with a cold
- herbs, spices, and other foods to help manage diabetes
- natural ways to overcome addictions to drugs, alcohol, caffeine, tobacco, and other addictive substances
- what to do to get a good night's sleep
- how to conquer your allergies

- what effects today's environment has on your immune system and how to defend your body against ecological illness
- power eating recipes to fight infection

These easy-to-follow strategies will allow you to incorporate these immune-building programs into your daily life.

If you want to start taking charge of your own health care for a change instead of leaving it to the medical profession (except in the case of dangerous illnesses, obviously), then this book is for you. It gives you tried-and-proven methods for multiplying your own immune strength—a real, hands-on approach to health care that provides solutions instead of just facts.

So, while I wish to see this wonderful volume treated with consideration and respect, I encourage you to use it freely as you need to. Don't be afraid to mess it up a little. Make it your own personal "yellow pages" health guide to remedy whatever might be ailing you.

John Heinerman

Contents

Anger 263

Hostility Can Ruin More than Your Day, 263 ✦ *Anger Injures Immunity, 264* ✦ *Anger: A Lethal Disease, 265* ✦ *How to Get Rid of Anger, 265*

Bubonic Plague 267

Is the "Black Death" Coming Back?, 267 ✦ *Plague Prevention: "Four Thieves Vinegar," 269*

Cancer 270

The Four Major Cancers, 270 ✦ *Is Cancer an Epidemic?, 270* ✦ *Herbs That Help Fight Cancer, 271* ✦ *Tijuana Cancer Clinic's "Recovery Diet," 276* ✦ *A Cancer Treatment Diet, 276* ✦ *How the Mind Can Help the Body Fight Cancer, 279*

Hepatitis 281

Knowing Your Disease Alphabet, 281 ✦ *A Canadian Doctor's Program for Treating Liver Problems, 282*

Tuberculosis 284

Resurgence of an Old Public Health Menace, 284 ✦ *Herbal Treatments for Tuberculosis, 285*

Summary 288

CHAPTER 8 ✦ "POWER EATING" WITH RECIPES TO FIGHT INFECTION 289

AIDS and Cancer 290
Allergies 292
Asthma and Bronchitis 296
Candidiasis 297
Chickenpox, Measles, and Mumps 301

Common Infections and How to Combat Them

IN REVIEWING the many different types of infectious diseases that afflict millions of people every month in this country, I decided to focus on just three major kinds in this opening chapter. All of them are pervasive and extremely difficult to control and properly manage. They are

1. The common cold
2. Influenza
3. Candidiasis (yeast overgrowth)

Quite possibly, these are the three most common infections that assault our bodies in one form or another, thereby weakening our immune defenses. The different microorganisms responsible for each of them may be found in the air we breathe, the water we drink, the food we eat, and the people we meet on a daily basis. Medical science hasn't found clear-cut and lasting cures for any of them, only temporary means at best for *trying* to hold them in check.

The many recommendations provided here have been proven to be efficacious about 85% of the time. They are all relatively simple to follow and, when prudently applied will give results with a minimum of discomfort. However, should your symptoms become critical or not go away in a reasonable amount of time, then prompt medical assistance should be obtained without further delay.

◆◆◆◆◆

THE COMMON COLD

Even a Doctor's Cold Can Be Cured Naturally

I recall an amusing incident a couple of years ago. I was playing golf with a doctor buddy at one of the local greens here in the Salt Lake Valley. Dr. G. had been repeatedly blowing his nose and clearing his throat in between our respective swings. I casually remarked, "Got a bad one, huh?" "Yeh," he growled in disgust. "Tried everything I can think of, but the damn thing just won't go away."

After hitting a beauty right in line with the hole I needed to get, I grinned and said, "You're the doctor." He retorted with, "Next thing I know you'll be quoting that scripture which says 'Physician, heal thyself.' " Then, needling me in a gruff but friendly way, he added: "You're the resident author here of self-help health books. Got any ideas?"

Well, after his putt, we sauntered on over to the next little knoll, chatting as we went. Dr. G. told me he'd had this cold "going on nearly four weeks." Aspirin, antibiotics, fluids, vitamins—nothing seemed to phase it. Finally, when I asked him how much sleep he'd been getting recently, he mumbled something about five hours a night.

"There's your prescription," I chimed. "Get 10 hours of good, solid sleep for about four to five days and you'll feel like a million bucks!" At first, he just kind of stood there in disbelief, not quite knowing what to say. "Just sleep is all?" he asked incredulously. "Sure," I said with a positive tone in my voice. "Why not? You've tried just about everything else and you still have your cold. What do you have to lose with this?" "Nothing, I guess," he responded.

I reminded him that often the simplest things are by far the best solutions to the most complex problems. "If I had suggested a long list of medications or food supplements, you probably would have accepted them more readily than something so apparently modest as sleep." He nodded in agreement. "This has *always* been the very *first* thing I recommend to anyone with a cold," I finished. "And it's *never* failed yet to knock out even the most stubborn germs!"

About a week later, he dropped by my research center for a quick hello and brief thank you. "You're right," he said before leaving the office. "I slowed down long enough to grab myself some extra zzzz's for a couple of days and that seemed to do the trick!" I didn't have the heart to tell Dr. G. that this remedy had come to me by way of the late Mrs. Marshall—once one of Jamaica's top folk healers and leading *voodoo* practitioners! Even the most broad-minded physicians have limitations to just how much they will or won't believe, and I wasn't about to test his any further.

Cracking a Cold's Secrets

In the last few years a great deal of research has been done on one of humanity's most irksome ailments. From mid-1980 to the beginning of this decade, scientists all over the country have been unraveling some of the mysteries surrounding the common cold. Here are some of the latest findings:

• Normal folks get 100 colds in their lifetimes, averaging two a year. Kids can catch as many as a dozen a year, though. The 1987 National Health Survey showed that colds cause almost 80% of 100 U.S. males and about 96% of every 100 females to miss at least two days of work or school annually.

• Colds are caused by viruses. These are small packets of genetic information enveloped in a coating of proteins that thrive in the relatively warm environment of the nose, about 91.4°F. The coat of each "cold" rhinovirus contains sites that can locate and attach themselves to cell "receptors" in the host, in this case in the upper respiratory system. There are more than 100 known strains of cold viruses.

• According to the January 1987 *Journal of Infectious Diseases*, proteins called kinins seem to be the chief cause of painful nasal congestion evidence of a nasty head cold. Released from plasma proteins activated by enzymes, kinins in the blood cause expansion of blood vessels, which permits fluid to leak into surrounding tissue. This fluid accumulation and its pressure on nerve endings is responsible for characteristic cold symptoms. Kinin levels increase as cold symptoms appear and then decrease as these same symptoms gradually fade away. And while kinin levels increased 20- to 80-fold in those afflicted with colds, there was *not* a corresponding rise in the level of histamines (proteins released by tissue cells during allergic attacks that also dilate blood vessels). This suggests that antihistamines are virtually worthless as far as effective cold remedies go.

• Colds slowed motor performance in a hand-eye coordination test but didn't affect performance in a visual search exercise. On the other hand, flu impaired the visual task but not the motor one. Relatively minor bouts of cold or flu can significantly hamper people whose duties require a high level of attention or hand-eye coordination.

• *Psychological Medicine* (Vol. 18, 1989, p. 65) observes that while the symptoms of cold and flu are greatest in the morning, the greatest impairment of performance takes place in the afternoon. And *The Milbank Memorial Fund Quarterly* (Vol. 30, Jan. 1952, p. 41) noted that colds in the early autumn were much milder than are those occurring in the later winter months, and that there are specific colds in the spring and summer months that require treatment *different* from those in the fall and winter.

• In the past scientific studies concluded that skin contact was the primary mode of transmission for the common cold. But no more, as Elliot Dick's research from the University of Wisconsin in Madison has shown. Now it's believed that *airborne* particles play a significant role in passing the infection along to others. In several early experiments, healthy poker players caught colds from their infected confederates, who sneezed and coughed periodically throughout several lengthy games. But in a final test, another dozen healthy players were put into a room where no aerosol transmission was possible. They used the same contaminated cards, chips, and pencils from previous games. Once every hour more freshly contaminated materials were delivered to them, but *none* of these players ever caught colds. Dick and his team concluded that the aerosol route spreads cold germs faster than skin contact does.

Ten Ways To Cope with a Cold

Now that we've learned some of the mechanics behind a cold's behavior, a variety of effective applications can be investigated here. All of the items listed have been successfully employed thousands of times over by those who've been bothered with colds. They are safe and simple when followed to the letter! The numerical rankings for each do not necessarily reflect their priority of importance.

1. Get plenty of rest. So says Walt Harrison, M.D., a pediatrician practicing in Jackson, Tennessee. "The drugstores are full of ineffective cold medicine," he reported. "But there's nothing like sleep—lots of it—to get over a cold."

2. Avoid prescription and over-the-counter (OTC) medications. "I think the worst thing we can do is put everybody on antibiotics for a cold," warned Dan Marshall, M.D., a staff physician at the University of Tennessee Health Services in Memphis. He told a reporter from the Scripps Howard News Service that "people think you can get a shot of penicillin, but antibiotics only work on bacteria and colds are only caused by viruses."

Furthermore, cold viruses keep changing every year. This constant evolution means that most cold and flu shots are rendered pretty much invalid when next year's new mutated strains roll around. As *Hippocrates* health magazine for November/ December 1988 correctly pointed out, you are better off catching a cold now and developing natural immunity against future infections "than the protection any vaccine could provide."

3. Do not eat in public places such as fast-food restaurants and the like. So wrote Victor G. Heizer, M.D., in his national best-seller of a half-century ago, *Toughen Up, America!* (New York: Whittlesey House, 1941). Food prepared by those who already have colds is one of the main ways in which these viruses are spread. This was amply demonstrated, he observed, in a highly interesting experiment conducted with apes. Some 15 healthy ones completely devoid of cold germs were isolated in separate rooms and attended by keepers who also were free of cold viruses. The apes were then fed one meal prepared by someone with an acute head cold. Neither the attendants nor the apes saw or came in contact with the infected person. Within two days *all* of the apes developed some degree of cold, from severe cases to coughs and 10-day sniffles.

Forks and spoons, warned Dr. Heizer, also transport cold viruses unless they are adequately sterilized. The same thing goes for cups and glasses, requiring a *minimum* of 5 minutes exposure to boiling water in order for the viruses to be completely killed.

4. "Make a conscious effort to keep your nerves steady; try not to worry!" Dr. Heizer advised. More up-to-date research has shown just how true this can be. A study of Western Electric employees in 1960 demonstrated that high job stress in some invited colds more easily than did low job stress in others. According to the *Journal of the American Medical Association* (Vol. 177, 1960, pp. 247–248) college graduates from business school moved directly into positions of company management, showed fewer incidents (89) of colds, than did high school graduates promoted from blue-collar factory work into similar management positions, who had far more colds (136 cases). The inevitable conclusion reached by Drs. W. N. Christenson and L. E. Hinkle, who conducted this research, was that the college graduates came from backgrounds that had already equipped them for the demanding rigors of corporate life, whereas the promoted blue-collar workers were suddenly thrust into the same environment and wholly unprepared for the greatly increased pressures that went with their new jobs.

More recently, Drs. George Solomon and John Morley, with the UCLA School of Medicine, have studied the interaction between stress and immune functions in healthy elderly people. In their research they discovered that the level of "natural killer" (NK) cells in the body depended a lot upon a person's emotional "hardiness" in response to life events. Now, NK cells are some of the system's most ardent fighters, helping to keep infection out of the body. Those elderly folks who didn't worry a lot, had the highest levels of NK cell activity, whereas those who were depressed or continually frustrated with life in general had the lowest NK cell counts and were sick more often. Thus, Dr. Heizer's advice is very timely for either preventing or treating a cold. Wakunaga's Kyo-Green (see the appendix) is good for this (2 tbsp. in 10 fl. oz. water).

5. The important thing with colds is to thin secretions; otherwise when they thicken, they tend to clog sinuses and ears. So reported Dr. Harrison of Jackson, Tennessee. Hot fluids seem to be especially valuable. Heading the list, of course, is grandma's proverbial chicken soup. In 1978 Marvin A. Sackner, M.D., of Mount Sinai Hospital in Miami Beach, Florida, found that hot chicken or fish soup did a fantastic job of clearing out mucus from the nasal passages of patients suffering from colds and related respiratory problems. Then a few years later, the *Mayo Clinic Health Letter* (September 24–28, 1984) gave a strong endorsement of its own for this very traditional remedy, saying that the soup ought to be homemade with spices like cayenne pepper, garlic and onions, a few vegetables such as carrots and celery, and some noodles but no meat. (See Chapter 8, pages 305-6, for a good fish soup recipe that should bring relief to even the worst congestion.)

Certain kinds of hot beverages are just as effective. A tablespoon of lemon juice and hot water with a tablespoon of honey is an old-fashioned standby. In the Ozarks they prefer a jigger of Southern Comfort with this remedy. I've occasionally mixed a couple of tablespoons of warm brandy with the ingredients suggested, which seems to have worked just as well.

The Chinese in Taipei, Taiwan, prefer drinking a cup of hot atractylodes tea to anything else for getting rid of a nasty head cold. The root of *Atractylodes lancea* can be found in the herb shops of any Chinatown district in larger metropolitan areas or may be obtained from Custom-Made Formulas in Salt Lake City (see the appendix). The Chinese I spoke with in Taipei prefer a slow simmer for the 2 tablespoons of the dried root in about a quart of boiling water on low heat for approximately 15 minutes, and then steeping it away from the heat for an additional 20 minutes or so. The spicy, bitter, and warmly stimulating tea is terrific for tightness of the chest when a cold enters its more severe stages. *Chemical & Pharmaceutical Bulletin* (Vol. 34, 1986, p. 3854) reported some time ago that this tea prevented gastric acid secretion stimulated by histamine in the stomachs of Shay rats, thereby demonstrating its strong antisecretory activity.

Mullein tea was a favorite of the late plant forager and prolific writer, Euell Gibbons. In his *Stalking the Healthful Herbs* (New York: David McKay, 1966), he lauded the fresh and dried leaves and fresh flowers as being wonderful for sore throat, hacking coughs, irritated lungs, and so forth. His recommendation was to add a tablespoon of the dried, crumbled leaves or 4 tablespoons of finely cut, fresh leaves to a pint of boiling water or white wine, and then simmer on low heat for 10 minutes. The tea was then to be strained through coarse cloth, sweetened with a little honey and a cup drunk every 4 hours or as needed. "I have tried this decoction and find it a pleasant, bland beverage that seems efficacious," he wrote. Also, he mentioned that the dried leaves could be smoked in a pipe to relieve lung congestion.

6. Stay away from dairy products, cheese, red meat, and anything with sugar or white flour in it, as these tend to produce unwanted mucus. Instead opt for foods that have *natural* sugars in them and can give the body energy—prunes and prune juice, figs, dates, cranberry or cranraspberry juice, any kind of green vegetable drinks (spinach, parsley, watercress, beet greens, etc., all make dandy "health" cocktails), cooked parsnips or carrots, pineapple and pineapple juice, citrus fruits and citrus juices, and so forth.

7. Wash your hands frequently! This may seem rather trite to some, but a number of eminent virologists, immunologists, and others believe that cold viruses can be easily passed on with our hands just as much as by our sneezing habits. The premise to their thinking is this: if you shake hands with someone who has a bad cold or handle what scientists term fomites (inanimate objects like a coffee cup, for instance) that the sniffler just handled, then when you touch your mouth, nose, or eyes, you transfer the infection to yourself.

8. Avoid crowds. You're more apt to catch a cold in public than at home. This is also true with children as well. Epidemiologists from the Centers for Disease Control, Emory University and the Georgia Public Health Department in Atlanta, compared the histories of 100 children age 2 or younger hospitalized for lower respiratory tract infections with those of some 200 healthy kids. They soon discovered that toddlers attending large day-care facilities were more likely to contract colds than were youngsters cared for at home or in small day-care homes. With an estimated 11 million children now being cared for outside the home each year, parents should make sure that they place their kids in facilities where *no more* than 6 children are cared for at a time. It also suggests that adults be more careful in the office, riding trains or subways to work, flying in fully loaded airplanes, or standing in long lines to buy tickets for some important event, for in all these situations can colds be more easily contracted than in less crowded environs.

9. Inhale *cool* air and avoid extremely warm air. Cold viruses seem to thrive better in overly heated conditions. Excessive warmth not only causes dilation of the blood vessels in the nose and lungs with resulting congestion in each, but also increases discharge of mucus and further loss of immune resistance. When I was in Sendai, Japan, several years ago, doing some research at the Tohoku Medical College, I noticed a virtual absence of colds in the populace during the winter months, even when the inside temperatures of many public buildings and private homes ranged from the shivering forties to less chilly but still somewhat cold mid-to-high fifties. Central heating (and air conditioning) are still lacking in many older structures. The only available sources of heat are often hearths filled with ashes and charcoal and the hot green tea that is sipped throughout the day. Sometimes a *kotatsu*, a low table with a heater attached underneath and covered with a quilt, is used to warm the hands and feet. Besides this, fuel has always been expensive and hard to come, so the goal has always been to "heat yourself, not the room." The result then is that cold air is continually being inhaled, and without any serious effects so far as I was able to discern.

Yet by the same token, one must be careful to not run the risk of getting hypothermia by unwise, long-term exposure to chilly conditions. That can be very dangerous, especially for the elderly. But upon my return from Japan, I began opening more windows in my apartment *during the winter months* and letting cold air circulate in those rooms (bedroom and study den) where

I spent the majority of my time. This several hours of frequent ventilation before closing the windows again, brought into my living quarters a cooler, but more exhilarating atmosphere and eliminated the old, stagnant, warmer air that used to make me feel tired and groggy. More important, though, I noticed *far fewer* respiratory problems than I had heretofore experienced. This is what finally convinced me that *some limited* exposure each day to *cooler* air was better for a person than was constantly warm air. Also, strange as it may seem, cold viruses don't proliferate so much in cooler air charged with negative ions as they do under warmer conditions burdened with positive ions.

10. Fortify the body with health food supplements. Probably the first things that come to mind after reading the previous sentence, are vitamins like A or C, kyolic garlic or white willow, or some wild cherry cough syrup—preparations that have historically been identified with treating the common cold. But while these things obviously have their place and are of some importance, they, nevertheless, are superseded by other things that many of us never identify as cold remedies. In his national best-seller *Food Is Your Best Medicine* (New York: Random House, 1966), the late Henry G. Bieler, M.D., pinpointed the liver *first* and the colon *second* in terms of focusing attention on how to deal with a nasty cold of any kind. It was essential to treat these organs, he maintained, if one expected to recover quickly; otherwise, something that could be easily remedied would continue to drag on for an indefinite length of time.

Two of the best herbs for the liver happen to be plant roots—dandelion and chicory. Health and specialty food stores sell different brands of herbal coffee substitutes with both of these featured as the chief ingredients. In the coarse, ground form, they are brewed just as coffee would be, but in the more convenient powdered form they can be made as quickly as instant coffee is. Four or five very warm cups daily on an empty stomach is recommended for the liver when you have a cold.

Juices are important too. Both carrot and tomato juice, either fresh or canned, really help to rebuild a weak liver. What I've found that's best is combining the roots with the vegetables for a really potent cleansing effect. This is done by mixing equal parts of carrot and tomato juice together in an 8-oz. glass and taking it with 2 to 3 gelatin capsules filled with equal parts of powdered dandelion and chicory roots. Many health food stores carry various brands of dandelion root, but chicory root in this form is much harder to come by. Custom-Made Formulas in Salt Lake City (see the appendix) can easily blend both roots together where such may not be readily available for purchase in other places.

There are laxatives galore to choose from for stimulating a sluggish colon when you have a cold. Metamucil is about the best you'll find in any drugstore. Its chief ingredient is a powdered herb called psyllium seed. Unfortunately, Metamucil also has a lot of sugar, which can be a drawback to shaking your cold. In health food stores, you'll find both single herbs and many herbal formulas for relieving constipation. A couple of the most effective are cascara sagrada and senna. They seem to work the quickest in the capsule form, which is also the handiest way to take them; figure about 3 capsules of either one twice or three times daily with at least 12 oz. of fluid. If you want a heavy-duty laxative, try 4 capsules of either herb with 8 oz. of prune juice into which has also been stirred a level teaspoon of wheat bran. Note, however, that this procedure is not recommended for expectant mothers.

Having adequately addressed the liver and colon, we finally should consider a few other supplements that definitely fall into the category of cold remedies. They are listed here with brief instructions for their use.

Vitamins A and C. Just about any brand will do, though food purists will insist that the health food store kinds are better. Still, it's really a toss-up between these or drugstore varieties. After all, what may or may not be natural is really in the mind of the consumer when it comes right down to it. Figure about 50,000 to 100,000 international units (I.U.) of fish or beta-carotene-derived A and about 50,000 milligrams (mg.) of C each day until your cold is conquered.

Zinc Gluconate. In a study done at the University of Texas at Austin, researchers identified two groups of people who had contracted typical colds. One set started taking zinc gluconate; the other received a standard placebo. After a week's treatment, 86% of the of the zinc gluconate takers had no more symptoms, but only 4% of the placebo group could boast the same. Zinc gluconate seemed to reduce the average duration of a cold from 10 down to just 3 days. "We're still not sure how it worked," said Dr. George A. Eby, one of the authors of the study. "But it's clear that it was effective. However, zinc gluconate must be *slowly dissolved in the mouth* rather than swallowed in order to be effective. The usual dosage is one 23-mg. tablet every 3 hours or up to 9 tablets a day. But because of the terrible taste—bitter and metallic—it may irritate the mouth and make you nauseous if taken on an empty stomach. Sipping some orange juice through a straw while sucking on one of these tablets will help to alleviate these minor problems.

Herbal Formulas. Some West Coast naturopathic doctors in Oregon and Washington have been prescribing Nature's Way Cold Care or Sinustop for some of their patients suffering from the common cold. An average of 4 capsules every 4 to 6 hours is what they've recommended where the best results have been achieved. (See the appendix.)

How Helga W. Got Rid of Her Cold

Helga W., a beautician residing in Racine, Wisconsin, responded to an article I wrote a few years ago about getting rid of colds. Here's what she did to shake her own cold symptoms:

> I've always followed the part you mentioned in your [newspaper] article about getting lots of rest. My grandma taught me the importance of that. I stay in bed for 10 hours at least, until I begin to feel better; then I get up and move around.
>
> You said hot chicken soup was good for a cold. Well, let me tell you that I use hot [clear] *cabbage* soup, instead, seasoned with lots of black pepper and a squirt of lemon juice. It really unplugs my stuffiness quite good!
>
> I don't use any herbs to speak of, but when I'm down sick with a cold I'll take a few teaspoon swallows of liquid kyolic garlic. Gosh, that stuff tastes awful if you don't put it into some capsules first. But it seems to work better than

any antibiotics my local doctor can give me. [Kyolic is available in most health food stores. See the appendix.]

You make a fuss about not eating dairy products and eggs 'cause they produce mucus you say. Well, when I'm sick like this I *always* drink a glass of *hot* milk—I mean *hot* both ways. I'll heat some up and then add a little dash of *extra hot* chili pepper juice or plain Tabasco sauce. It sure burns like hell going down the throat, but somehow seems to clear up the stuffiness in my throat and lungs. I usually take this at night just before I go to bed.

I'm not much into taking pills, even if they're vitamins and good for you. Instead I get my [vitamin] C from hot lemonade and my [vitamin] A from hot, [clear] fish chowder soup. I also find that if I'm really plugged up, that some strong, hot coffee will help me to breathe much easier! Maybe you can use these things in one of your books or articles later on.

◆◆◆◆◆◆

INFLUENZA

A Disease Worse than World War I

If there's only one thing that you'll remember from this section, let it be this sobering warning: if you have the flu, then you had better treat it just as seriously as if a doctor diagnosed you as having bubonic plague or cancer! In other words, unlike the common cold, *influenza can be very deadly* if not properly attended to!

History is on my side in this alarming pronouncement. It is truly *America's forgotten pandemic* as Alfred Crosby of the University of Texas has correctly titled his recent account of this terrible epidemic which swept through America with lightning speed in 1918 (*America's Forgotten Pandemic*, London: Cambridge University Press, 1989). According to Dr. Crosby, it killed *more* people faster than any other single disease in the history of humankind, the Black Death not excepted! Some 5,100 died in just half a month in October in Philadelphia alone, where a shortage of embalmers and grave diggers threatened to make matters even worse. In just a single day, believe it or not, 528 bodies piled up awaiting burial; many corpses, in fact, had to be stacked up in street gutters for several hours before being properly disposed of. What started out as 2,899 cases in August jumped to 10,481 in September and then skyrocketed like crazy in October with 195,876 fatalities; in the last four months of 1918, a quarter of a million people died. In all over a half-million Americans succumbed to influenza in ten months, in the most lethal internal convulsion since the Civil War when 498,000 soldiers died in a four-year period.

Ironically, this terrible epidemic was spread by our American doughboys sent to Europe to fight against the Germans. By the summer of 1918, when the latest batch of our troops landed in France, plenty of flu got off with them. From France it spread west to England and south to Spain where it killed 8 million Spaniards. It soon struck eastward into the ragged ranks of Kaiser Wilhelm's army in Germany, leaving tens of thousands "too exhausted or dead to hate," as Konrad Adenauer (then mayor of Cologne) put it. On it swept, to imperial Russia, China, and Japan, then down to South Africa, and across to India (where 12 million people died of it) and eventually to South America. In all, over 25 million deaths were directly attributed to this viral holocaust.

Without meaning to be an alarmist, I'd like to remind you that what "goes around, comes around." It seems that history is starting to repeat itself so far as this frightening infection goes. *The New York Times* (January 12, 1990) reported that most of Texas was struck exceedingly hard with "a particularly dangerous form of influenza" that doctors hadn't seen before. In the Houston area alone, a quarter-million people became very ill as a result of it. Dr. Paul Glezen, chief epidemiologist at the Influenza Research Center at the Baylor College of Medicine in Houston, was quoted as saying that this new strain *was the most virulent form* he'd ever seen. Then, less than a month later the February 5, 1990 issue of *Newsweek* magazine stated that between 50 million and 60 million American citizens would be affected by this incredibly mean form of the A-Shanghai flu virus before it finally faded away in the spring.

Every year more aggressive and nastier strains of influenza make their appearance in this country. Several leading epidemiologists at the Centers for Disease Control in Atlanta, Georgia, have shared their private concerns with me about a possible strain coming soon that would wreck health havoc with our entire society. As one scientist to another, they explained that flu viruses are getting genetically smarter and evolving more rapidly than the time it normally takes to reformulate flu vaccine. They felt that if greater attention isn't paid to this problem right now by federal and state health agencies, then a repeat of the 1918 disaster could still occur within this decade.

What You Need to Know About the Flu Virus

Influenza isn't your garden variety common cold by any means. It's as different in its attack on the immune system as, say, a mugger in a dark alley is to an attack by a gang armed to the teeth in a deserted park. Understanding something about its brutal behavior is the first step in curbing some or all of its systemic violence.

Influenza virus falls into two major types: A and B. Although B is the less virulent of the two, both will make you sick in much the same way. And while there are dozens of different flu strains, only a few do the most damage each year. For instance, in the winter of 1989, Type B and two strains of Type A were making millions of people very sick—A-Taiwan in about half the states, A-Sichuan in about 10 states, and Type B in virtually all states. But despite the wide variety of strains, the symptoms always remain the same.

Flu victims typically experience a sudden onset of fever, with temperatures around 101°F, or higher in young children. This is the body's way of defending itself; hence the trademark high fever that common colds generally lack. Like some other respiratory infections, flu is characterized by a sore throat, a dry cough, chills, weakness, loss of appetite, and incredible aching of the head, back, arms, and legs. Unlike other respiratory infections, though, it often can cause malaise—a general depression that often marks the onset of an illness. "You basically feel like you've been run over by a Mack truck," CDC influenza surveillance officer Walter J. Gunn told a *USA Today* reporter on February 10, 1989. "You feel like this is the sickest you've ever been in 10 years."

Scientists give the various viruses responsible for causing flus a host of different names. In the last decade we've seen such strains as Hong Kong, Sichuan, Taiwan, Leningrad, and Ann Arbor. The names themselves are pretty meaningless, however: flus are named after the place where the virus was first isolated, not the place of origin. Many of those strains originating out of the Far East, though, are usually of the A type and more aggressive than B type. In the past Type A used to hit mostly young to middle-aged adults and the elderly, while Type B usually showed preference for young children. But since the 1989 flu epidemic, both types are now hitting all age brackets. Furthermore, Type B is showing signs of increased hostility, leading some scientists to speculate that it will eventually become just as mean and nasty as Type A has always been.

The word "influenza" is an Italian word meaning influence—of the stars or the weather or a dozen other erstwhile-suspected causes. The flu has been around since the time of Hippocrates. Anthropologists who believe in the "theory of evolution" know that influenza viruses are some of the fastest-changing organisms around. In fact, it would be fairly safe to say that the flu virus is one of mother nature's best "quick-change" artists around.

Influenza, not to be confused with the common cold or the grossly misnamed "stomach flu," is extremely difficult to pin down because of its migratory habits. Flu viruses travel around the globe, constantly evolving as they go. Mutations cause tiny changes on the viruses' outer surfaces which confuse the body's immune system. Antibodies produced in earlier years may not readily recognize and fight off a newly modified virus. More disturbing and certainly devastating, is the appearance of a flu virus totally unlike anything ever isolated before, something so different and out of the ordinary that epidemiologists are required to identify it as a new "subtype" of some kind. It seems that these wholly new forms occur when the genes from an animal flu virus somehow merge with those of a human flu virus. Now your typical flu virus that's just undergone a few minor changes—and still looks vaguely familiar to the body's preprogrammed defenses—often encounters a mild counterattack. But a new subtype will launch an immediate full-scale infection before the body's immune defenses have a chance to gear up for retaliatory action. The last new subtype to do this was first isolated in Hong Kong (hence its name) in 1968. When it reached our shores, close to 60 million people experienced absolute misery that winter.

What's especially frightening about the flu's natural unpredictability is that of an *increased danger* from newer human-animal subtypes. "These bizarre subtypes we're now seeing more of," one scientist from the Centers for Disease Control in Atlanta told me recently by phone, "are genetically awesome. There's no way in the world that we're going to be able to develop vaccines fast enough to cope with them. In fact, by the time we get one vaccine out, it has already become obsolete when next year's flu season rolls around. Look at what happened to us in the spring of 1987. We thought then that the latest strain of Hong Kong flu would be the main culprit the following winter. Well, we were right about it being Hong Kong, but by the time it hit, mutations had changed the virus's appearance so much that most of those who'd been immunized for it got sick anyway. And things are going to get a lot worse in this respect, before they get better!"

It may still be somewhat premature to predict that the flu virus will someday become as frightening a health threat as the acquired immune deficiency syndrome (AIDS) epidemic now is, but all evidence *does* point in this direction. Sooner or later, a couple of subtypes will be evolving somewhere in the world with the same deadly consequences as the variant that hit the world in 1918. When this health nightmare occurs, present fears about AIDS will all but vanish, as the mounting mortalities from these "super flu" subtypes dominate the news in staggering numbers well into the hundreds of thousands! This is no idle threat designed to get your attention! Influenza is serious business. As newer and deadlier subtypes keep evolving, our personal risks of survival will be decreasing. Making drastic changes in our diets is one way of averting death by influenza!

The Free Radical-Flu Connection

A recently published study in the May 26, 1989, issue of *Science* suggests for the very first time that influenza's symptoms aren't caused directly by the virus itself but, rather, result from the action of oxidizing free radicals produced within the immune system. Dr. Hiroshi Maeda, a biochemist at Kumamoto University Medical School in Japan, and his team discovered that the levels of free radicals generated by immune cells taken from influenza virus-infected mouse lungs increased with time after infection. They also noticed that T lymphocytes increased in number, suggesting that elevated free radical production by immune cells, possibly primary T cells, contributes to influenza pathogenesis.

For those unfamiliar with free radicals, suffice it to say that they are highly reactive compounds containing unpaired electrons that steal electrons from other molecules and cause extensive tissue damage throughout the entire body. Previous studies have shown an overreaction of the immune system contributes to flu symptoms, and other research has amply demonstrated that immune cells produce free radicals under certain stressful conditions.

Durk Pearson and Sandy Shaw are college graduates with backgrounds in biochemistry and biology. In 1982 they wrote a best-selling book entitled, *Life Extension* (New York: Warner Books, 1982). In Part IV, Chapter 3, of their massive work, they identified certain foods high in free radical activity. Heading their list were broiled, fried, and deep-fried foods, especially meats. And, believe it or not, hamburgers/cheeseburgers are loaded to their buns with destructive free radicals! This is due to a combination of factors: the initial grinding process, long-term refrigeration, and rapid frying on an open grill where plenty of oxygen can combine with the cooked protein. This destructive cross-linking is also evident in fried eggs and toasted bread. As they noted in Part II, Chapter 7, these scavenger molecules produce mutations in your body deoxyribonucleic acid (DNA) that can lead to cancer; can make blood clots abnormally by destroying the body's ability to produce a natural anticlotting hormone called prostacyclin (or PGI_2); may cause brain damage in the elderly; and have been implicated in arthritis, emphysema, cerebral hemorrhage, and the wrinkling and aging of the skin.

Besides completely avoiding beef, pork, and chicken during your bout with flu, dairy products and eggs are also definite no-no's as well. It seems that these foods contain a particular enzyme known as xanthine oxidase, which is chiefly responsible for the generation of free radicals. Dr. Maeda's team discovered that this enzyme's activity dramatically increased in both influenza-infected mouse lung cells and infected mouse serum.

Can the simple process of dietary elimination work positive results when the flu is going around? Experiments conducted at our Anthropological Research Center here in Salt Lake City (see the Appendix for address) seem to suggest yes. In one of our simpler studies, we solicited the services of seven college students, three male and four female. When the Taiwan Type A flu strain finally hit Utah in mid-January 1989, we interviewed all of them and found that six had not as yet contracted it (only one female had and she was excluded from the study).

We asked these half-dozen test subjects to go about their normal daily routine, with just one exception: the three men were to include in their diets as much animal protein and dairy products as possible for one month while the three women were asked to abstain from such staples for the same length of time. Special meal diaries broken down into breakfast, lunch, dinner, and snacks were supplied by us and filled out every day by each subject.

Five of the six came down with the flu during the next 30 days (one of the women was fortunate enough not to get it). Each student doctored himself or herself as they thought best. I purposely refrained from recommending herbs or any supplements so as not to invalidate any of our findings. After the meal diaries had been collected and each subject carefully interviewed, several amazing things turned up. First, the three men who had subsisted frequently on animal protein, diary products, and eggs, contracted the worst symptoms and took between 7 to 10 days to get over them. On the other hand, the two women who avoided all meat, eggs, milk, butter, cheese, and yogurt, reported lesser miseries and recovered within 3 to 4 days. Second, the lone woman who did *not* contract influenza during the entire month, recorded consuming a number of spicy ethnic foods in her meal diary. Especially evident was cayenne pepper, garlic, ginger, and thyme in the variety of Mexican, Chinese, and Vietnamese foods that she dined on every so often. All four of these spices are antioxidants, meaning that they curb the activity of free radicals or destroy them outright.

Also, many of these ethnic foods she consumed were very

high in sulphur and copper. Increases in the dietary intake of both of these trace elements tend to dump more of another trace element, molybdenum, into the urine. And when molybdenum is depleted from body tissues and blood supply, then xanthine oxidase activities substantially *decrease* within the intestines and liver. With her much lower xanthine oxidase levels, she, unwittingly, had created an internal environment without too many free radicals. This is probably why no influenza virus had much of a chance to survive in her system for very long.

How I Cured Myself of the Flu in Singapore

In the early spring of 1986 I left Utah for a trip to various locales scattered around the Pacific Rim. The weather in Salt Lake City at the time of my departure had been in the low teens, and it was quite stormy as well. Hence, my body had become acclimatized to very chilly and damp conditions, but found itself about 17 hours later suddenly thrust into the very warm and balmy climate of Hong Kong. This plus the fact that I didn't get much sleep during my brief two-day stay there apparently set the stage for what happened when I arrived in Singapore, where the temperature was about 80° F.

At the tip of the Malay Peninsula in the South China Sea sits the tiny city-state-nation of Singapore. With an area of just 238 square miles and a population of only 2.5 million people, Singapore is smaller than Indianapolis and less populous than metropolitan Cleveland. And with 76 percent of its people ethnic Chinese, Singapore remains what it has been since 1819 when Sir Stafford Raffles founded the city—an outpost of foreign customs, foreign money, and foreign dynamism conveniently perched at the epicenter of the Southeast Asian tropics.

I checked into the Raffles Hotel, one of the few colonial-era buildings remaining. This stately, four-story, white-stucco affair, framed by swaying palms and a lovely inner courtyard full of all types of native flora, was home to some of the century's best known writers. A local British resident later informed me that the room in which I was then staying for about a week was the very same one that the popular writer Somerset Maugham had occupied while turning out short stories about the passions of British Army colonials.

My second day in Singapore greeted me with a strange tickling in the throat, only to be accompanied later by an insatiable desire to get warm—and this in already warm weather. Some hours later a vise started gripping my temples, and not too long thereafter, every muscle and joint in my body ached so bad it felt as if I'd been kicked and stomped all over by a mad Missouri mule. That same day, the tickling in my throat traveled up to my sinuses and then down again into my chest where it sat like a half-ton gorilla, substituting its own voice for mine. My eyes turned glassy and I then wished that I was back home in my own bed and could have pulled the covers up and slept until the crocuses bloomed. Additionally, a raging fever and acute diarrhea both hit me, at once, making me wonder if I was ever going to survive. I later discovered that I had picked up A-Hong Kong and, boy, was it a doozy.

In a strange, faraway land and without any vitamins or herbs that I was used to taking for a condition such as this, I felt helpless. But since "necessity is the mother of invention," I decided to make the best of what was available there in the hotel for me and managed rather nicely after all. The people at Raffles, the hotel where I was staying, especially the concierge and those in the kitchen, tried to accommodate me in every way possible.

The first thing I did to ward off my chills was to eat a large bowl of a soup they had on the menu then. One of the kitchen staff later supplied me with the initial ingredients and instructions for preparation. Rather than place it in the recipe chapters, I've decided to include it here instead.

◆◆◆◆

Lotus Roots and Chamomile Soup

1 section of pork knuckle	½ oz. chamomile flowers
1 section of lotus root	¼ cup of red jujube dates
1 slice of ginger root	6 cups of water

1. Slice down skin from lotus root. Cut into pieces. Soak in saltwater to clean mud out. Then scrape clean and scald with boiling water for about 5 minutes. If lotus isn't available in your area, substitute ½ cup of chopped

watercress, omitting the saltwater soaking, scraping, and parboiling. I later found out that lotus is high in vitamin C.

2. Soak the jujubes overnight, then wash clean. These long, dark reddish brown fleshy drupes are common throughout China, Japan, India, Malaysia, Australia, and tropical Africa. They are usually available in food or herb emporiums in the Chinatown districts of larger American cities. If unavailable, ⅛ cup of chopped black mission figs and ⅛ cup of dromedary dates may be substituted.

3. Bring pork knuckle to boil in the water. Reduce heat to medium and add all other ingredients *except* the chamomile. Cover and cook for 1 hour. Then remove lid and add chamomile; cover again and simmer an additional 10 minutes. The pork knuckle adds flavor and makes the lotus root runny and juicy. Serves four.

This soup really warmed my insides up nicely, and I slept undisturbed for about 5 hours.

When I awoke my chills were gone, but I still had a king-size headache and my body felt as if it had just been in a rugby match or ice hockey game. In spite of a definite physical weakness, I managed to put on my swimming trunks and go to the hotel's sauna room, where I stayed for almost half an hour. The steam sure felt good and my headache and body pains diminished quite a bit. I repeated this procedure again later that night.

I discovered that hot ginseng root tea, with a little chamomile added, worked wonders for my chest and sinuses. My British friend procured some coarsely cut Korean ginseng root from a local Chinese herb pharmacy, and the hotel kitchen provided a metal quart pitcher full of boiling water to which I added one generous handful of ginseng root and about 1 tablespoon of chamomile flowers. I put a flat dinner plate on top of this pitcher and weighed it down with a heavy glass ashtray so everything could steep better. Several large glasses of this stuff later had me expectorating all kinds of awful looking mucus.

I don't quite remember just when my temperature shot up, but nothing seemed to cool me down. The concierge suggested that I try their "Singapore Sling" from the bar—a drink for which the Raffles Hotel has become famous internationally. As a Mormon, I usually abstain from all manner of liquor, but, in this case, felt it to be justifiable, seeing how sick I was at the time. It took only one and a half glasses to bring my fever down. The bartender was gracious enough to provide me with the instructions for making it.

◆◆◆◆◆

Raffles' "Singapore Sling"

2 fl. oz. (about ¼ cup) gin

juice of half a lemon

1 tsp. powdered sugar (honey can be substituted)

½ fl. oz. cherry-flavored brandy

enough Canada Dry to nearly fill a 12-oz. glass

enough ice cubes to fill a 12-oz. glass

1. Put all the ingredients, except the brandy and the ice, into a capped shaker and shake vigorously by hand for about 20 seconds. Then pour the contents into the ice-filled glass.

2. Next, slowly pour the brandy over the back of a soup so that it lays on top. A few finely diced chunks of fresh pineapple can also be added for decoration.

◆◆◆

I found for my condition that it was better to keep the brandy floating on top, rather than mixing it in with everything else. I slowly sipped the brandy off with a straw before drinking everything else. My temperature returned to normal within just a couple of hours.

Two other things that plagued me throughout my worst day were constant diarrhea and stomach problems. To correct the loose stool, I phoned the concierge and had him ask the kitchen to boil up some ordinary white rice, but to save the liquid for me, and to discard the rice. They kept me well supplied with rice water, and I must have drunk four or six glasses in a couple of days' time before my diarrhea finally quit and my stool became firmer again.

Besides all of these different liquids that I was taking, the only real solid food my stomach could keep down was fresh papaya. I had that for breakfast, lunch, and dinner the following day, when I started to show signs of improvement. By the third day, I was able to handle mangoes and bananas as well. I also drank them in juice form from the bar whenever I could.

My full recovery, although I was still weak, took about three days in all to accomplish. But the remedies, with some slight modifications since then, have proven to be a boon to many of my friends, colleagues, and students who've had the flu themselves. To the herb soup, steam bath, hot herb tea, cold alcoholic beverage, rice water, and tropical fruits, I'd like to add those items previously recommended for treating a cold: sleep, no drugs, no eating out, no stress, elimination of mucus, no meat or dairy products, clean hands, isolation, cool air, and nutritional supplements. This is, by far, the best program I know of for treating influenza of any kind.

◆◆◆◆◆

CANDIDIASIS (YEAST OVERGROWTH)

An Epidemic in Disguise

How can a common yeast, *Candida albicans*, that thrives in most of us as part of our natural body flora, wreak so much havoc in the minds and bodies of millions of sufferers? Billions of friendly bacteria help the immune system to keep this yeast under control. Candida is an organism that lives with us and in us. And considering how incredibly rapidly yeast antigens can be reproduced, there probably are millions of strains of candida, each differing slightly from one another. Touch a doorknob, shake hands with a friend, kiss someone you love, sleep in a hotel bed, and have sexual intercourse with strangers, and your chances are very good of picking up new strains all the time.

But such constant exposure to the yeast doesn't always mean that it will produce a serious health problem. Illness only comes about when a *particular* immune system cannot cope with a *particular* strain of candida. However, even in the event that one does unhappily fall victim to candidiasis, there's usually a bright outlook for recovery when the correct things are done to hold it in check.

According to University of California at San Francisco immunologist Alan Levin, the health of close to a third of the

American population is adversely affected in some way by candida allergies. Orian Truss, M.D., an internist in private practice in Birmingham, Alabama, has investigated the behavior of this particular yeast in nearly 3,000 patients for better than two decades. His conclusion is that candida is implicated in a wide variety of human ills, ranging from depression and hormonal disturbances to allergic reactions, childhood learning disabilities such as autism, and autoimmune disorders like lupus or Crohn's disease.

Unfortunately, a real Neanderthal attitude still persists with most of the American medical community in regard to yeast infection. They seem to think that candidiasis hypersensitivity is just another health fraud being perpetrated upon a gullible public. But nothing could be further from the truth. Health care professionals who have become acquainted with Dr. Truss's research, like William G. Crook, M.D., of Jackson, Tennessee, have been able to assist thousands of people in the last decade who suffer from candidiasis. He, like a growing number of doctors, has been able to cross over from traditional medical boundaries to find new, holistic treatments for this hidden and pervasive epidemic.

The Facts About Candidiasis

A lot of *mis*information has been spread about yeast overgrowth in the last few years due to consumer hysteria and those who've written popular articles and books on the subject without being fully qualified to do so. Only health professionals who really have a good grasp of the disease and fully understand all of its ramifications are in a position to advise. It is from their works rather than the literature geared for the layperson that the following data have been procured.

1. Candidiasis is not transmittable. Specialists who have thoroughly researched it know that while the candida organism itself is transmittable from one person to another, the actual illness is not.

2. Drugs and diet shift the candida balance ever so slightly, thereby inducing illness. Physicians familiar with candida know that prescription and over-the-counter medications, along with certain chemicals in our food supply, upset normal behavior of candida, rendering it from a relatively harmless to very harmful state. Dr. Crook blames the antibiotics and growth hormones routinely administered to cattle, swine, and poultry as causing toxin-producing yeasts to multiply within the body. Dr. Truss blames penicillin, birth control pills, cortisone, and childhood immunizations, which suppress the immune system's ability to fight yeast infection.

3. Diets high in carbohydrates and sugars dramatically increase candidiasis hypersensitivity. These foods exacerbate the physical and mental problems associated with yeast infection. They also can produce a cross-sensitivity to other models and fungi. Dr. Truss discovered that that moldy environments and foods containing yeast and molds (cheese and blue cheese dressing, for instance) likewise initiated—or heightened—patients' symptoms.

4. Candida often disrupts multiple body systems. Consider the case of one young woman whom Dr. Truss treated back in 1970. Her medical history revealed that she suffered from chronic candida vaginitis since her teens, chronic constipation, occasional oral thrush, and a blind spot in one eye. He placed her on a low-carbohydrate, low-sugar, yeast-free diet and prescribed Nystatin, the standard drug of choice for treating candida. Besides all of these conditions clearing up, her multiple sclerosis (MS) also went into complete remission as well. When she went off the drug for a while, all these physical problems (including the MS) returned, but cleared again as soon as she went back on this antifungal medication and anticandida diet. This case serves as a classic example to show just how many different body systems can be affected by a single strain of yeast.

5. Allergies to food, plants, animals, household chemicals, personal toiletries, smoke, pharmaceuticals, and the environment in general are often induced or else aggravated by candidiasis. Treat the yeast infection, Dr. Truss said, and usually the allergies will clear up of their own accord.

How Shirley L. Coped with Her Candidiasis Problem

Shirley L. is a thirtysomething computer programmer at a U.S. government laboratory. She works in a department staffed mostly by men. As just one of a trio of women there, she's had to put up with her share of sexist jokes and macho thinking.

Early on in her career she discovered that she had yeast infection. "I read up on Candida from all the books and magazine articles that I could lay my hands on," she told me by telephone a while back. "I went to this M.D. who put me on Nystatin right away, but soon even that stuff wasn't good enough to control the infection. Next I sought out a homeopathic doctor, who had me taking a strong herbal liquid from West Germany under my tongue several times every day. That helped for a couple of months, but soon the damned stuff [meaning her candidiasis] flared up again, and I mean really bad this time!

"Then came the heavy vitamin therapy from an orthomolecular practitioner. Again, it went into remission for a longer period. I finally thought I had brought it under control. But boy! Was I ever surprised as hell when it raged back with greater intensity the third time round. To me it seemed like everytime I tried something different and it went away for a while, and then came back again, it returned much stronger each time. I couldn't figure out what was going on, and almost convinced myself, 'Shirley, old girl, there's nothing you can do about it, so just learn to live with the monster inside of you.'

"That is, until I heard about this little skinny fellow from India, who was teaching yoga classes. Well, he interviewed me for a short time and basically said that he wasn't going to give me anything to take. Boy, was that ever a switch! Instead, he just laid his hand on my forehead and then against my chest and said, 'The medicine I'm going to give you will heal you here and here.' Then for the next several days, he took me through some intensive sessions of deep-breathing, stretching, and meditation exercises that really calmed me down.

"I couldn't believe it when I returned to work just how great I felt. Oh yeh, I still have to put up with the same old sexist crap from a bunch of guys who really haven't fully grown up yet.

But I no longer let them get to me. I've discovered that my daily half-hour workouts [morning and evening] with yoga really have put my mind and heart at ease. And you know what else has happened in the process? My candidiasis has pretty much gone away *of its own accord*! Now ain't that wild? I think the on-the-job stress I was encountering all the time had a lot to do with my problem. But now I pretty much have things under control, even without always avoiding foods that may sometimes aggravate my yeast infection. Probably, if I watched what I ate a little more closely, then I'd have this thing licked for sure! But yoga has *definitely* helped me a lot!"

An Anticandida Diet That Really Works

The best advice offered on a particular problem obviously should come from an expert on the subject. You would no more ask your pharmacist to take waist measurements for a new pair of slacks than you would a plumber to check the oil in your car engine. For this reason, three different physicians who work extensively with patients suffering from candidiasis were individually consulted about the food recommendations made to help hold this problem in check. Luc De Schepper, M.D., practiced in Santa Monica, California, for a while and wrote a book entitled *Candida, The Epidemic of This Century* (West Lake Village, California: L.D.S. Publications, 1986). Dennis Remington, M.D., is a Mormon physician practicing in Provo, Utah, who also has authored a work entitled *Back to Health* (Provo, Utah: Vitality House International, 1986). The third doctor consulted was Orian Truss, M.D., who practices in Birmingham, Alabama. Between what the three of them provided, this author was able to construct an effective and worthwhile antifungal diet.

Dr. Schepper maintains that the first line of immune defense against candida is diet. Dr. Remington concurs by stressing the importance of (1) avoiding foods that feed candida and (2) avoiding foods that can contribute further yeast to the body. Dr. Truss insists that potential candida victims need to (1) avoid eating raw and cold foods and (2) avoid consuming leftovers. All three physicians encourage their patients to frequently rotate their diets, because by eating the same foods over and over again they can acquire food allergies symptomatic of candidiasis.

First Month Diet

1. Whole Grains. Hot or cold breakfast cereals permitted:

All-Bran	Puffed Wheat/Puffed Rice
Cracked Wheat	Quinoa (an Inca cereal)
Fiber One	Roman Meal
Grits	Shredded Wheat/Spoon-Size S.W.
Millet	Wheat Hearts
Oatmeal/Oat Bran	Wild Rice

Other whole-grain foods allowed are muffins, biscuits, pancakes, waffles, rice cakes, whole wheat tortillas, and corn tortillas. Also popcorn, amaranth, and whole wheat pasta products (noodles, macaroni, spaghetti, and lasagna) may be consumed. The American Dental Association found that popcorn is very helpful in getting rid of thrush (oral candida) and proclaimed it to be a safe and nutritious snack—if eaten without butter or salt. Amaranth is a little known grain once used extensively by the ancient Aztecs of old Mexico. It's exceptionally high in protein value: 16% versus 12% for wheat, 10% for rice, and 9% for corn. A combination of amaranth and corn flour gives 100% of three essential amino acids—lysine, tryptophan, and leucine. *Bread-stuffs made with baker's yeast should be avoided!*

2. All vegetables (except iceberg lettuce). The list includes

Asparagus	Cauliflower
Avocados	Collards
Banana squash	Eggplant
Beet greens	Green beans
Bell peppers	Kale
Broccoli	Okra
Brussels sprouts	Parsley
Cabbage	Parsnips
Carrots	Peas

Potatoes	Tomatoes
Spinach	Turnip greens
Summer squash	Yams
Sweet potatoes	Zucchini squash

Boiling *isn't* the best way to prepare many of the items. Either *lightly steam* or briefly *microwave cook* them so they're still crunchy. Also, *baking* for some of these vegetables is good too. These three methods don't cause significant losses of vitamins and minerals as lengthy boiling would; they also seem to kill the candida fungus as well.

3. Many Legumes. Brief descriptions of some are as follows:

Black beans: small, oval, tender, and mushroom-flavored.

Black-eyed peas: medium, oval, and nutty crunchiness.

Chicpeas: round, nutty flavor, and chewy firmness.

Fava beans: large, flat, oval, firm texture, dainty taste.

Kidney beans: dark/light red, white, oval, and soft, bland taste.

Lentils: small, disk-shaped, subtle flavor, firm texture.

Lima beans: large, white, oval, mild taste, soft texture.

Mung beans: white, tiny, sticky when cooked or sprouted.

Navy, white, Great Northern beans: small to large, mild, firm.

Pinto beans: small, oval, mild flavor, soft texture.

Split/whole peas: yellow or green, soft texture, grainy flavor.

Soybeans: firm, round, bland tasting.

Slowly baking or gently simmering are the best ways to prepare legumes to bring out their distinctive flavors with minimal loss of valuable nutrients. Legumes also contain protease inhibitors (PIs). These PIs interfere with enzymes that are known to produce malignant tumors. It's also believed that these same substances may exhibit some antifungal activity, thereby limiting the spread of candida.

4. Unprocessed nuts and seeds (except peanuts and peanut products). The following are permitted

Acorns	Pecans
Almonds	Pinenuts
Brazil nuts	Pistachio nuts
Butternuts	Poppy seeds
Cashews	Pumpkin seeds
Chestnuts	Safflower seeds
Filberts	Sesame seeds
Hazelnuts	Squash seeds
Hickorys	Sunflower seeds
Macadamia nuts	Walnuts

Both Drs. Remington and De Schepper insist that *commercially* salted and roasted nuts and seeds should *not* be consumed, since the oils in which they're cooked are unhealthy and tend to promote candidiasis. Peanuts and peanut products need to be avoided because they are very susceptible to the deadly aflatoxin mold. Not only does aflotoxin promote cancer, but when it intermingles with candida albicans, very serious health consequences may result. Certain enzymes common to seeds, when injected into animal models previously inoculated with melanoma cells, prevented them from spreading. A similar effect keeps candida spores from rapidly multiplying.

5. Certain spices. These can be used for flavor or supplementation.

Allspice	Cinnamon	Lemon grass
Almond	Cloves	Mustard
Anise	Garlic	Onion
Bay		

The January 1983 *Indian Journal of Dermatology* reported on a young Indian army soldier who was treated for sporotrichosis on his left ring finger, forearm, and arm. He acquired this fungi from contact with brush scratches or sphagnum moss. Physicians used raw garlic juice to cure him. The adjoene in garlic inhibits fungi by damaging its cell walls. A 1945 issue of *Food Research* (Vol. 10, pp. 273–281) showed that many of the spices listed, especially cinnamon and cloves, inhibited the spread of many different yeasts, including two species of candida. Kyolic garlic can be substituted in place of raw garlic.

6. Butter and cold-pressed oils. These are allowed:

Avocado, Linseed, Olive, Safflower, Sunflower, Walnut

According to the *Journal of Nutrition* (Vol. 110, 1980, pp. 1555–1572), high levels of oil used by the fast-food industry in deep-frying suppressed the reproduction by budding of tiny white blood cells from the lymph nodes, spleen, thymus, tonsils, Peyer's patches, and bone marrow—all vital parts of our lympathic immunity. Also diets high in deep-fried foods "reduced the killing of ascites tumors by splenic T-cells." *Deep-fried foods should be avoided by candiasis sufferers.*

7. All fresh- and saltwater fish (with fins and scales), lean beef, veal, lamb, and rabbit (except poultry and pork). De Lamar Gibbons, M.D., spent almost two decades practicing medicine among the Navajo Indians in southeastern Utah. During that period, he discovered virtually *no* cancer or candidiasis cases among them. According to information supplied by the *Salt Lake Tribune* (November 29, 1987), he attributed this remarkable phenomenon to their complete abstinence from poultry—"Navajos don't eat chicken or turkey!" The December 11, 1987 issue of *Science* reported that when cells containing *Candida albicans* were injected into mice, tumors developed earlier, grew faster, invaded surrounding tissues more quickly, and metastasized to the lungs sooner than did ordinary tumors induced by cells lacking yeast particles. More recently, scientists have isolated an oncogene in chickens, which is responsible for tumor development in humans. (Oncogenes are genes that contribute to the cancer process.) Based on the evidence, it seems that this yeast species expedites the progress of cancer and that the consumption of chicken, likewise, increases the risk as well.

8. Use only goat's milk and avoid dairy products and eggs. Dr. De Schepper calls dairy products, cheese of all kinds, cottage cheese, and even eggs some of the "main culprits" in promoting the growth of yeast. Clearly, they ought to be avoided at all costs.

During this initial four-week diet program, the following items should also be avoided: any kind of sweets, white flour products, yeast-containing foods and food supplements (B-complex vitamins and brewer's yeast), alcohol, all fruit juices and fruits (fresh, canned, or dried), coffee, obvious fungal foods (mushrooms), sprouts, processed meats, condiments (catsup, mustard, pickles, mayonnaise), colas, soft drinks.

Finally, be sure to rotate your foods frequently. The easiest way to pick up food allergies is to eat the same things repeatedly. For instance, don't have oatmeal for breakfast or tunafish sandwiches for lunch, three times in one week; vary the foods to be consumed at these meals and dinner so that potential allergies don't develop.

Second Month Diet

1. If the candidiasis condition has substantially improved, then certain previously eliminated foods can be *gradually* added back. Dr. Remington recommends yeast breads: 1–2 slices daily for a week. If no problems are experienced continue eating it; if problems occur, again eliminate it from the diet. Do this with other foods, too.

2. Add back only fresh fruit and just one kind at a time. Overly ripe and canned fruits should continue to be eliminated, because of possible fungal contamination or addition of white sugar. Some fruits may require peeling or thorough washing to reduce intolerance to them. Avoid dried fruit because of the sucrose it contains.

3. Add back natural sweeteners such as honey, blackstrap molasses, and pure maple syrup, but still avoid white sugar products! Honey is a strong antifungal agent. An offering of honey, piously buried in Paestum in a sacred chamber 2,500 years ago, never decayed and was still recognizable in 1957, according to A. H. Gardiner's *Egyptian Grammar* (London: Oxford University Press, 1966, 3rd ed., p. 27). Honey contains hydrogen peroxide, which explains its anticandidiasis and antibacterial activities, noted the *Journal of Pharmacy & Pharmacology* (Vol. 36, pp. 283–284) in 1984.

4. Carefully add back just those types of cheese which your system can handle, but avoid moldy ones like bleu cheese or Roquefort.

5. Continue adding other foods on an "as needed" basis, but continue to avoid alcohol and deep-fried food. After a month on this diet, your body should feel a lot better and be in decent shape to do a little experimenting to see which foods agree with you and which ones don't.

Supplements for Fighting Candida

A Seale, Alabama, physician by the name of Calvin L. Thrash, Jr., M.D., recommends the following several supplements to all of his candidiasis patients with good success. Here is a recent experience which he shared with me through a mutual friend, Charlie Fox of Mission Viejo, California.

"Early this year [1990] when I was on the West Coast, I saw a lady with a severe yeast problem—almost unable to eat anything, lots of gas, bloating, discomfort, poor digestion, etc. She had tried everything, including Nystatin, with minimal help. We told her to take the liquid kyolic garlic, three teaspoons three times daily, along with diet, and some other suggestions. She called me a few months later to say that in just a couple of weeks time her symptoms were gone. . . . At the end of two months of kyolic her cholesterol had dropped [from 350] to 220! She said that it had never been that low in her adult life [she is presently 45 years of age]. She said while kyolic was expensive, it was definitely worth the price." (See the appendix for information on where to obtain kyolic garlic in case your local health food store does not carry it.)

Two other supplements important in the battle against yeast infection are vitamins A and C. Holistic-minded doctors usually prescribe about 25,000 I.U. of A and up to 10,000 mg. of C to their patients suffering from candidiasis.

Another equally important but little understood nutrient is copper. While the body of a healthy adult contains barely 1/50th of a teaspoon of copper—just a dusting as it were—any less than this can severely impair a person's ability to fight off even the most common infections.

Biochemist Mark Failla at the USDA's Vitamin and Mineral Lab in Beltsville, Maryland, has studied the effect of a marginal copper deficiency on immune response in rats. Failla raised two sets of rats, one fed a diet with 50–60% of the copper needed for optimal growth, the second with a diet adequate in copper.

When he introduced *Candida albicans* into the rat's bodies, he observed a significant difference in their immune systems' reactions. In the copper-deficient group, the rats' white blood cells were unable to kill the yeast as efficiently as those of the copper-adequate rats.

When the researchers then fed the deprived group adequate copper for one week, the cells began to combat the yeasts as effectively as those in the group that had been fed a copper-adequate diet from birth.

The immune system in both rats and humans needs copper for the proper functioning of neutrophils, specialists in the body's antibacterial army of white blood cells. Neutrophils move from the blood through vessel walls to get to sites of injury or infection where they literally eat foreign cells.

Dr. Failla's research suggests that marginally adequate copper may debilitate the invisible army that guards against microbial invasion such as in the case of candidiasis. The National Research Council recommends 2 to 3 mg. of copper per day in the average diet; unfortunately, most diets contain far less than this. The best way to get more copper into the body isn't necessarily through supplementation, but by eating more foods rich in this trace element: oysters and other seafood, liver, cocoa, blackstrap molasses, nuts, and wheat bran.

Summary

1. Colds and flus are caused by viruses. They thrive in warm, damp conditions. Sweating and inhaling cool air may help overcome them

2. Plenty of sleep is the best prescription medicine for both.

3. Mental and emotional stress worsens cold, flu, and candidiasis.

4. Warm and cool liquids are important in treating colds and flus.

5. Avoid meat, bread, dairy products, eggs, sweets, soft drinks, and fried foods in the event of a cold, flu, or yeast infection. However alcohol is useful for the first two.

6. The body needs to be fortified with supplements (vitamins A and C) and food rich in one trace element (copper).

7. Free radicals are implicated in cold and flu, while candidiasis mimics the symptoms of other diseases and may eventually lead to cancer.

8. Antibiotic drugs hinder more than help all three common infections.

9. Pushing the body beyond the limits of its endurance is *never* a good idea.

10. Keeping the bowels open and regular is very important to good health.

◆◆◆◆◆ 2 ◆◆◆◆◆

Autoimmune Diseases: When the Immune System Runs Amok

AN AUTOIMMUNE CONDITION is one in which the body becomes allergic to itself! To understand how this is possible, consider what happens in the case of an organ transplant. The recipient's body will automatically trigger a rejection of a vital organ from another body, in this case the donor's. Such rejections are instigated by substances called antigens; the human leukocyte antigen (HLA) is responsible for this action and has been implicated in a number of autoimmune diseases. Basically HLA and similar antigens are usually the result of severe stress or viral infection to the body or both, in which case the immune system goes berserk and starts attacking or rejecting healthy areas of the body.

Autoimmune diseases, as a group, reports *Science* for June 15, 1990, "affect 5 to 7% of the population," often with very severe disability and, therefore, are a major cause of chronic illness. Morphologically, these disorders are marked by excessive production of white blood cells in the lymph nodes and spleen and normally accompanied by prominent centers of reactions. The course of the conditions in many of these particular disorders is progressive, unrelenting, and prolonged as a rule. The following list of "autoimmune diseases" was compiled from Brunson's and Gall's *Concepts of Disease* (New York: Macmillan, 1971) and Lendon Smith's *Feed Yourself Right* (New York: McGraw-Hill, 1983), as well as the aforementioned article in *Science*

Addison's disease/chronic adrenal insufficiency

Ankylosing spondylitis

Celiac disease/gluten-sensitive enteropathy

Chronic ulcerative colitis

Crohn's disease/regional enteritis

Diabetes mellitus/insulin-dependent diabetes

Graves' disease/hyperthyroidism

Myasthenia gravis/Hoppe-Goldflam disease

Pernicious anemia

Psoriasis

Rheumatoid arthritis

Scleroderma/dermatosclerosis

Systemic lupus erthythematosus

◆◆◆◆◆

ADDISON'S DISEASE/CHRONIC ADRENAL INSUFFICIENCY

This autoimmune disorder is of insidious onset, being induced by immune proteins called antibodies attacking the adrenal glands. The results are hormone imbalances that lead to darkening of the skin, abdominal pain, and occasionally coma. Other more common characteristics are weakness, fatigue, listlessness, anorexia, weight loss, nausea, and vomiting. It's interesting to note that viral infections sometimes occur in both the medulla and the cortex (the inner and outer layers) of the adrenals. Each of these glands fits like a cap over both kidneys and may be adversely affected by urinary tract infection.

Natural Supplements for Preventative Care

Since many advanced cases of hypoglycemia eventually turn into Addison's disease, greater attention should be directed toward controlling this low-blood-sugar problem. (See Chapter Three for more information on how to deal with hypoglycemia.)

To combat urinary tract infection, the following several substances are especially useful: cranberry juice, goldenseal root and juniper berry One 8-oz glass of Ocean Spray cranber ry juice daily is suggested with a meal. One capsule of Wakunaga goldenseal root (see appendix) on an empty stomach is also useful. And 2 cups of juniper berry tea always seems to curb kidney infections. To make the tea, bring a quart of water to a boil. Then add 2 teaspoons of the dried berries. Cover, reduce heat to lower setting and simmer for 5 minutes. Remove from stove and steep for half an hour. Strain, sweeten with honey, and drink. Vitamin C (3,500 mg.) and fish-oil vitamin A (about 50,000 I.U.) should also be taken to stop infection in this part of the body as well. Raw adrenal gland supplement is also advised for Addison's disease.

What a Tampa Doctor Does for His Addison's Patients

A certain Tampa, Florida, doctor I know, who specializes in what he describes rather laconically as "that pooped feeling," recommends high-cholesterol foods for those suffering from the more medically correct diagnosis of "energy exhaustion."

"In this day and age, too much emphasis is being put upon *low* cholesterol this and *low* fat that," he lamented to me one day in the spring of 1988. "That may be okay for those with plugged arteries and all, but I seriously question the medical wisdom in it for everyone."

My physician friend sees on the average of between 7 and 10 "energy exhaustion" patients a day. Some are full-blown Addison's cases, but the majority tend to be borderline or complete hypoglycemics. "You can't do without cholesterol in some forms for such cases," he advised me.

"Take the case of a middle-aged gentleman I was treating just the other day," he continued. "This guy had been going downhill energy-wise, for some time, since his wife got on an anticholesterol health kick. And while she may have been doing his arteries a big favor, she was unwittingly damaging his adrenal gland in the process.

"So I sit down and explained to them both, but particularly to her (since she cooked all of his meals), just how badly his body demanded cholesterol. I said that it was an important source of the natural adrenal steroid hormones that help give us a feeling of energy and strength I cited hydrocortisone the glu costeroids, and DOCA—that salt- and water-balancing steroid. Most of this medical talk, I'm afraid, pretty much went right over their heads.

"But I finally got down to brass tacks by telling his wife that she needed to feed her hubby *more* not less cholesterol-rich foods. I began the list by recommending certain fatty freshwater or saltwater fish, either baked or steamed. I followed this up with guacamole dip made from ripe avocados and nuts like Brazil, which are also high in natural fats.

"I suggested she be imaginative with salads, but to use generous amounts of olive oil. I even recommended that he eat a slice or two of seven-grain or stone-ground whole wheat bread each day smeared with *real butter* of all things, instead of some whimpy cholesterol-free margarine. I've even suggested an occasional beef cube steak for breakfast for some of my patients. In every single instance, where they follow my advice, their energy levels soon come back. This is what happened with this particular fellow once his wife got her act in the kitchen together!"

◆◆◆◆◆

ANKYLOSING SPONDYLITIS

This is a progressive, inflammatory kind of arthritis believed to be of genetic origin, but usually triggered by sudden stress or a hidden virus. About 500,000 Americans (mostly men) are afflicted with it. It first strikes the spinal column and nearby structures; the bones may join together (a process called ankylosis). Hip, shoulder, neck, ribs and jaw joints are often afflicted as well.

Symptoms include nagging pain in the hips, neck, or lower or middle back, which worsen with bending. Stiffness and lower-back inflammation might appear, often at the joint where the tail bone meets the pelvic bones. Spine and chest motion can be difficult and painful. Pain often comes and goes, so some victims are fooled into thinking they've "slipped a disc" or strained their backs. In the more advanced stages, the spine becomes forwardly flexed, forcing the victim to walk with head downward.

The disease was relatively unknown until the late Norman

Cousins, the former editor of *Saturday Review* magazine came down with it and wrote a narrative of his suffering that became a worldwide best-seller, *Anatomy of an Illness* (New York: Bantam Books, 1980). He and his wife had gone to the Soviet Union in the summer of 1964. While there he encountered various types of stress—anxiety, air and water pollution, and horribly bad food—which adversely affected his body. Upon arriving back home to Connecticut (where he then resided), he could feel something was very wrong with him. A week later he was hospitalized with this disease.

Positive Attitude Plus Vitamin C Equals Effective Treatment

While receiving medical care for his worsening condition, Cousins did some things on his own which, in the end, were the real factors in his eventually getting well again. Rather than being exotic solutions, they were simple attitude readjustments of the mind and heart. Along with vitamin C, they became the chief means of curing his devastating health problem.

1. Negative thoughts cripple, but positive emotions help heal! It dawned upon Cousins that if negative energy produces negative chemical changes in our systems, then positive thoughts and feelings should produce positive chemical changes. The will to live, faith, hope, confidence, love, and laughter were things he discovered that elicited positive changes in his medically impossible condition.

2. Attitudes determine just how intense physical pain will be. Cousins's ceased taking the aspirin and phenylbutazone that the doctors were doping him up with in a vain attempt to control his terrible pain. He said that the bones in his spine and nearly every joint throughout his body felt as though he had been hit and run over by a Mack truck. But he wanted to initiate other things which could possibly alleviate some of his pain; hence, he began a diligent effort to develop

   a. A strong determination to *not* let this disease get the best of him

   b. An absolute faith and confidence in himself and his own inner abilities to do something about the situation

    c. A sure hope that everything he was trying would work out

    d. A greater love for himself, family, and fellowmen than he previously had

But the last goal he had set for himself, the ability to laugh, was the hardest of all to come by. "Nothing is less funny than being flat on your back with all the bones in your spine and joints hurting," he wrote. What was he to do? Help came to him from the least expected quarters.

3. Prolonged laughter relieves pain better than aspirin could. One day, while laying in his hospital bed in complete agony, one of the old "Candid Camera" classics came on the TV set he was watching in his room. The unrehearsed reactions of people to certain deliberately rigged situations prompted him to start laughing like crazy. Thirty minutes later when the program ended, he discovered that his pain had also substantially decreased as well. This set him to thinking about the possible benefits that laughter might contribute to his deteriorating condition. So, he made arrangements to be transferred out of the hospital and into a setting that would be conducive to his recovery. He then ordered all of the old "Candid Camera" segments, Marx Brothers films, and Three Stooges comedies that he could lay his hands on, along with a projector to show them. His attending nurse was instructed in how to run the machine properly. With her help everyday he would watch about 10 minutes of side-splitting screen comedy and enjoy "at least two hours of pain-free sleep." That was repeated several times throughout the day. When he got tired of these, she would switch to different humor books and read out of them a while with the same anesthetic effects. *This, above anything else, he attributes to getting well.*

4. Massive amounts of vitamin C given intravenously also helped. Imagine the astonishment of Cousins's personal physician, when he was informed that his patient wanted about *25 grams* of vitamin C to be routinely administered over a period of several hours through slow intravenous drip. Cousins noted that his doctor's eyes opened wide when he first proposed this idea to him. However, the doctor was willing to accommodate his patient anyway he could, but suggested starting out with smaller doses: 10 grams the first day, 12.5 grams the second day, 15 grams the third day, and so on until the end of the week, when they reached the full 25 grams. By then his laugh therapy was in full swing and he was entirely off all prescription medication, including sleeping pills. He reported that his periods of pain-*free* sleep were becoming "increasingly prolonged" and that movement had begun to return to his thumbs, fingers, neck, and knees. His overall recovery took an additional couple of years until total physical mobility had been achieved.

Certainly this highly unorthodox program may not work for everyone else similarly afflicted. First, he tackled the problem in its beginning stages. Second, there was *a powerful change in personal attitude.* Third there was his removal from his noisy and depressing hospital setting to a quiet and cheerful hotel environment instead. And, finally, there were massive doses of ascorbic acid regularly *administered by a qualified doctor!*

◆◆◆◆◆

CELIAC DISEASE/GLUTEN-SENSITIVE ENTEROPATHY

My good friend, Lendon Smith, M.D., classifies this as an autoimmune disorder in his book, *Feed Yourself Right.* Better known as celiac disease, it's brought about by an intolerance to wheat and rye protein, more specifically, an acute sensitivity to gluten. Symptoms are those often characteristic of malabsorption: large, pale, bad-smelling stools, abdominal swelling, poor growth, and weight loss.

More common in young children from infancy to 10 years old than in adults, the condition reflects an inflammation of the child's small intestine by gluten, which, in turn, completely interferes with normal digestion. The partially digested food passes out in bowel movements, thereby depriving the system of essential vitamins, minerals, amino acids, and especially fats.

In advanced stages, other symptoms may be present. The child or adult could experience anorexia nervosa (self-induced weight loss by voluntary starvation), vomiting of partially digested food, acute diarrhea marked by greasy, hard-to-flush stools, and a pronounced potbelly. However, reaching this crisis stage is rare, since most cases are detected early on and can be properly treated.

Cardamom: An Effective Treatment

A pediatrician who works at the Boston Children's Medical Center in Boston, Massachusetts, once told me that *the first mandatory rule is to place the child (or adult) on a gluten-free diet for life!* Once this very necessary step has been taken, the youngster (or, more rarely, a grown-up) speedily improves.

Different books are available through most health food stores that carry gluten-free recipes. There are also gluten-free breads and rolls sold in some of these stores or in supermarkets in some major metropolitan areas. Consulting with local health food store owners, nutritionists, and pediatricians should help you find those books and foods most helpful to celiac victims.

When I was doing some ethnomedical research in different parts of Indonesia in 1986, I met a doctor in the large city of Surabaya by the name of Singh Rhee, M.D. He acquainted me with the spice, cardamom. The seed is slightly sticky, brown-black, warmly aromatic, and with a vague hint of eucalyptus. It is an essential ingredient in curries and pilaus, especially those from northern India and Pakistan.

Dr. Rhee has treated a number of Australian and New Zealand children afflicted with celiac disease by administering powdered cardamom (1 to 2 capsules) on a daily basis; sometimes he even recommended adding it to cooked cereal. The result is that they can tolerate gluten a lot better.

◆◆◆◆◆

CHRONIC ULCERATIVE COLITIS

The major symptom is diarrhea (occasionally bloody), often a dozen to two dozen times a day. Also characterized by mild to severe abdominal cramps; futile, urgent efforts at defecation; tenderness in the lower quadrants of the abdomen; and sometimes anemia.

Chronic ulcerative colitis can start as early as childhood or a little later in adolescent years. Often the chief causes are the same as those for asthma—genetic, emotional, and nutritional. One doctor discovered a higher than anticipated incidence of asthma, eczema, and hay fever in a group of his patients with ulcerative colitis. When these systemic allergies were brought under control, the colitis cleared up, suggesting a common origin for all of them.

Five Easy Ways to Combat Chronic Ulcerative Colitis

The following simple recommendations are most efficacious:

1. Avoid refined carbohydrates and dairy and corn products. No white sugar, white flour, milk, cheese, butter, yogurt, tacos, tortillas, corn oil, or corn should be consumed in the first couple of weeks. But once the colon has calmed down and the stool has returned to fairly soft consistency, then yogurt, cottage cheese, goat's milk, and whey powder may be added back into the diet.

2. Frequently consume those foods that promote soothing healing. Bananas, ripe papaya and ripe mango, and ripe melons (cantaloupe, casaba, honeydew, and watermelon) are very good. Also, drink two herbal tea combinations at separate times on an empty stomach—they really do promote rapid healing of the colon. The first of these is comfrey root—marshmallow root. In a pint of boiling water, add 1 level teaspoonful of each root (dried, coarsely cut) and simmer for 5 minutes on low heat, then remove and steep for 1 hour. Strain, sweeten with honey or molasses, and drink 1 cup twice daily. The second calls for equal parts of chamomile and yarrow to be added to a pint of boiling water; remove from heat, stir, cover, and steep for 45 minutes. Strain, sweeten with pure maple syrup and drink 1 cup twice a day. Also in larger quart amounts, each combination can be introduced as a soothing enema when lukewarm. Certain juices are of considerable value here, too—papaya juice, mango juice, pineapple/papaya juices (equal parts of both mixed together), but *avoid* citrus juices as they tend to aggravate colitis.

3. Eat foods that give considerable energy *and* stop diarrhea. A millet–brown rice combination is one of the very best dishes for promoting energy and stopping diarrhea at the same time. Cook both grains with extra water, drain off, and drink the liquid.

4. Take nutritional supplements. Kyo-Dophilus (2 capsules) (see Wakunaga in the appendix), vitamin B-6 (50 mg.), Pines' Wheat & Barley Grass (6 tablets daily; see the appendix), high potency B-complex (100 mg.), calcium (800 mg.)–magnesium (400 mg.) combination (2 tablets daily), zinc (25 mg.), vitamin A (25,000 I.U.), powdered vitamin C (Quest Electro-C; see the appendix), and pantothenic acid (100 mg.).

An "Okie" Remedy

At the end of some of my books or magazine and newspaper articles, I often ask readers to send in their favorite remedies. Well, just like the popular country-western hit goes, "I'm an Okie from Muskogee . . . ," a reader from Muskogee County in western Oklahoma responded in a letter to me dated August 21, 1983:

> Read your piece on heart care in one of our local papers here. Must say it made a lot of sense, though I hope I never have to use any of it myself. But it's good to know jest [sic] in case I might ever need to follow any of it.
>
> In your asking for things that are good to use when you get ill, I have something to share with you that my grand-pappy used for many years for his colitis. Maybe some folks out there can benefit from it, I hope.
>
> Doctors he consulted couldn't help him too much with his problem. Not until a local bartender suggested that he try some kalua-and-cream drink mix *without* the alcohol did he begin to experience any noticeable relief to speak of. Sometime after this, he discovered that by boiling up a little shredded coconut meat in a tiny bit of water *and then adding* it to his kalua-and-cream drink did it seem to help his colitis even better.
>
> I can't remember just how often he took this combination, but think it was at least once a day, probably in the afternoon when it bothered him the most.
>
> Jest [sic] sign me "a friendly Okie from neighborly Muskogee"—J.R.

◆◆◆◆◆

CROHN'S DISEASE/REGIONAL ENTERITIS

A lengthy study recently published in *Digestive Diseases and Sciences* (November 1987) on Crohn's disease, attributed this idiopathic inflammatory bowel disorder to certain immunologic defects in the body's mucosal immune system. The misguided actions of T cells are believed to be the real culprit behind the origins of intestinal inflammation in this autoimmune disease. However, certain infectious agents can also produce near identical inflammation of the gastrointestinal (G.I.) tract as well. Examples of such mimicry may be found in the G.I. infections caused by mycobacteria and yersinia microorganisms. More striking though in this uncanny similarity to Crohn's disease is the inflammation caused by the strain of chlamydia producing a particularly aggressive and nasty venereal disease known as lymphogranuloma venercum, which is becoming more widespread of late. Still, an erratic suppressor T cell is blamed for calling in those immune elements that actually cause tissue injury in Crohn's disease.

A Change in Diet Alleviates Symptoms

Several different approaches can be taken toward making this autoimmune disease go into remission. All that's needed is just a little patient experimenting and the determination to stick with those things that alleviate your symptoms.

Dietary Management: In one study of 33 patients with active Crohn's disease, remission was produced in as soon as 2 weeks through elimination diets; all medications were withdrawn during this time. Foods were then slowly reintroduced one per day; reactions were recorded and confirmed by retested several weeks later. Of 29 patients who completed reintroduction of foods into their diets, all discovered specific foods that precipitated their symptoms.

According to *Human Nutrition & Applied Nutrition* (November/December 1984), half of the patients were intolerant of more than three foods. The foods most frequently provoking symptoms were wheat (69% of the patients); dairy products (48%); yeast (31%); corn (24%); potato and tap water (17% each); and banana, tomato, wine, and eggs (14% each). Remissions were maintained in 22 patients for 6 to 32 months *without* drugs so long as they avoided most of the foods just listed.

Another study reported in *Gut* (October 1985) showed that there is really no justification for limiting dietary fiber in patients with Crohn's disease. Patients with Crohn's disease who had been following a low-residue diet were randomly assigned to either continue their low-fiber diets or to return gradually to their normal Italian diets. There was no difference in outcome between the low-fiber and high-fiber groups as judged by symptoms, need for hospitalization or surgery, or new complications. But most in both groups avoided dairy products, legumes, and isolated fruits and vegetables.

Remedial Measures: An old Hawaiian folk healer from Molokai I once met treated those who came to her with Crohn's disease with slices of ripe papaya for breakfast every morning. This eliminated the need for periodic injections of vitamin B-12.

In the event that colic should occur, she would have her patients sprinkle some cinnamon or ginger over their fruit, which always seemed to work.

She would treat the inevitable diarrhea that occurs every so often in Crohn's disease in one of two ways. Either she would give patients a cup of cooked rice water to drink several times a day, or she would combine a cup of papaya juice with ½ cup of seawater and 2 tablespoons of lemon juice.

Sometimes fevers occur in children afflicted with this autoimmune dysfunction. To correct this, she would dilute some concentrated papaya juice with a little *ice*-cold water and have the kids slowly sip it.

Weight loss and lack of appetite are also occasionally associated with Crohn's disease. To encourage heartier appetites, she would serve up simple stews made from lamb or goat meat to which had been added cut chunks of *green* papaya, cut whole lemon (skin and all), diced sweet potato, and pinches of spices such as coriander, ginger, marjoram, and savory.

◆◆◆◆◆

DIABETES MELLITUS/INSULIN-DEPENDENT DIABETES

Diabetes has been accurately described as an "underestimated disease," because of the tremendous damage it can cause to the heart, eyes, muscles, and kidneys. Though few may know it, diabetes is the nation's number one cause of kidney disease and blindness, besides accounting for a large number of heart disease, stroke, and loss of limb cases. That's why if it is left unattended for very long, it can wreak havoc beyond estimation.

There are two types of diabetes:

Type I (Insulin Dependent). The pancreas ceases insulin production (the hormone that enables the cells to utilize glucose properly). Often called juvenile or sudden-onset diabetes because it primarily strikes people under age 25 and accounts for about 10% of all cases in America. With sudden-onset diabetes, the victim can get very sick, very fast. *Science* (May 13, 1983) described this type of diabetes as an autoimmune disease and the *Annals of Allergy* (November 1987) presented evidence on how the immune system of a young diabetic goes berserk and destroys the individual's vital beta cells in the pancreas where insulin is produced. Three other journals in 1979—*New England Journal of Medicine* (May 24), *Science News* (June 2), and *Scientific American* (November)—furnished conclusive evidence that Type I is induced by a virus! Symptoms include constant urination and bedwetting in an otherwise dry child, excessive thirst and consumption of large volumes of water, fatigue, irritability, and sweet or fruity breath (due to the presence of acetone). In the more advanced stages coma, dehydration, and labored breathing all become dangerously evident.

Type II (Noninsulin Dependent). The beta cells in the pancreas lose their ability to respond to insulin. This type is often referred to as "borderline" diabetes and has the potential to be far more sinister than the first one, simply because it isn't taken as seriously. This maturity- or adult-onset kind accounts for the other 90% of diabetics in this country. My colleague, Lendon Smith, M.D., refers to diabetes as really being a *combina-*

tion of different illnesses involving the body's sugar metabolism. And Robert C. Atkins, M.D., a New York City physician, asserts that hypoglycemia or low blood sugar is one of those diseases behind the majority of Type II cases. Excessive consumption of white sugar–white flour products, both doctors say, is the leading cause of this. Typical symptoms include losing weight without trying to; continual thirst; chronic fatigue, mood swings, and frequent forgetfulness (all classic signs of hypoglycemia); frequent urination; and progressive nervousness, growing insomnia, hypertension, and obesity (in many other cases).

Diabetes Responds to Nutritional Regimen Treatment

One of the very best management programs I've ever seen for Type I diabetes, was devised by a St. Petersburg, Florida, mother for her 6-year-old daughter who contracted the juvenile-onset kind when she was 5. In February 1990 at the Juvenile Diabetes Research Center on the campus of the University of South Florida in Tampa, her girl's condition was evaluated with at least four dozen other diabetic children of similar age. It was discovered that she got by nicely with just 14 units of insulin administered daily (7 units per injection), whereas **all** of the other kids averaged 34 units per day (17 units per shot). Also she looked healthier and felt better than the rest of her age group did, which frankly amazed the doctors investigating each child's progress.

Now I've known the parents for more than a decade, and was especially pleased when they consented to share with me the nutritional program they built from scratch for their daughter, Sarah Ann. Here are the main highlights of her regimen:

1. *No* **red meat, just** *fresh* **fish.** Louise either broils or stir-fries grouper, king fish, trout, tuna, salmon, shrimp, shell fish, or whatever may be in season at the time.

2. Whole grains, especially buckwheat. "I recently read an article," Sarah's mother informed me by telephone, "that suggested buckwheat was excellent for diabetics, so we are feeding our daughter more of this. I usually fix it as a side dish much as you would brown rice and serve it with many of our meals. I also make regular cereal and pancakes of it as well. We've noticed Sarah's sugar levels have become more stable since she's been eating buckwheat."

3. Green beans and green bean juice. "We had heard from an old Amish folk healer in the nearby Amish community at Sarasota that green beans really brought sugar levels down," Louise said. One day I went to the store and bought *three pounds*, which my daughter consumed raw in *four days* time. She constantly was snacking on them after she came home from school at 3:00 P.M. Now I monitor her blood sugar levels three times each day, and was there ever a difference! Several days before she went on this green bean binge, her sugar levels were running 212 and over, but since then they've dropped to between 80 and 100, which doctors say is preferable." Besides consuming them raw, Sarah also drinks them in juice form.

4. Raw almonds and raw hazelnuts. "For some reason," Louise continued, "when Sarah puts these in her pocket and snacks on them while she is in school, her blood sugar is stabilized a lot more."

5. Blackberry leaf tea sweetened with stevia. "I make plenty of this herbal tea for our family of five, which we drink with nearly every meal instead of juice or water or milk," she added. "I add a few broken leaves of stevia, a natural sugar substitute that is unbelievably sweet. I use the powdered form of stevia in my cookies, pies, and so forth." (See the Appendix for Custom-Made Formulas as a potential source for this plant sweetener from mainland China.)

6. Consistency in the eating schedule. "If Sarah sticks to her appointed schedule for eating, everything goes fine," she said. (8:30 A.M. breakfast, 11:00 A.M. lunch, 3:30 P.M. snack, 6:30 P.M. dinner, and 8:30 P.M. bedtime snack.) "But if she misses just one of these, then it seems like everything is thrown out of kilter."

7. Exercise. "My daughter gets plenty of aerobic exercise in the swimming pool of our back yard," she pointed out. "And since the back of our property abuts Tampa Bay, she enjoys walking and running on the small beach we have here. My husband and I, along with my older daughter Amy and son,

Ronnie, each take turns massaging Sarah's feet every night for about 5 minutes. For some reason still unknown to us, this helps her to sleep better."

8. Nutritional supplements. Sarah Ann, age 6, takes the following health food supplements each day:

GTF chromium	200 mcg. four times daily (any local health food store)
Guar gum	2 capsules three times daily (any local health food store)
AquaVite	2 tablets three times daily (see appendix for Great American Natural Products, Inc.)
Super herbal C	300 mg. eight times daily (see appendix for Great American Natural Products, Inc.)
Garlic	500 mg. twice daily of kyolic (health food stores or see appendix for Wakunaga)

Many of the aforementioned items would benefit Type II diabetes as well. However, oral antidiabetic medications for this kind, and even insulin injections for Type I in adults, can prove to be especially hazardous in certain instances. Robert C. Atkins, M.D., of New York City, who trained to be a cardiologist years ago, believes that prescription drugs such as Orinase, Tolinase, and Diabinese, among others, can sharply increase a person's risk of cardiovascular death. He supports his belief in this regard by pointing to the *Physicians' Desk Reference* and the package inserts for each drug—in both instances, the adverse side effect of potential heart failure is clearly evident. And the January 1990 issue of *Pediatrics* reported that, due to their mothers' daily insulin injections, children of Type I diabetic women experienced double the risk of birth defects.

Type II diabetes may be suitably managed with the following conventional and sometimes unconventional methods. From among them different programs can be worked out to fit individual health needs.

1. Be a nibbler and snack often. Research has shown that wolfing down one or two large meals a day can set your insulin awry, whereas "snacking" on four or five smaller meals tends to keep it more level.

2. Stay with a high carbohydrate and fiber (HCF) diet. James W. Anderson, M.D., has been on the staff of both the Veterans Administration Medical Center and the University of Kentucky College of Medicine, both in Lexington. He put a dozen, nonobese, insulin-treated diabetic men on control and HCF diets to determine which worked the best in reducing insulin requirements. Four subjects had insulin-dependent (Type I) diabetes mellitus and eight had noninsulin-dependent (Type II) diabetes mellitus. The average age was 53 years. For a week they first received control diets, consisting of highly refined foods either made out of white flour (bread, rolls), white sugar (desserts, soft drinks), or both (pies, cakes) or else highly processed (breakfast sausages, luncheon meats) or overly cooked (mashed potatoes). Then he switched them to HCF diets for the next two weeks. During this period the men subsisted on whole-grain cereals, bran cereals, whole-grain breads, vegetables, legumes, and fresh fruits. It was soon discovered that the insulin requirements necessary to maintain satisfactory glycemic control were *73% lower with HCF* diets than with control diets, according to *Annals of Internal Medicine* (Vol. 98, Part 2, 1983, 842–846).

Sample Menus For Diabetics

The following sample menus are frequently prescribed by Dr. Anderson for his diabetic patients with very good results. Because most of them also needed to lose weight, each menu was limited to just 1,800 calories. These menus will give you a rough idea of how to formulate your own daily meal plans to manage Type II diabetes successfully.

More recent, corresponding work by nutritionists at the University of Toronto has shown that the higher the intake of phytic acid (in legumes) and lectin (in cereal grains, legumes, and other plant foods), the lower the blood-glucose levels. Seven different legumes (including beans and chickpeas) initiated a much slower, wonderfully lower rise in blood sugar. In a follow-up experiment, 10 healthy volunteers ate unleavened bread made from navy bean flour—with and without the beans' usual phytic acid. Believe it or not, their blood-glucose responses were 52% higher after they had consumed the bread *without* phytic acid in it.

According to reports in *The American Journal of Clinical Nutrition* (April 1986 and January 1987), parboiled, cracked wheat or bulghur (a traditional Middle Eastern staple) and pumpernickel bread (a popular whole grain rye bread of Northern Europe) were two of the best grain foods to keep glucose levels down. Also, when Australian aborigines and South Pacific islanders strayed from their traditional high-fiber foods such as cassava, coconut, roots, berries, and leaves, and instead consumed a lot of refined Western foods, they soon developed Type II diabetes. Once they returned to their healthier, native staples, practically all symptoms of their diabetes eventually disappeared.

Herbs, Spices, and Plant Foods That Help Manage Diabetes

Information supplied by Bep Oliver-Bever from her *Medicinal Plants in Nigeria* (Lagos: Nigerian College of Arts, Science and Technology, 1960), article in *Journal of Ethnopharmacology* (1980), and *Medicinal Plants in Tropical West Africa* (1986) provide a short but highly effective list of certain medicinal herbs, spices, and plant foods that are very useful in the management of Type II diabetes.

Onions. Several powerful sulphur components in Bermuda and green onions remove compounds from the pancreas that activate the production of insulin. These sulphur constituents actually stimulate the production of more insulin which has been shown to produce "a marked fall in blood sugar plus an increase of serum insulin levels" in fasting human subjects.

Garlic. The sulphur-bearing compound, allicin, in garlic "produced a significant drop in the fasting blood glucose levels" of a dozen subjects in clinical trials. Kyolic garlic can be taken with meals rich in carbohydrates. (See appendix, p. 328.)

Pau D'Arco (Taheebo). Fluid extracts of a West African species of this particular herb were tested in mongrel dogs and found to produce "powerful hypoglycemic responses" within just a matter of minutes. Ten to 12 drops of pau d'arco, twice daily, beneath the tongue is the suggested dosage (Alta Health Products features a very strong liquid concentrate of pau d'arco for such purposes. See the appendix for further details.)

Fenugreek. Israeli researchers have isolated coumarin and nicotinic acid from fenugreek seed, which accounts for its remarkable antidiabetic effects. A tea made from the seeds and consumed every day is said to lower blood sugar nicely. To make the tea, add 1 teaspoonful of seeds to a pint of boiling water; cover and reduce heat, simmering for a few minutes. Then remove from heat and steep half-an-hour.

Cinnamon, Nutmeg, Turmeric, and Bay Leaf. Recent research has demonstrated that certain spices hold new importance in their ability to lower elevated blood-sugar levels. According to Dr. Richard Anderson at the USDA's Human Nutrition Research Center, four particular spices affect insulin, the hormone that directs cells to absorb blood sugar. Insulin works less efficiently with age, thereby permitting sugar to remain in the blood at high levels. Untreated, this can lead to diabetes. Well, Anderson and his team applied 22 different spice extracts to rats' cells and measured their individual insulin activities. Cinnamon, nutmeg, turmeric, and bay leaf solutions yielded the greatest effect, more than tripling insulin's normal activity level. He thinks these spices would be useful in the diets of diabetics.

Trace elements such as chromium, zinc, manganese, vanadium, magnesium, and tyrosine are good in regulating Type II diabetes.

◆◆◆◆◆

GRAVES'S DISEASE/HYPERTHYROIDISM

In four out of five instances, especially in women, an overactive thyroid gland is the result of Graves's disease. First Lady Barbara Bush's recent illness has focused greater public attention on this disease, which affects over a million Americans each year. This autoimmune disorder is brought about when some of a person's white blood cells produce a protein that stimulates the thyroid gland.

According to Dr. Manfred Blum, an endocrinologist at New York University Medical Center, symptoms characterizing Graves's disease include rapid and irregular heartbeat, weight loss despite increased appetite, anxiety, insomnia, trembling hands, excess sweating, frequent bowel movements, and menstrual irregularity. Muscle weakness and wasting may occur, and the thyroid gland may become noticeably enlarged. In close to half the cases of Graves's disease, another common symptom is bulging of the eyes. Swelling of the tissues in the eye socket causes the eye to protrude. The eyeball becomes dry and gritty, and eye movement is restricted. Blurred or double vision may result.

Iodine Treatment Slows Overactive Thyroid

The horseshoe-shaped thyroid gland implicated in this disease is located in the front of the neck just below the larynx or voice box. This gland produces thyroxine, a hormone that regulates the body's rate of utilizing nutrients and expending energy: the more hormone, the faster the rate.

Treatment of Graves's disease involves decreasing the amount of thyroxine that the thyroid gland produces. The most common method of accomplishing this is to increase the amount of iodine taken into the body. Dr. Blum explained that when this trace element is absorbed by the thyroid, it slowly reduces thyroid tissue and activity.

The richest sources of iodine happen to be certain seaweeds such as dulse, Irish moss, and kelp. The best way to use them is in a liquid form, with the exception of kelp, which can be used in coarse granules or else powdered to season a variety of foods with instead of black pepper or salt. Pure Herbs of Madison Heights, Michigan (see the appendix), has incredibly strong fluid extracts of dulse, Irish moss, and kelp, which can be used by those suffering from Graves's disease with fairly good results.

Such fluid extracts are to be taken sublingually (beneath the tongue), 8 to 10 drops at a time on an empty stomach, twice daily. Also two Pure Herbs formulas, HIK/W and VM/W, may also be used, since both are high in iodine derived from dulse and kelp.

How Mrs. B. Brought Her Overactive Thyroid Under Control

Around 1956 I was living with my family in Provo, Utah, where my father then operated his own business, Cottage Book Shop. I attended Maesar Elementary School and had as my fourth grade teacher, a woman I'll call Mrs. B.

Some 14 years later, when I moved back to Provo from Idaho Falls, Idaho, to take some classes at Brigham Young University, I worked part-time in the funeral business selling prearranged funerals for Berg Mortuary. In the beginning I called upon all my old school teachers then still living, most of whom had retired. Among these was Mrs. B.

During our pleasant visit together reminiscing over old times, she informed me that she had contracted Graves's disease just a few years earlier. This episode stands out in my memory because of the somewhat dark humor that I had attached to it during my visit with her. At one point in our conversation, I remember kidding her about being ready for a funeral plan since she already had Graves's disease and, with one foot in it, needed something to cover all of these future expenses adequately.

This wisecrack, of course, didn't help me to make a sale that day, but my good-natured teacher took it well enough and was not to be offended by my remarks. She, however, did tell me how she had brought her own hyperthyroidism under control.

She went to a local health food store and bought a large jar of kelp tablets and started to take them each day. Her regimen was one tablet with each meal or three tablets daily. In about two months, her quick heartbeats, weight loss, worrying, hand shaking, profuse perspiration, and numerous trips to the toilet had greatly subsided. Also, she said the inflammation within her eyeballs, causing them to protrude noticeably, had diminished quite a bit as well. She attributed these reversals to the kelp tablets, which were a rich source of iodine that her body badly needed.

◆◆◆◆◆

MYASTHENIA GRAVIS/HOPPE-GOLDFLAM DISEASE

This condition is marked by a chronic and progressive muscular weakness, usually beginning in the face and throat. Unlike similar problems, however, it isn't accompanied by a wasting of the muscle tissue. It is believed to be caused by a defect in the conduction of body bioelectrical energy through the nerves and into the muscles.

The thymus gland situated in the base of the neck and involved in the development of normal immunological functions frequently becomes enlarged when this disorder occurs. Often a benign tumor is the main culprit behind the abnormality of the thymus; sometimes surgical excision of the growth results in improvement of myasthenia gravis, but other times it doesn't seem to help very much.

Vitamin and Mineral Treatment Helps Muscles Contract

My colleague, Lendon Smith, M.D., believes that certain minerals and vitamins are helpful in getting the receptor sites at nerve-muscle junctions in the head, neck, and diaphragm more responsive to the neurotransmitter, acetylcholine, which prompts muscle contractions in these areas. I've added suggested daily dosages to some of them.

Manganese	15 mg.	Vitamin E	400–800 I.U.
Vitamin C	2,500 mg.	Brewer's yeast	¼ tsp.
B-complex	2 tablets	Rex's Wheat Germ Oil*	1 tsp.
Vitamin D	400 I.U.	Liquid lecithin	1 tsp.
Calcium	600 mg.		

*Must be purchased at a veterinary supply house; all other items can be obtained at any local health food store. (See Quest Vitamins in the appendix.)

A Veterinarian's Remedy That Really Works

During my youth in Provo, Utah, I became acquainted with a number of elderly people by virtue of where we then lived and because of my father's bookstore. On our particular block, there were mostly businesses and only a few other houses. There weren't any other youngsters my age or my brother's age with whom we could play or visit, just a lot of elderly folks. So they became our friends instead.

Near us was a gentleman of advanced years by the name of Dr. Vance. My father sometimes took us to see him if we had something wrong with us. Dr. Vance had unusual remedies that always seemed to work. However, he wasn't your typical everyday, garden-variety physician. You see, Dr. Vance was a DVM, not an M.D.—that is, as a doctor of veterinary medicine he was more used to seeing four-footed and hooved patients than the two-legged, shoe-and-sock wearing kinds.

Once, when I happened to be at his place for some reason, there was a plump, middle-aged woman ahead of me who wanted to see him for some malady affecting her face and throat. Soon the good doc came into his front office and proceeded to conduct a lengthy interview with her right there in front of me, as was his usual custom. During the lengthy conversation, I kept hearing two words come up which he used to describe her affliction. I couldn't remember the first part, but gravis definitely stuck in my mind as I quickly associated it with the word gravity in order to remember it better. Years later when diseases and remedies became my own fields of expertise, I finally was able to get down the myasthenia portion as well.

Finally, he left the room and returned with a square tan and green metal can, adorned with silhouettes of farm animals and clearly labeled in bold letters, "Rex's Wheat Germ Oil." He told her to take 2 tablespoonfuls every day for the first couple of months, then to cut back to just 1 tablespoonful every other day.

Her first reaction upon seeing the container suggested that she wasn't about to take medicine intended for cows and horses. But he reassured her that it wasn't medicine, but unrefined wheat germ oil rich in vitamin E that would resolve her muscular condition nicely. She paid for the stuff and left. A while after this when I saw Dr. Vance again for something else, I inquired about "the heavy lady with the gravis." He said her facial paralysis had completely disappeared and that now she was able to swallow normally.

◆◆◆◆◆

PERNICIOUS ANEMIA

Pernicious or megaloblastic anemia is characterized by large germ cells in the bone marrow and by their large progeny in the peripheral blood supply. Biochemically, it is of diverse origin, since it could result from blocked DNA synthesis of any cause. Clinically, the cause is almost invariably deficiencies of vitamin

B-12 and/or folic acid. But deficiencies of both vitamins usually occur from inadequate ingestion, inadequate absorption, inadequate utilization, increased requirement, increased destruction, or increased urine-fecal excretion, alone or in combination.

The following symptoms usually mark the presence of pernicious anemia: paleness of skin, weakness, and breathlessness (common anemic symptoms); palpitations; nosebleed; pins-and-needles sensations of the hands and feet; sore, thick, reddened tongue; appetite loss; weight loss; and skin yellowness (indicating jaundice). More advanced cases exhibit difficulty in walking, nausea and vomiting, impotence or frigidity, mental confusion, and possible coronary failure. An abnormally low amount of white blood cells (leukopenia) and greater susceptibility to infections (especially of the genitourinary tract) may also characterize sufferers of this disease as well.

A Homemade Tonic

The *three* most important nutrients considered essential for treating pernicious anemia are iron, vitamin B-12 (cyanocobalamin), and folic acid. An incredibly iron-rich drink can be made from the following ingredients combined in a food blender:

2 cups (16 fl. oz.) distilled water

1 level tbsp. Pines's Organic Beet Powder (see the appendix)

1 Tbsp. crude blackstrap molasses

2 Tbsps. dessicated liver (previously juiced) or 1 Tbsp. liver powder

1 tsp. powdered watercress (see the appendix, Great American)

1 tsp. Kyo-Green (see page 328)

3 Tbsps. chopped black mission figs

Certain vegetable juices are also incredibly rich in iron as well. Consider juicing and blending these together: spinach, celery, parsley, beet greens, and carrot tops. Add 2 Tbsps. chopped pineapple for flavor.

According to *The Pharmacological Basis of Therapeutics* (5th ed.; New York: Macmillan, 1975), vitamin B-12 may be found abundantly in certain organ meats like lamb and beef liver, kidney, and heart, and clams and oysters. Moderate amounts occur in nonfat dry milk; some seafoods like crab, striped bass, salmon and sardines; and egg yolk. Minimal amounts are present in muscle meats, other seafoods such as lobster, scallops, flounder, haddock, swordfish and tuna, and some cheese (Limburger). (Note: 10 micrograms (mcg.)/100 gr. of wet weight constitutes an abundance of B-12; moderate amounts vary from 3 to 10 mcg./100 gr. of wet weight.)

Folic acid is ubiquitous in nature, occurring in practically all types of foods. However, those foodstuffs with the highest folic acid content of dry weight include yeast, liver, and fresh green vegetables. Some fruits are also relatively high in this vitamin as well. They include 1 avocado (124 mcg.), 1 cup boysenberries (83.6 mcg.), 1 cup pineapple juice (57.7 mcg.), 1 cup of strawberries (26.4 mcg.), 1 medium ripe banana (21.8 mcg.), 1 tangerine (17.1 mcg.), and 1 pear (12.1 mcg.)

Somewhere between 50% and 95% of the folic acid content of foods is usually destroyed by protracted cooking or by canning. This is probably the main reason why folic acid deficiency is so common in people today.

Dr. Vance's Anemia "Cure"

The health drink previously given for pernicious anemia originated with that old Provo, Utah, veterinarian who lived near us. Dr. Vance, as he was known by everyone, had successfully treated anemia in sheep, goats, and horses with a novel "salad" combination consisting of carrot tops and coarsely chopped carrots, some slightly stewed black figs, and a ladleful of blackstrap molasses mixed in with everything else. The animals to whom he fed this curious mixture took to it like "a cat does to milk," he was fond of saying.

Later, when treating people out of his home, he slightly altered this by juicing the carrot greens and roots and figs, then pouring them into an electric blender with the molasses. He recommended that his patients with pernicious and regular anemia, drink an 8-fl.-oz. glass of this concoction every morning before breakfast.

♦♦♦♦♦♦

PSORIASIS

Psoriasis is one of those diseases that seems to keep coming back in those unfortunate enough to be afflicted with it. It's characterized by eruptions on the skin of red circular patches of all sizes covered with dry, silvery scales. The patches enlarge slowly, forming more extensive patches. Psoriasis appears mainly on the legs, arms, scalp, behind the ears, and lower part of the back.

About 2% of the white population in America is troubled with this disorder. Quite often, psoriasis is present with another autoimmune disease, rheumatoid arthritis. The two, somehow, seem to go hand-in-hand.

A One-Week Cleansing Program

First, a week-long cleansing of the body is in order. This is best implemented with certain fruit (pineapple, papaya, and cranberry) and vegetable (carrot and mixed greens combined) juices. Also red raspberry leaf and red clover blossom teas are helpful to drink as well.

Normal bathing or showering routines should be temporarily suspended. Instead, the skin should be lightly sponged off with mineral water or seawater. Frequent exposure to the sun or ultraviolet light can reduce the scaliness and redness. A modified version of Paavo Airola's famous skin formula is recommended externally: 2 Tbsps. each of safflower, olive, and almond oils, with 1 tsp. of Rex's Wheat Germ Oil (obtained from a local veterinary supply house). Mix ingredients together and refrigerate. Apply small amount to afflicted areas *in the evening* before retiring.

Daily supplements should include 1 Tbsp. Rex's Wheat Germ Oil, 3 Tbsps. lecithin granules, 50,000 I.U. vitamin A, 800 mg. magnesium, 1 tsp. flaxseed, 3 tablets high-potency B-complex, and 4 sarsaparilla capsules.

Pioneer Remedies for Psoriasis

During my childhood in Provo, Utah, our family resided within the ecclesiastical boundaries of a Mormon meeting house known as the Provo Fourth Ward. Directly across the street from this old historic building lived an elderly, heavy-set lady who walked with a limp and had a crotchety personality to boot. She was a descendent of one of the first settlers of Utah, and proud of it.

Now this Sister Smith (as I'll call her) was plagued from time to time with psoriasis and used two different herbal compounds to relieve the swelling and itching. The first of these was a tea made with equal parts of burdock, cleavers, sarsaparilla, and yellow dock. To about a pint of boiling water, she would add half teaspoonfuls of each, turn the stove off, cover the pot with a lid and let the mixture steep for 45 minutes or so. Then she'd strain the tea and drink a cup several times daily on an empty stomach.

Her second remedy was an ointment that she applied to her skin with great success. One day she let me watch her prepare the concoction.

First, she carefully measured out 1½ teaspoonfuls each of *fresh* comfrey lead, chickweed herb, marshmallow leaf and flower, and marigold flowers. She snipped each of these ingredients into tiny pieces with some large scissors. Next, she slowly melted on low heat in a porcelain saucepan about 7 ounces (or 200 grams) of ordinary Vaseline or petroleum jelly. After it was reduced to a liquid, she then added the cut herbs and brought everything to a rolling boil. She then turned the heat down and let the contents gently simmer for about 15 minutes. She made sure, however, to stir it well with a wooden ladle.

She then poured the mixture through fine gauze and pressed out all of the liquid from the herbs. The mixture was then poured into empty baby food jars and sealed once it had sufficiently cooled.

◆◆◆◆◆

RHEUMATOID ARTHRITIS

Of the estimated 32 million arthritis cases in this country, about 7 million (of which three quarters are women ages 36–50) of them are rheumatoid in nature, with the rest being the more common kind, osteoarthritis. Rheumatoid arthritis appears to develop in those who have an inherited susceptibility to the disease. Whatever it is that exploits this vulnerability—undoubtedly a virus or bacteria—initiates the problem by disrupting the immune system.

Victims of rheumatoid arthritis (RA) first experience swelling and pain in one or more joints, lasting up to 1½ months as a rule. Sometimes the condition moves around the body in a hopscotch fashion—the wrists and knuckles usually are involved, the knees and joints of the ball of the foot are often involved, while only parts of the fingers are affected. Nodules the size of a pea or mothball sometimes form beneath the skin.

Other RA symptoms besides those of the joints themselves are evident. Problems like muscle aches, fatigue, morning muscle stiffness, and even a low fever indicate the presence of RA. After resting or sitting a while, the entire body feels stiff and difficult to move. After a period of loosening up, motions become easier and less painful. Patients often have problems with fluid accumulation, particularly around the ankles. Sometimes, RA may attack other body tissues, including the whites of the eyes, the nerves, the small arteries, and the lungs; a mild form of anemia is also quite common.

RA: The Immune System Gone Wild

To understand RA is to understand something about the immune system itself, for RA is the classic case of immune functions gone completely awry. Normally, when bacteria or viruses enter the body, our immune system marshals a swift-moving and powerful army of cells that identifies, deactivates, and ultimately digests the invaders (also called antigens). Infantry cells called lymphocytes possess the ability to distinguish "self" cells (those belonging to the body) from all other matter. They meet the invading antigens and crank out antibodies for a counterattack.

As the antibodies lock onto and immobilize these antigens, a blood-serum material known as "complement" joins with the antibody-antigen pair to form a complex. Next to enter this internal fracas are scavenger cells called phagocytes, which have been genetically programmed to complete the cleanup process. They engulf the complexes, then deliver them to lysosomes— tiny sacs inside the phagocytes filled with potent enzymes. There the complexes are shredded and digested.

However in RA, a monkey wrench of some kind has been thrown into the body's finely tuned immune machinery. Instead, the defender cells suddenly turn against "self" cells, those of the synovium (the thin membrane lining joint interiors). Potent antibodies badly damage the membrane, producing painful inflammation.

The scavenger cells too can go haywire; when they consume the complexes, the walls of the lysosomes (or sacs), for some strange reason, become greatly weakened. The highly potent digestive enzymes break through the walls with great intensity and rapidly pour into a natural lubricating substance called synovial fluid, which constantly bathes the joints. Saturated with the enzymes, the fluid begins to eat away the synovial lining and the cartilage. A jagged growth called pannus appears, damaging the cartilage and increasing inflammation.

Detecting trouble, new lymphocytes and scavenger cells rush into the war zone. But they aren't functioning properly either; they also begin attacking "self" cells. What should have been a battle against invaders is now a full-scale civil war. These skirmishes result in joint warmth, swelling and pain in those suffering from RA.

This terrible autoimmune reaction is believed to be caused by either a virus or a bacteria. In June 1981, I attended a meeting of the Arthritis Foundation in Boston, Massachusetts. There I heard researchers say that the Epstein-Barr virus (EBV) lurks in millions of people for long periods of time, but can suddenly become activated enough through stress to initiate the devastating processes that inevitably lead to RA. (EBV causes one form of cancer and has been present in the majority of AIDS cases.)

Other scientists are of the opinion that bacterial infection is behind the occurrence of RA. Roger Wyburn-Mason, M.D., of the United Kingdom claims that a parasitic amoeba is behind RA, having discovered it in the tissues of all his patients suffering from this crippling affliction. He believes that many people already have low-grade pathogenic amoeba in their intestines and colons. He thinks that 50% of all residents of the British Isles and about 75% of those living in the Southern states here, have these infections.

There is strong evidence in favor of this view. Peter Utsinger, M.D., a director of the immunological laboratory at Philadelphia's Germantown Hospital, studied hundreds of patients who had intestinal bypass surgery to lose weight without having to diet. About 25% of all those submitting to this particular surgery developed dermatitis and many of the symptoms so typical of RA. This surgery appears to overwhelm the digestive system, causing the circulating blood to absorb bacteria from the bowels that would normally stay there. These putrefying organisms then trigger the formation of antibacterial antibodies, which in turn link up with this bacteria and travel throughout the body. They eventually settle into joints, organs, and tissues, causing damage.

Based on these facts, it would appear that natural anti-inflammatory agents and herbal antibiotics would be a very useful holistic approach toward the successful management of RA in general.

Five-Step Plan for Treating Rheumatoid Arthritis

A number of things can be done to remedy RA. They include certain dietary restrictions, nutritional supplementation, behavioral modification, mild exercise, and some environmental considerations.

1. Dietary Restrictions: Allergy is an important factor in both RA and osteoarthritis. Hypersensitivity to certain types of foods can accelerate the pain and swelling associated with this disease. Marshall Mandell, M.D., and Anthony Conte, M.D., published research in the *Journal of the International Academy of Preventive Medicine* in June, 1986, on the role of allergy in arthritis. In double-blind studies with arthritic sufferers, they discovered that soy powder–flour was the leading cause of inflammation and pain recurrences (70.3%); while coffee, eggs, milk, and white sugar products each affected 60.6% of the test subjects; with apples, beef, lettuce, and oranges being the last most frequent offenders (50%). Another doctor by the name of Childers, who himself suffered from RA, omitted potato, tomato, eggplant, and green bell peppers from his diet and soon discovered that his pain and inflammation had gone.

Reports published in *Clinical Ecology* (October/December

1984) and *International Archives of Allergy & Applied Immunology* (October 1985) mentioned that RA patients demonstrated food intolerances for corn, wheat, red meat, milk, and cheese. The importance of restricting certain foods from the diets of RA sufferers is best illustrated in a placebo-controlled, blind study of dietary manipulation published in the February 1, 1986 issue of *Lancet*. The experiment was conducted at the Department of Rheumatology, Epsom District Hospital in Epsom, Surrey, England. For a week, 49 RA patients were given an elimination diet containing just foods very likely to be well tolerated. The percentage of patients with severe pain during the day decreased from 36% to just 4%. The average duration of typical morning stiffness decreased from 53 minutes to only 10 minutes. And the average number of painful joints decreased from 22 to 18. Over the next five weeks, foods were slowly reintroduced to the patients' diets and those causing reactions were eliminated. At the end of six weeks' time, 75% of RA patients rated their condition as better or much better. Blind clinical and lab assessments also showed significantly more improvement than during a six-week placebo period. The medical journal concluded that dietary manipulation is of positive benefit to RA patients.

2. Nutritional Supplementation: Indian researchers screened a series of Ayurvedic drugs for their antiarthritic effect and reported in 1956 that out of all of them, licorice root proved to be the most effective, when given as a tea. South African pharmacologists with the University of Witwatersrand in Johannesburg reported that stinging nettle lowers the uric acid content of the blood and prevents further calcification of the joints of RA patients. The nettle was consumed fresh as a boiled or steamed potherb or else taken as a medical tea several times daily.

Back in 1984, teams of researchers at the University of California at San Francisco and Massachusetts General Hospital in Boston, investigated a strange protein called Substance / P, which increased the severity of arthritis in lab rats. The researchers studied normal rats and rats in which arthritis had been artificially induced, and found that they could increase the severity of this disease simply by injecting Substance P into joints. They soon discovered that when capsaicin, the chemical constituent that makes chili peppers exceedingly hot, was injected into the animals, it alleviated their joint tenderness to quite an extent. Capsaicin inactivated pain fibers in these rodents' nerves by inducing a burning sensation in them. This confirms the validity of an old Southern folk remedy for using cayenne pepper as a food seasoning and also taking it in capsule form (6 to 8 daily) to relieve RA misery. (Note: Cayenne pepper is decidedly hypoglycemic and should be used cautiously by those with low blood sugar.)

The oriental approach to RA with herbs is quite effective. The *Kitasato Archives of Experimental Medicine* (Vol. 55 1982, pp. 39–45) gave clinical evidence to show that a combination of peony root and angelica root nicely suppressed all symptoms of arthritis. The Japanese administered this in the form of a tea. To 1 quart of boiling water, add equal parts (2 Tbsps. each) of coarsely cut, dried peony and angelica roots. Cover, and simmer on low heat for 10 minutes; let steep an additional 50 minutes. Strain and drink 1 cup three times daily on an empty stomach or as needed.

I recall some years ago lecturing at a large health convention in Toronto, Canada. During the course of my remarks, I casually mentioned that a water extract of yarrow flowers could reduce arthritic inflammation. Almost immediately a hand shot up and when called upon to speak, a rheumatologist from one of the local hospitals arose, visibly angry at me. "I think it's terribly irresponsible of you to make statements like this without evidence to back them up," he said and then promptly sat back down again. Whereupon, I sifted through the papers in the folder that lay open before me on the lectern and called his attention to the "Isolation of the Anti-inflammatory Principles from Achillea millefolium," which appeared in the August 1969 *Journal of Pharmaceutical Sciences.* Arthritis induced in animal models, I pointed out, decreased by 35% and was attributed to a protein-carbohydrate complex within the plant itself, which was "retained at the site of inflammation for tissue repair." He said nothing more after this.

Prickly ash bark, myrrh gum, and cherries also are excellent for reducing the pain and swelling accompanying different forms of arthritis, like RA, osteoarthritis, and gout. They can be taken separately in capsule form or, as in the case of cherries, consumed fresh. Custom-Made Formulas of Salt Lake City has periodically made small amounts of a special antiarthritis preparation consisting of all three ingredients for some doctors and their patients (see the appendix). Also, the *Indian Journal of Medicinal Research* for June 1966 reported that a pharmaceutical preparation of garlic killed the virus or bacteria responsible for causing RA in some patients. A product of equivalent strength is available here in most health foods stores or nutrition centers under the name of kyolic garlic (see page 328).

Other items useful for RA are salmon or fish oil dietary supplements and *medical grade* DMSO (Dimethyl Sulfoxide). About 4 capsules daily of the fish oil is suggested. On the other hand, caveat emptor ("let the buyer beware!") when it comes to obtaining *the right kind* of DMSO. The purer *medical grade* is *not* found in health food stores or doctor's offices as a rule, but can only be obtained from veterinary supply houses or veterinarians themselves. To use *any* kind of industrial-grade DMSO is to run the risk of putting dirt and other impurities into your blood stream. Medical grade DMSO should be administered *only under knowledgeable supervision.*

Certain vitamins and minerals are also helpful. The benefits of vitamin A present in the fish oil can't be underestimated. Vitamin E (400 I.U. daily) and selenium (100 mcg. daily) are of definite therapeutic benefit. And so is the trace element copper. Seafood, especially oysters, clams, and scallops, is very high in copper, along with most legumes (especially chick peas and lentils), nuts (especially Brazil, pecans, and filberts), raisins, blackstrap molasses, and avocado.

Externally, copper works wonders too with RA, osteoarthritis, ankylosing spondylitis, rheumatic fever, and sciatia, according to the medical journal, *Agents Actions* (November– December 1984). One colleague, Thomas Nufert of Thomas Laboratories in Hayward, California, did considerable research into copper's anti-inflammatory properties. The result was a product called ARTH-RELIEF, which thousands of arthritis sufferers and some doctors have used over the years with success. It's now marketed by Bronson Pharmaceuticals in La Cañada, California (see the appendix for further information).

Finally, a regimen of calcium (750 mg.), magnesium (250 mg.), pantothenic acid (100 mg.), and vitamin C (2,500 mg.) taken daily with meals should be seriously considered, too. Additionally, some doctors have reported limited success with New Zealand green-lipped mussel, but other health professionals who've prescribed the same thing told me that it didn't perform that well with their RA patients. Perhaps, individual responses are elicited because of the many different body chemistries involved.

3. Behavioral Modification: Certain scientists intimately familiar with the mechanisms by which stress can induce certain illnesses are convinced that anxiety, overwork, and insomnia make it much easier for viruses and bacteria to cause the joint infections that ultimately lead to rheumatoid arthritis. Such a one was the late Hans Selye, M.D., of McGill University in Montreal, whom I had the good fortune of meeting in 1980. This world-renowned authority on stress told me that if RA patients had kept careful diaries of daily events in their lives for the year *preceding* their first encounters with this disease, most of them would have discovered just how many stressful moments had occurred in that year leading up to their arthritis attacks.

He showed me various studies to this effect. In one study a "life chart" was created for RA patients who were asked to keep track of the onset of their attacks. With the data recorded on the chart, a 62% relationship between arthritis attacks and some stressful event was found. In a second study of almost 300 patients, almost half of them noticed that physical and/or emotional stress set off their attacks. In men, it was job stress, and in women, it was both job and domestic anxieties. In women over age 40 RA was almost always correlated with some kind of stress. A fourth study indicated that "decent" folks, who always seemed nice on the outside but in reality, kept their feelings pent up inside of them, were invariably *prime candidates* for RA. Another rather bizarre but highly interesting paper which Dr. Selye showed me proved that people who are downright psychotic *never* get rheumatoid arthritis! A final study of eight identical twins—one of each pair with RA and the other without—stated that 80% of them had felt the awful impacts of varying psychological stresses just before the onset of their disease; the non-arthritic twins had no stress in their lives whatever.

Probably one of the best solutions to removing heavy stresses from someone's life is a complete change of scenery. Nowhere could that be more strongly evidenced than in the life of Civil War veteran, Josiah Copley, Jr. Enlisting in the 21st Illinois Volunteers in midsummer of 1861, he saw fierce action at the Battle of Chicamauga (near Murfreesboro, Tenn.)—certainly one of the bloodiest engagements of the entire war, with casualties exceeding 34,000 on both sides. Young Copley was taken prisoner in the late fall of 1863 and was transported with thousands of others to the terrible Confederate prison in Andersonville, Georgia, which had been appropriately nicknamed "Death Camp" by those who managed to survive it. Of the some 32,000 Union prisoners incarcerated there, about 3,000 died every month from malnutrition, swamp fever, scurvy, dysentery, exposure, and starvation.

When he went in relatively healthy, he weighted about 185 lb, but when released at the close of the war, "he was little more than a skeleton" of his former self, weighing a pitiful 92 lb! During his tenure there, he contracted severe rheumatoid arthritis and what would today be categorized as chronic fatigue syndrome. His was a dual affliction: not only was he unable to move without great pain and suffering, but he didn't even have sufficient strength to go to the outhouse by himself! His manic depression bordered on insanity. The only thing which physically saved him was a *complete* change of scenery. As his biographical sketch relates: "Josiah recuperated on a farm in Kansas, the green pastures and quiet groves seeming like heaven after the hell of Andersonville!" It took him almost three years to regain completely his former weight and cheerful disposition, and to become entirely free of arthritis and constant fatigue.

Contemplating nature in all of her pastoral beauty, especially that which is green in color, has been repeatedly demonstrated to *significantly reduce pain!* A University of Delaware scientist investigated two groups of patients recuperating from cholecystectomy in a suburban Pennsylvania hospital between 1972 and 1981. Twenty-three surgical patients assigned to rooms with windows looking out on a beautiful assortment of trees had *shorter* postoperative hospital stays, had *fewer* negative evaluative comments from nurses, took *fewer* analgesic drugs to curb their pain, and had lower scores for minor postsurgical complications. On the other hand, reported *Science* (April 27, 1984) patients with nothing but boring views of a red brick wall had longer hospital stays, complained more often, needed far more pain-killing drugs, and had higher scores for postsurgical complications, which led the author of the study to conclude that "the natural scene" was much more therapeutic than was the monotonous scene of "a largely featureless brick wall."

In the book, *The Pleasure Connection* (San Marcos, California: Synthesis Press, 1987), two registered nurses (Dera and James Beck) discuss the advantages of imagination where actual wilderness trips aren't always economically feasible or physically possible. They tell the reader to imagine himself or herself among the tall pines of Oregon and Washington or deep in the majestic redwood forests of northern California. They then proceed to describe step-by-step what the reader should be imagining next: babbling brooks, pastured meadows, warbling birds, gentle breezes, and so forth. From these meditative efforts, a biochemical balance called the *parasympathetic response* is achieved, in which the entire body is able to relax. Endorphins secreted by the brain soon deliver a state of euphoria and freedom from pain to the entire system. These endorphins also reduce blood pressure, slow heart beats, calm the digestive processes, relax muscles, and permit the body to repair itself. Self-imagining the *green* things of nature, they point out, seems to bring about the highest production of endorphins possible within the body.

This then is what RA patients ought to be doing more of themselves in order to relieve their pain and misery. If it worked for Josiah Copley, Jr., and Pennsylvania hospital patients, then it will definitely work for you!

4. Mild Exercise: Exercise has become a key component in the effort to bring relief to millions of arthritis sufferers throughout America. In 1981 the Stanford Arthritis Center developed an exercise regimen that was eventually picked up by the Arthritis Foundation and used in many of their chapters around the country.

One of the first things dispelled is the myth that exercise would wear out the joints of arthritis victims a lot faster. But recent research has shown that just the opposite is true. In fact, clinical evidence indicates that arthritis pain is reduced by as much as 25% in individuals who take part in simple exercises.

Interestingly, it isn't so much the exercises or relaxation techniques that reduce the pain as it is the psychological effects of people gaining a feeling of control over their lives. Exercise helps arthritis sufferers to set goals and accomplish things they didn't even know they could accomplish.

In one case, an elderly RA patient was unable to visit her new granddaughter because she couldn't walk up a stairway of 17 steps. The woman set a program for herself of gradual climbing, even when it took her almost 30 minutes to complete the task. But at the end of six months she was finally able to negotiate all of the stairs with *minimal* pain. The end result was getting to see her grandchild on Easter Sunday.

The first type of simple exercise is to move the affected joints through their various range of motions. This keeps the joints from losing their functions. Moving the shoulders about even with a few simple shrugs or just drumming the fingers one by one on a flat surface prevents them from losing their mobility. All that is really necessary is just to move every joint through the range of motion it's supposed to move through two or three times a day.

The second exercise calls for strengthening the muscles in order to help the joints become more stable. This consists of light isometrics in which the arthritic person contracts each muscle for 6 seconds without moving the joint. Muscle strength can be maintained by doing this as little as half-dozen times each day; it really doesn't take a lot of time or effort as some might think it would.

The third step is performing an endurance exercise for about a half-hour each day. Walking, swimming, bicycling, and jogging on a minitrampoline are all recommended. These exercises can be done comfortably and only three or four times weekly for beneficial effects.

Ballroom dancing is making a comeback in some health circles with arthritis victims. Consider the screen actress, Cyd Charisse, who danced opposite Gene Kelley and Fred Astaire and starred in such musical hits as *Singing in the Rain*, *Silk Stockings*, and *Brigadoon*. With the help of her rheumatologist, Dr. James Day of the University of Colorado Health Sciences Center, she found that dancing greatly alleviated the morning stiffness, inflammation flare-ups, and chronic pain of her RA.

5. Environmental Considerations: A change of climate can definitely help your arthritis. So said Joseph Lee Hollander, M.D., an eminent rheumatologist with the University of Pennsylvania Hospital. In his laboratory RA patients lived comfortably for long periods of time in a 15-foot-square, pleasantly furnished room called the Climatron, where scientists created different types of climates.

At the start of each patient's residence in the Climatron, all the climate factors were kept at a constant level to help patients become adjusted to the room. After patients had been in the chamber for about a week, doctors began manipulating the "climate," such as increasing then decreasing barometric pressure, and increasing then decreasing internal humidity. Other variations on these two themes were also employed as well.

Research showed that a combination of falling pressure *and* rising humidity rather than these factors alone, "significantly worsened" existing conditions of arthritis. Also that RA victims living in the upper Midwest and northeastern United States were more prone to misery than were those living elsewhere in the country. Not surprisingly, doctors discovered that "the best refuge for arthritis is a warm, stable, dry climate," which is what Arizona can offer.

A Miami rheumatologist has successively treated swollen joints with soft laser light that's 65 times *weaker* than supermarket checkout scanners. Still other people have sat for hours in abandoned mines in Basin, Montana, because the natural radon emissions seem to help their RA a lot. Finally, acupuncture has proved useful for many arthritis sufferers.

◆◆◆◆◆

SCLERODERMA/DERMATOSCLEROSIS

Scleroderma means "hard skin." The skin of sufferers becomes stiff and tight, especially on the face, arms, and fingers. It is due to poor circulation through the small blood vessels, which leads to scarring of the skin. If the skin becomes tight like a drum, the hands could then become stiff.

Dermatosclerosis (its other synonym) isn't really arthritis as such, but it can lead to deformities resembling those of true arthritis. Actually, when scleroderma joint tissues are examined under a microscope, some signs of a true arthritic condition are apparent.

Scleroderma patients generally have Raynaud's phenomenon as well. This is a condition characterized by color change in the fingers, going from white to blue to red, after exposure to cold weather. The scleroderma process often involves other organs, too, besides the skin. Frequently the G.I. tract is involved. The esophagus or gullet can develop changes similar to those of the skin and the swallowing wave can be seriously interrupted. The stomach and small bowel may both become dilated, and outpouchings of a special sort can develop in the colon. Scarring of the lungs may, likewise, occur and, in some patients, the kidneys become abruptly involved in hypertension and kidney failure.

Scleroderma usually strikes women and some men in their forties and fifties. Many experience considerable mental anxiety over their "mummylike" skin. Calcium deposits beneath the skin also lower their self-esteem.

How to Impose Circulation and Relieve Symptoms

The most important corrective measures to be taken for scleroderma seem to be improving blood circulation and attitude readjustment. Herbs like cayenne pepper and ginger root are ideal for improving blood circulation. Powdered cayenne can be used as a seasoning on foods or else taken in capsule form (about 3) each day with tomato or V-8 juice. Ginger root can be taken in capsules as well (2 each day) or made into a tea—1 Tbsp. fresh, grated root steeped in 1 pint boiling water for 30 minutes. The grated root can also be used in certain culinary preparations as well. Calcium (1,000 mg. daily) and vitamin C (2,500 mg. daily) are also ideal to take to improve blood circulation and the health of capillary walls.

Brisk 10-minute rubdowns with the hands, a dry natural bristle brush, or even a dry towel all help to stimulate the circulation. Sometimes, though, a little bit of oil or cream is necessary on those portions of the skin which have become "mummified," so as to not further aggravate the condition.

Oriental stretching exercises are one of the most useful things to do preserve skin tone and joint mobility. Any instructor in the martial arts can help a person learn some of these simple techniques. Another method is to place the hand flat on a table and pressing until the fingers are straight, making a fist, and then cocking the wrist to stretch the joint further, and so forth, should be repeated several times daily.

Saddle Soap: An Effective Remedy

Sometimes the dangdest things turn out to work exceedingly well for the most unlikely health problems. This can certainly be said about the use of ordinary saddle soap to treat the hardened skin, which becomes tight as drum on the face, arms, and fingers, of those suffering from all the classic symptoms of scleroderma.

It was old Dr.Vance, that Provo, Utah, veterinarian who first brought this most unusual remedy to my attention. He discovered that by gently rubbing the surface of such mummified skin with a little saddle soap, it would restore some of the resiliency just as it would with hard, dry leather.

A cowboy who once worked on my ranch in southern Utah further corroborated this by telling me that his grandpa used the same stuff on his arms, hands, and face as he did to soften up his boots, chaps, and saddle. Saddle soap may be obtained from any farm or ranch supply house or place specializing in leather goods. Use as directed on the package label, remembering that it needs to be gently *massaged into* the skin and left there *without* being washed off for a while.

◆◆◆◆◆◆

SYSTEMIC LUPUS ERYTHEMATOSUS

Systemic lupus erythematosus (SLE) is a mouthful, indeed. "Systemic" refers to the many parts of the body that may become involved in this form of arthritis, more often thought of as a "connective-tissue" or "collagen" disease than anything else. The "lupus" part, quite literally, means "wolf." And the term "erythema" refers to the red color of the rash. Lupus or SLE is a highly variable disease. Some with it aren't even aware that they have it and require no treatment, but others may come down with a major illness.

SLE affects mostly women and can damage the skin, joints,

and internal organs. Early signs include fever, weakness, fatigue, appetite or weight loss, and rashes that appear on the face, neck and arms, aggravated by sunlight. It can even be inherited from parents who already have it or some other form of arthritis. Consider the case of television actress, Victoria Principal, a major star on the popular program, "Dallas." Her mother has lupus and her father osteoarthritis. In 1983 she began showing all the early signs of lupus herself, including frequent problems with her immune system. But she worked out a program to bring it under control.

More recently, Elizabeth Taylor contracted this deadly autoimmune disorder. Taylor was diagnosed as having it on Friday, May 25, 1990 at St. John's Hospital in Santa Monica, California. This, plus a serious bout with pneumonia, almost killed the legendary star.

A Holistic Approach Controls Disease

The first thing Ms. Principal did was to take time out from her hectic filming schedule to rest. She took short 45-minute naps several times daily during a 12- or 14-hour day of shooting. Second, she learned to relax through Eastern meditation. Soft background music and internal imaging together with a lot of determination and self-discipline helped. Third, she avoided junk foods and instead now subsists on fresh fruits, nuts, seeds, berries, yogurt, cottage cheese, vegetable juices, cooked vegetables, salads, legumes, and a few whole grains. Fourth, she avoids the sun *only* when it seems to cause a flare-up of her symptoms.

In Ms. Taylor's case, doctors have worked hard to rebuild her already-weakened liver. Massive doses of vitamin B-complex were injected intravenously. And because of yeast infection covering her mouth and throat, she was placed on Nystatin and an anticandida diet (see first chapter for more details). They have also kept her out of sunlight since the slightest amount can cause immediate rash.

Supplements useful for lupus include vitamin E (1,200 I.U.), pantothenic acid (75 mg.), PABA cream (externally), selenium (150 mcg.), vitamin C (7 grams), and slippery elm bark (4 capsules)—all taken daily. (See Custom-Made Formulas and Great American Natural Products in the appendix.)

Summary

1. Autoimmune diseases result in a flawed immune system that attacks the body itself instead of harmful viruses and bacteria.
2. The majority of these diseases are often virally induced.
3. Stress and poor dietary habits are two major contributors to these diseases.
4. Symptoms for each vary, but inflammation and pain are the most common.
5. Attitude changes play a big role in the treatment processes for each.
6. The methodical elimination of aggravating foods is another step.
7. Fresh and natural foods (nonallergenic) should be consumed more.
8. More frequent, smaller meals each day are better than three big ones.
9. Climate is a factor to be reckoned with in many such diseases.
10. Most autoimmune diseases overlap each other and have corresponding symptoms, which make correct diagnosis more difficult at times.
11. Supplementation should include items that do the following:
    a. Reduce stress.
    b. Reduce pain and inflammation.
    c. Improve digestion.
    d. Facilitate better body waste elimination.
    e. Produce strength and energy.
    f. Lubricate joints and muscle tissue better.
    g. Destroy disease-inducing viruses and bacteria.
12. Other therapeutic considerations such as massage or acupuncture deserve to be well explored and implemented if necessary.

••••• 3 •••••

What to Do About "Immune Blackouts"

"Immune blackouts" are a lot like the engine performance of your average car—any single factor or combination of several can greatly reduce its normal functioning. Dirty points, wet plugs, loose wires, weak battery, or something as simple as being out of fuel can contribute to lower than expected results from a poorly maintained vehicle.

Now the dictionary defines a blackout as a period in which an event or action is *temporarily* suppressed, *momentarily* dulled, or *briefly* extinguished for one reason or another. In the health application here, it's intended to mean those problems that may lead to a less ambitious or lazier immune system—one that, in a sense, is running on less than optimal energy.

In other chapters, we have considered a variety of factors which might also qualify to some extent as promoting "immune blackout." But for our purposes here, the focus is more specific and concentrated on those several problems which truly sap immune strength and steadily undermine the vitality of our natural defense forces. They are:

Alcoholism	Hypoglycemia
Anxiety attacks	Insufficient sleep
Drug addiction	Smoking and passive smoking

♦♦♦♦♦♦

ALCOHOLISM

How Alcohol Wrecks Immune Health

Next to the heart, the liver is probably the second most important organ in the body. It's responsible for myriad functions, including the following:

- Its more than 1,000 enzymes build chemicals our body needs and detoxify harmful ones.
- It makes proteins from nutrients absorbed from the small intestine and sends them all over the body, *especially to the lymphatic system*, to build cells. (White blood cells, part of our frontline immune defenses, originate in the lymph glands.)
- It stores consumed sugar in the form of glycogen until needed for energy.
- It converts beta-carotene from consumed vegetables into antiviral and antitumor vitamin A.
- It stores vitamins D and B-complex and iron (the last two of which are important in the regulation of some autoimmune diseases).
- It breaks down alcohol and fat and helps keep the brain alert.
- It manufactures urea waste which is then eliminated by the kidneys.

But consumption of alcohol wrecks many of these normal functions, thereby throwing the immune system off kilter. Cirrhosis, caused mainly by alcohol, is the third most prevalent killer for people under age 65 and the fifth most common disease for people under 40. Numerous epidemiological studies have determined that the liver cannot adequately filter out harmful microorganisms from the body when alcohol is present in any great quantities. A report in the December 1, 1985 issue of *Cancer* noted that when wine was drunk by those also consuming pork, they became more susceptible to hepatitis B virus than did those *not* drinking alcohol with their meals.

An April 5, 1971 article on "The Alcoholism of Eugene O'Neill" in the *Journal of the American Medical Association* stated that even after O'Neill became a teetotaler, he was still more susceptible to cold and influenza viruses than the average citizen would have been. In time, "he succumbed to pneumonia in a Boston hotel." Alcoholics, whom I've profiled in past health surveys which this research center has conducted, showed a greater tendency toward bacterial infections than did another nonalcoholic group of comparable age, weight, and height.

Other clinical evidence points out that the minute quantities of arsenic and sulfites present in wine and beer have the potential to induce bronchospasms; asthmatics should, therefore, avoid commercially made alcoholic beverages. (Home brews don't seem to present the same problem, but still may not be too good for the liver.) Women who drink run a greater risk of contracting breast cancer than do women who don't. This is because alcohol suppresses the production of "killer" cells normally generated by the immune system, to fight cancer in the body. Alcohol also upsets our limbic system (particularly the hippocampus), a set of brain structures that are known to influence our moods. In his book, *Head First: The Biology of Hope* (New York: E. P. Dutton), author Norman Cousins repeatedly presents strong clinical proof to show that anxiety and depression really flatten our immune systems.

In other words, alcohol *and* the barroom environments in which it is served greatly agitate our individual mood centers, which are somehow wired to our endocrine defenses as well. The sulky, brooding feelings generated by the liquor and the music, in turn, suppress the production of key immune components needed to keep body defenses strong. Under these types of negative influences, it isn't hard to figure out why an unnoticed but very real "blackout" of natural immunity can occur.

Fighting Alcoholism with Good Nutrition

No herb, mineral, or vitamin can compensate for personal inability to quit drinking altogether! Definitely, counseling and support groups such as Alcoholics Anonymous are needed. Recognition of suppressed guilt and inadequate sexual practices are two very important things which the reforming alcoholic must come to grips with as a rule; so, too, must he or she with the undeniable realization that *alcoholism is a disease*, plain and simple! These are some of the things that New York psychiatrist Hamilton employed with playwright O'Neill which helped him stop drinking within a matter of weeks. Once these things are successfully accomplished, then a sensible nutritional program can begin.

Medical colleagues of mine who've worked extensively with recovering alcoholics, have collectively provided me with the following helpful data. They suggest that a diet for an alcoholic consist of complex (or whole-food, high-quality) carbohydrates in the forms of fresh fruit, lightly steamed or raw vegetables, legumes, and whole grains. They also specify fiber (bran or wheat germ) and protein (preferably baked, broiled, or steamed fish instead of so much red meat or chicken).

Items to be eliminated from the diet obviously include alcohol, as well as sweets and caffeine. All of these, they insist, can adversely affect blood-sugar levels, which, in turn, can trigger an obsessive-compulsive behavior response and can lead to addiction again. In addition to three meals a day, nutritional snacks (fruits, nuts, cheeses) should be taken about two hours after every meal and before bedtime to help prevent blood-sugar problems (especially hypoglycemia).

As a healthier diet is pursued, the following items should be totally eliminated or else greatly minimized:

Refined foods—white flour, white rice, white pasta

Processed foods—sausages, bacon, cold cuts, hot dogs

High salt/sugar foods—canned foods, condiments

Junk foods—potato chips, "fast" foods like hamburgers

Adhering to these simple rules, they say, will guarantee recovering alcoholics that their addictive disease will *never* return!

Boosting the Body's Immunity

Since the liver seems to sustain the most damage from excessive alcohol consumption, common sense dictates that it should receive priority attention. Goldenseal root (see appendix) is excellent for banishing harmful microbes that may still be lurking in the liver somewhere. About 2 to 3 capsules daily to begin with are recommended; this can later be reduced to just 1 day after about three weeks. (However, goldenseal root exerts a hypoglycemic affect on some people.)

Dandelion and chicory roots make wonderful tonics for the liver. I recommend that they used in some type of beverage rather than in capsule or tablet form for this purpose. Equal parts (1 Tbsp.) of both added to a quart of boiling water, covered and simmered for 5 minutes, then steeped for 40 more minutes, makes a dandy tea; drink 2 cups of the strained tea sweetened with a little pure maple syrup. Some companies, such as Nature's Sunshine Products of Spanish Fork, Utah, make a product called Herbal Beverage, consisting of such roots. There are similar products that can be obtained from just about any supermarket that have these herb roots and certain roasted cereal grains in them. These natural "coffee" substitutes are easy to fix—just add a level teaspoonful to a cup or mug of hot water, stir, sweeten with honey, and finish off with a touch of cream or canned goat's milk for a fantastic beverage that not only tastes great but is good for the health of your liver as well.

The following nutrients are of considerable benefit in the renewal of health in recovering alcoholics:

L-Cysteine. Cysteine is a powerful water-soluble, sulfur amino acid. It plays a potent role in energy metabolism by being converted into glucose, if necessary. Undoubtedly it's most thrilling and satisfying role within the body occurs in the liver. Here it assists the small but ubiquitous protein glutathione to detoxify carcinogens and other potentially harmful chemicals. Throughout the rest of the body, it functions as the major antioxidant scavenger of free radicals. Cysteine (created when two cysteines bond together and hydrogen remains) occurs naturally in wheat germ, granola, oats, egg yolks, cayenne pepper, garlic, onion, mustard leaves, cabbage, brussels sprouts, cauliflower, broccoli, and horseradish; duck liver is incredibly high in cysteine, with a lesser amount occurring in avocado. The Brain Bio Center managed by C. C. Pfeiffer, M.D., and E. R. Braverman, M.D., in Rocky Hill, New Jersey, regularly prescribes 500 mg. twice daily of L-cysteine, in company with selenium (about

90 mcg. daily is suggested). (Selenium is important in the prevention and treatment of infectious hepatitis. Alcoholics consistently show much lower selenium levels than nonalcoholics do.)

Glutathione. This detoxifying amino acid is synthesized from cysteine. Some perceive it to be the single most important constituent of the body's toxic waste disposal system. It helps the body essentially four different ways, all of them protective: (1) as an effective antioxidant against free radicals; (2) as an antitoxin in the liver; (3) as a necessary immune component for the production of lymphocytes, phagocytes, and macrophages (all of which attack and destroy invading bacteria); and (4) finally, as a structural protectant of red blood cells. The liver seems to manufacture glutathione whenever extra cysteine is present; so the more cysteine-containing foods consumed or L-cysteine supplement taken, the greater will be your blood and liver glutathione levels as well.

Vitamins B-6 and C. Both work in harmony for the normal conversion of cysteine and the production of extra glutathione. About 5 mg. of B-6 and 1,500 mg. of C are recommended on a daily basis for this.

Vitamin E. Also involved in glutathione metabolism. One teaspoonful of Rex's Wheat Germ Oil from any veterinary supply house is recommended daily or 1,500 I.U. in capsule form.

Magnesium and Zinc. Magnesium (500 mg.) and zinc (25 mg.) are also necessary each day for normal glutathione metabolism.

Chronic Alcoholism Cured by Diet and Meditation

Harvey G., a prominent West Coast attorney, was interviewed a couple of years ago by me and several other social scientists, as part of an ongoing research program we were conducting with recovered alcoholics. We were interested in how successes like Harvey's were achieved.

> My old man was an alcoholic. I guess I started doing some serious social drinking my last year in high school and my

first several years in college. The frat brothers I ran with in those days loved to party on the weekends. I won't say we were typical of [John] Belushi in *Animal House*, but we were wild and crazy enough in our own way.

The stress of the [law] firm I was employed with only added to my problem. By the time a full partnership was offered to me, it felt like the walls were closing in around me. Booze became my escape mechanism from the real world of pressures out there. If it hadn't been for the threat of losing my family and job at the same time, I doubt I would have faced up to my terrible dilemma as strongly as I did.

For me AA [Alcoholics Anonymous] wasn't the answer. In fact, it was more a joke than anything else. One thing I noticed early on was that my eating habits had become atrocious. You know the typical hurried breakfast—coffee and doughnut on the run. And while lunch wasn't always at McDonald's, it was just more time to discuss courtroom strategies for impending cases with colleagues or clients. I drained more than one Pepto-Bismol bottle each week to cope with mounting heartburn. I actually felt better when I didn't eat at noon, to tell you the truth. Dinner was the only time I could really relax, but I usually was so tired that I'd doze off in the armchair or watch TV after the usual meat-and-potatoes ensemble.

Some guy talking on the radio one morning said that breakfast was the most important meal of the day. So I started paying more attention to that. I began getting up earlier to eat a bowl of cooked cereal or to have some poached eggs on seven-grain toast. I quit the coffee routine and instead starting drinking chamomile tea, because it tasted and smelled so pleasant.

After ten days or so of this, when I started noticing how much better I felt and more energy I had, I extended the renovation to include lunch. Green stuff became the order of the day, so much so, in fact, that I was sometimes ribbed by others about suddenly turning into a rabbit. But I soon discovered that salads not only digested better for me, but also seemed to give me that extra boost of energy I needed in the afternoon hours.

And you know what? With these adjustments in the way I ate, my need for drinks dropped correspondingly. Oh sure, I still needed a highball or a couple of martinis late in the day, but not as many and not as often. It wasn't too long before they became more objects of distraction than anything else. I mean like stirring them while discussing legal matters with others, much as you might use a fork to play with half-eaten potato salad. Pretty soon more drinks were going to waste than being put down the old hatch.

Dinner has stayed pretty much the same, though. I mean it isn't easy to go completely healthy, so I compromised by making the first two meals of the day better and keeping the delicious 'sins' of dinner in place. This pleased my wife who wasn't too crazy about learning to cook strictly vegetarian meals.

Another thing I did, though, was to lay off the sweets and soda pop. I noticed every time I ate or drank anything sweet my craving for alcohol would substantially increase. Since I'm not a biochemist or nutritionist, I can't exactly tell you why this happened. But I know it was easier for me to 'go sober' when my intake of sugar dropped tremendously.

Finally, there's the meditation thing I got into. It was the last little push I needed to completely lick this thing for good. I know there's different kinds. I use TM [transcendental meditation] myself. It seems to work for me okay. I do about 10 minutes of the mind-clearing thing and thought focusing twice a day. It's sort of like having a masseur or masseuse gently massage your mind for you.

◆◆◆◆◆

ANXIETY ATTACKS

Two Classic Cases of "Immune Blackouts"

The great Indian philosopher and political leader Mahatma Gandhi once said, "There is nothing to fear, but fear itself." And the New Testament informs us that

> there is no fear in love; but perfect love casteth out fear; because fear hath torment; [and] he that feareth is not made perfect in love. (I John 4:18)

The above two examples are illustrative of the frequent "anxiety attacks," from which many of us periodically suffer. Upon thorough analyses, one discovers that a lack of self-confidence, a tendency to be possessive and in control, an inclination toward psychosomatic behavior, and an inherent weakness for being influenced by *perceived* situations or rumors are all underlying causes to this particular form of "immune blackout." In each and every instance, rectifying these various problems leads to an obvious absence of such stressful moments.

Case 1: Mass Psychosomatic "Influenza"

In an intriguing article in the Monday, March 12, 1990, issue of *The New York Times*, reporter Tim Golden asked the obvious question, "Was it all in their minds?" He was making reference, of course, to the sudden onset of a bizarre illness among 34 Triborough Bridge toll workers, all of whom were mysteriously strickened with sudden, flulike symptoms that had lead bridge officials to at first suspect possible environmental contamination of some kind. But after spending hundreds of thousands of dollars on all kinds of environmental testing, they came to the ultimate conclusion that this large outbreak was commenced or prolonged by nothing more than psychosomatic factors.

Bridge officials and doctors who worked intensively on the case believe that at least one or two toll workers actually became sick from some type of undiscovered environmental cause; however, the rest of those involved in the outbreak were subject to psychological causes such as suppressed fear, hysteria, and genuine concern for those who *did* get sick. Scientists refer to this malady as "epidemic psychogenic illness" or "epidemic stress syndrome." As part of the syndrome, groups of people under considerable stress suffer real but largely subjective symptoms— dizziness, nausea, headaches, and eye irritation—for which no clear medical cause can be found.

The symptoms appear and then subside rapidly, but sometimes can recur. They are contagious virtually by rumor: when others under similar stress hear about or see evidence of the illness, they too can suddenly fall ill. While apparently more common among grade school choirs and high school marching bands, the phenomenon has been documented among telephone operators, assembly-line workers, and others who perform simple, repetitive tasks at a fast pace. Doctors say public fears of environmental pollution can actually contribute to the problem. And, for some unexplained reason, women are about twice as likely to fall ill as men. Could it be that they are more inclined to believe rumors than their male counterparts?

Psychological Solutions to Group Stress

Psychologists, who were hired by bridge authority management to investigate this epidemic stress syndrome along with epidemiologists and toxicologists, came up with some workable solutions to this puzzling outbreak. First, they had to convince toll workers that there was *absolutely no* contamination by coffee grounds, coins, uniform laundering, heating ducts, air vents, and drinking water.

Second, they had to demonstrate to toll workers that this sudden outbreak was due more to psychological factors than anything else. They accomplished this with the aid of union officials and senior management. Union officials persuaded most of the recovered workers that they believed the malady was mentally induced. As further proof of this, bridge authority senior managers joined toll takers in their booths full time. The result was that *none* of the managers came down with dizziness, lightheadedness, headaches, nausea, chest tightness or chest pain, and sore, dry throats as the workers had done. A combination of several methods finally convinced most of the afflicted workers that their sudden illness had, indeed, been more in their minds than anything else.

Case 2: Suspicion Induced "Common Cold"

Another variation of "epidemic stress syndrome" may be found in the more personal experience of someone I know, whom I'll call "Sally." I've known Sally and her family for several years now and have become very close friends with all of them. Sally is 44, remarried, with an adult child, several teenagers, and a preschooler still at home.

Now Sally has always been of the suspicious type, constantly imagining things that were never there. Her biggest emotional turmoils of late have been about her three sons. Her eldest, now in his twenties, believes that he is mature enough to make decisions himself without always having to inform her about every little thing he does. Sally interprets his silence on these matters as evidence that the poor kid is engaged in illegal activities of some kind. "If it was legal, then you'd have nothing to hide by telling me," she often shouts. And the familiar comeback from him is, "Oh, mom, give me a break."

Her two younger teenage sons, models of everything decent and virtuous in 14- and 16-year-old boys, also have come under her attack. And this because they haven't hugged or kissed her as much of late as they used to. "We're teenagers, mom, not little boys," they try to tell her, but without much success.

Well, during the first two months of 1990, this woman came down with all of the symptoms of a common cold, which no one else in her family got. Her head ached often, but no sinusitis was present. She coughed and sneezed quite a bit, but no mucus was evidenced. Her body felt weak and tired in spite of resting a lot in bed. Her lingering "cold" caused her to seek counselling from a local church group with the rest of her family.

How to Overcome Fear-Based Sickness

The young lady who conducted their therapy session had just graduated from the University of Utah with a degree in psychology. She patiently listened to all sides of the issue and to everyone's opinion, before giving some of her own. From members of the family who were there, including Sally herself, I obtained the following synopsis of what their psychologist told them.

The very first thing she advised Sally to do was to get a medical checkup to see if she had hypoglycemia. The counselor thought that this could very well be one of the main causes of her many unfounded suspicions.

Second, Sally was informed that she was being too possessive of all her children and trying to exercise control over them in ways that were not healthy or socially accepted. She was reminded that kids needed to have certain freedoms, and that parents needed to have more confidence in their children than they ordinarily do.

Third, Sally was encouraged to develop more self-confidence. By bolstering her own self-worth and capabilities, she was told, she would be able to shake many of her fears.

Fourth, it was suggested that her children and husband more actively demonstrate their love for her, through frequent verbal acknowledgments as well as through actual embraces when they felt so inclined. By exhibiting patience, they would naturally encourage her to change more as well.

It took about a month for these recommendations to take effect. But one of the first noticeable results was a disappearance of her "common cold" symptoms. Her headaches cleared up, her frequent coughing and sneezing ceased, and she felt more energetic than she had heretofore done. The obvious reason for her recovery was that these were allergic reactions, mainly induced by the fears she felt regarding members of her family. Once *positive* thoughts and feelings replace negative ideas and emotions, an individual begins to feel better and symptoms such as these quickly evaporate into thin air.

As an anthropologist who has studied many different cultures worldwide, I've come to discover that anxiety attacks are no respector of race or religion. For instance, the widespread health phenomenon known as "susto" which occurs throughout much of Latin America, "is a culturally patterned sick role in individuals who are unable to fulfill their normal social obligations." It's marked by fear and classic "cold-influenza"-like symptoms. For the most part, only psychological counseling can effectively remedy such temporary "immune blackouts" as these.

◆◆◆◆◆

AMPHETAMINES

What You Need to Know

These compounds stimulate the central nervous system and induce a transient sense of well-being, self-confidence, and alertness. Among those using amphetamines are people who work irregular hours (members of the medical profession, truck drivers, students) and athletes and others who must put forth almost superhuman physical effort during particular periods. Kitty Dukakis, the wife of the 1988 U.S. Democrat presidential candidate, checked herself into Edgehill-Newport, a swank Rhode

Island treatment center for alcohol and drug dependency, because of her 26-year bout with amphetamines.

Heavy use of amphetamines, however, leads to a paranoid psychosis with feelings of persecution, delusions of reference, feelings of omnipotence, and formication hallucinations (imaginary snakes or insects such as spiders crawling on or under the skin). Moreover, their consistent use tends to run the body ragged and wear down internal glands such as the adrenal, thymus, pituitary, and pineal, which are intricately connected to the immune system as well. As a consequence, amphetamine users tend to get sick more often with colds and flu than those who do not depend on such drugs.

Natural Alternatives Provide Energy Boost

Safer alternatives for revving up our mental and emotional engines would be black and green teas from the Orient, various tea combinations containing perky spices (like those put out by Celestial Seasonings), yerba maté (from Paraguay and Brazil), hot chocolate, and cocoa. I've discovered that oatstraw or bedstraw tea (2 Tbsp. in 1 pint boiling water and steeped for 30 minutes, then strained and consumed) to which has been added some drops (3–5) of peppermint oil (while the liquid is still hot) really gives a nice pickup to the body. Also, some (but not all) herbal energy supplements work well too, because they contain kola nut. (See the appendix for Great American Products' "Super Energy" formula.) Most of these items can be readily obtained from local supermarkets or health food stores.

Follow the drug detoxification program outlined at the end of this section.

◆◆◆◆◆
CAFFEINE: THE QUICK FIX

Quite a few doctors believe that coffee and cola beverages are highly addictive due to their "quick-fix" caffeine contents. Lendon Smith, M.D., one of America's leading health authorities, confessed to having been addicted to coffee so much that "I was drinking it from the pot—there has to be something wrong with someone who drinks coffee from the pot!" Realizing it had become a strong habit-forming substance in his life, he gave it up entirely and opted instead for healthier coffee substitutes like Pero, which consists of roasted cereal grains and herb roots instead.

The extent to which caffeine addiction can go, beyond just grouchy people who've missed their morning coffee by chance, is best illustrated by what happened in the state of Ohio during the 1977–78 blizzard, which piled up snow for almost three months and paralyzed travel everywhere. Supply trucks couldn't get to the thousands of local stores in those areas blanketed the hardest. A manager of one of these small country grocery stores reported that his patrons accepted the ordeal in the beginning. No one complained as he sold out of the fruit, vegetables, bread, milk, and other perishables, and even many of the boxed and canned food items that usually get replenished every couple of months. But just as soon as he ran out of bottled and canned Coca-Cola and Pepsi-Cola, his customers turned irate as hell, cussed him up and down with every profane word an old salty sailor might use, and *even threatened* his life several times! "What's the world coming to?" asked the *Cincinnati Enquirer*, which reported this rather bizarre story.

How Caffeine Addiction Upsets the Immune System

Aside from how caffeine stimulates the brain and nervous system, is what it can do to the immune system. Research shows that the entire endocrine system is disoriented completely by excessive amounts of caffeine in the circulating blood plasma. Some glands produce too little of a vital substance, while other organs produce too much of something else. "You either have not enough or else more than needed," one pharmacologist told me about this xanthine alkaloid. Caffeine addiction, in his opinion, turned body immunity into something of a teeter-totter—immune functions either become overworked or else underplayed and suppressed.

Besides natural "coffee" substitutes, there are a few other herbal beverages as well. Some of the more popular ones feature ginseng root in naturally carbonated water. These are marketed under such snappy titles as "Ginseng Rush" or "Ginseng Up" (probably to capitalize on the popularity of 7-Up) and are available in glass or plastic bottles and snap-top aluminum cans. Also, some of the larger health food stores in cities like Los Angeles, Boston, or New York carry natural fruit-flavored brands with different herbal ingredients in them. One of the more popular ones features ginseng root and wild black cherry extract in a Perrier-type water. Those who've quit their colas have found these to be satisfactory alternatives.

How a Waitress Quit the Coffee Habit for Good

I met Ruth W., a thirtysomething waitress in a south side Chicago hash house some years ago while lecturing at an annual convention of the National Health Federation. I had stopped in for a quick hamburger . . . (Yes, Virginia, there are moments that even the healthiest of us commit occasional dietary indiscretions!)

Our short conversation soon turned to the reason a Salt Laker would be in the "Windy City." Upon learning of my interest in herbs and general health matters, Ruth remarked, "Oh, yeh! I used an herb to kick the coffee habit for good." I asked her which herb it was and she replied, after a moment of deep thought, "I believe it was valium."

This prompted a laugh from me and the correcting statement, "You must mean valerian, because there isn't any herb called valium." "Yeh, that's what it was," she responded. Ruth drank a warm cup of the tea each morning and afternoon. "Smells awful," she said with a look of disgust on her face. "But you force yourself to like it after a while."

To about 3 cups of boiling water, she would add 1 level tablespoon of the dried, chopped root. She'd then cover the pot and simmer the mixture on low heat for 10 minutes, and then steep it for an additional 30 minutes. "Really helped me get rid of the caffeine blues."

◆◆◆◆◆

CRACK AND COCAINE

Not much needs to be said about the enormously widespread appeal of cocaine and several of its by-products. In 1984 *Science Digest* estimated that 4–5 million Americans tried cocaine "*at least once a month!"* Since then, this figure has nearly doubled, according to the latest statistics supplied by the federal government. Marvin Snider, director of preclinical research at the National Institute of Drug Abuse in 1984 called cocaine our *worst* chemical epidemic known to man, making it an "even more powerful drug than heroin." Crack, a more insidious form of cocaine, is in *every* American community, according to what California probation officer, Tom Wright, told *Life* magazine in January 1989.

Customary symptoms of cocaine and its by-products include rapid mood changes (sudden elation, inappropriate laughing, unexpected crying, and depression), sudden need for money (to feed the drug habit with), intoxication (but without the smell of alcohol), inability to concentrate or perform simple manual labor, desire and need to be alone, and so on. In the more advanced stages of cocaine addiction/crack addictions, outbursts of violence and sexual degradation become more frequent. A cocky, daring, and foolhardy attitude is also evident. Coronary arrest, strokes, and convulsions increase as well. Those using coca paste can suffer from paranoia, excitability, hallucinations, and delusions.

How Cocaine Affects the Immune System

Cocaine acts on three neurotransmitters: norepinephrine, serotonin, and dopamine. But the one that really delivers cocaine's ultimate punch is dopamine. Dopamine-releasing neurons concentrated in an area called the midbrain (laying at the base of the brain), are involved in behavioral arousal or motivational states. Without these important cells, we would not longer respond to events and other stimuli that are rewarding and pleasing, as is the case with victims of Parkinson's disease.

In his recent book, *Head First: The Biology of Hope*, author Norman Cousins has collected together a wide body of recent scientific evidence to show that the brain, the endocrine system, and the immune system are inexplicably wired together and in constant states of interaction with each other. This means that neurotransmitters like norepinephrine and dopamine invariably bind to receptor sites on immune cells scattered throughout the body. In other words, cells from the brain are naturally equipped to carry on biochemical communication with our immune cells. These split-second "conversations" are terse and to the point. But cocaine prolongs the time that dopamine, once released into a synapse, has to "talk" to an immune cell. Ordinarily, when dopamine has delivered its message, it is then reabsorbed or taken up again by the sending cell within the brain. Cocaine, however, blocks this re-uptake mechanism, causing this neurotransmitter to hang on to its immune receptor longer than necessary. This lengthened clinging produces obvious euphoria, but at the same time upsets the delicate balance between brain and immune functions. The result can be an immune system more dependent on a longer-surviving "feel-good" neurotransmitter than what is really necessary. A comparable analogy would be a friend or relative (dopamine) who drops by for a short visit (your immune cells). Timed just right, the visit (chemical interaction between the two) produces perfect harmony, but an unwelcomed overstay (cocaine-induced dopamine clinging) can cause more excitement (euphoria) than what you (your immune system) might be accustomed to.

The most evident symptom of cocaine abuse is a terrific elation followed by a severe depression when more needs to be snorted through the nostrils. This back-and-forth whipsawing of the immune system either produces too many infection-fighting cells or else too few of them, as the case may be. Little wonder then that most cocaine users have really screwed up immune systems. When comedian Richard Pryor, accidentally burned himself in 1980, doctors found it very difficult to reverse the rate of infection in his body; massive amounts of antibiotics had to be intravenously administered just to keep the actor alive. It was believed that his prior use of cocaine had a lot to do with this particular "immune blackout."

The Betty Ford Drug Rehabilitation Center—part of the Eisenhower Medical Center at Rancho Mirage, California—opened on October 3, 1982, and has since then treated over 6,000 patients for dependencies on alcohol, cocaine, and prescription drugs. Among the celebrities who've been patients there are Chevy Chase, Mary Tyler Moore, Liza Minnelli, Elizabeth Taylor, Robert Mitchum, Tony Curtis, and Johnny Cash.

Consult the drug detoxification program outlined at the end of this section for rehabilitating your immune system. Some of the data given came from therapists who work at this facility.

As far as I know, there are *no* safe alternatives to cocaine or crack. However, check under *Marijuana* in this section for several *legal* options.

Oscar's Treatment For Crack/Cocaine Addicts

"Oscar" isn't his real name, but this 47-year-old self-styled holistic healer is for real, and so is his unlicensed drug rehab "clinic" in the Castro district of San Francisco.

I met Oscar at the annual Whole Life Expo where I was a speaker. He didn't exactly project a picture of success with his psychedelic T-shirt, small goatee, dragon tattoo on his arm, and four or five tiny earrings in one lobe. In fact, I thought he looked more like the junkies he treats than any kind of healer. But, obviously, looks can be deceiving. This fellow *gets results* with the remedies he uses, and that's what counts as far as I am concerned.

His own research with many crack and coke users showed that an increase of the water-soluble amino acid L-tyrosine within the brain exacerbates the drug's effects. So, logically, he attempts to reduce the intake of those things that increase the amount of tyrosine in the brain.

Oscar told me about one patient, a 27-year-old Latino male working as a salesclerk in a prominent clothing emporium. The fellow had been snorting coke off and on for about ten months. The first thing Oscar did was give him a list of foods that either contained tyrosine or else increased its presence in the brain.

By altogether eliminating these from his diet and quitting the cocaine, the man soon noticed a reduction in symptoms typical for this drug. Topping Oscar's list of *forbidden* foods is anything with the new artificial sweetener, aspartame (also known as NutraSweet) in it. Aspartame contains phenylalanine, which increases brain tyrosine like crazy. Other foods included pork, cottage cheese, ricotta cheese, wheat germ, turkey, duck, and wild game.

♦♦♦♦♦

HEROIN AND ITS BUILT-IN "SAFEGUARDS"

Of the more than 25 alkaloids obtained from the opium poppy (*Papaver somniferum*), the most significant one is morphine and its acetylated by-product heroin.

Heroin behaves very differently in the system from cocaine. For one thing, it doesn't have the instantaneous effects that the latter does—cocaine and crack hit the brain a lot sooner and then wear off more rapidly. But heroin is an easier habit for addicts to sustain—the lulling effects of a dose may last for several hours. Symptoms are also different as well. Drug Enforcement Agency officials, state troopers, county sheriffs, and city police officers don't encounter the same level of violence that they do with cocaine and crack addicts. For heroin has built-in pharmacological controls that are more apt to put a user to sleep, whereas cocaine will keep its victim in an agitated state of insomnia. Also, far less heroin is used in the same period that cocaine would be. Rats given free access to heroin were found to limit themselves voluntarily to smaller amounts that wouldn't debilitate their bodies.

Heroin Creates Havoc in the Immune Gene Pool

As a consequence, the immune system doesn't receive the biochemical "slapping" from heroin that it does from cocaine. However, greater havoc in the immune gene pool can progressively occur over an extended period of time, resulting in irreversible chromosomal mutations. Investigators at the Human and Behavioral Genetics Research Laboratory of the Georgia Mental Health Research Center in Atlanta studied the chromosomes in antiviral white blood cells of heroin addicts and nondrug users, as the cells underwent their normal division processes. Under ordinary circumstances, such chromosomes have the ability to repair themselves after being damaged in some way. But in the heroin addicts more DNA damage than in nonaddicts was readily evident, based on findings of significantly increased chromosome damage in their white blood cells and of their much lower ability to repair DNA damage. Among heroin addicts there was a substantial increase in the number of "poor" repairers of genetic material; the poor repairers displayed only one quarter the capacity of the nonaddict group members to repair damaged DNA. Interestingly, among the nonaddicts who smoked, *none* were classified as "high repairers."

Natural Substitutes That Help Kick the Heroin Habit

While heroin and morphine have recently attracted some interest by the medical community in relieving pain in cancer patients, their uses should be curtailed otherwise because of the long-term genetic damage involved. Other natural and safer replacements for heroin include fluid extracts of wild lettuce from France and a strong Ayurvedic preparation of oat tincture from India, both of which not only help to kick the opium habit in general, but also tend to relax and stupefy the system to some degree much as heroin would. When a fluid extract of valerian root is combined with the other two (lettuce and oats), a very sedative and analgesic effect, which *does* not interfere with normal white blood cell division, is noticed. (See the appendix on page 327 for pure herbs tinctures.) About 10 drops under the tongue twice daily of these *three combined* is suggested for withdrawal *and* substitute replacement. (See Custom-Made Formulas in the appendix, for a company which can make this combination to order.) Prickly ash bark and juniper berries are good for helping to repair short-term genetic damage. Make them as a tea—1 Tbsp. of each in 1½ pints of hot water, covered and steeped for an hour before straining. Drink a warm cup of it twice daily in between meals.

How a Heroin Junkie Recovered by Using Herbal Remedies

Oscar told me of an episode involving a 31-year-old Cuban whom he called Raoul. Raoul had once been a hopeless heroin addict, but now to all appearances seemed to be fully recovered.

Oscar's approach to this case had been essentially a threefold one: (1) a sweating, cleansing herb (*Vernonia cinerea*) in the form of a tea, (2) an herb (turmeric) in capsule form to help detoxify the liver, and (3) an herbal tea (*Viola odorata*) to help quiet the nerves.

Raoul boiled up 1½ pints of water every morning to which he added 2 level tsp. of coarse, dried, ash-colored fleabane plant. After simmering 2 minutes and steeping another 40 away from the heat, he strained the contents into another receptacle and drank 1 cup of the *warm* tea every 4 hours. Before lunch, he would then take up to 4 capsules of powdered turmeric. In between, he would occasionally sip a warm cup of wild violet leaves (to which he sometimes added an equal part of chamomile flowers) to soothe his jangled nerves. To make this tea, add 1½ Tbsp. of fresh violet leaves to a pint of boiling water and let it steep for 12 hours in a pot covered with a lid. This three-step program helped Raoul put heroin behind him.

◆◆◆◆◆

"ICE"—THE DRUG FROM HELL

Considered to be just as addictive as crack cocaine but far more pernicious in its effect upon the body in general and immune system specifically. Looking like chunks of rock salt or shaved ice, this Asiatic variation of speed or methamphetamine, yields incredibly quick highs and awfully hellish lows within a matter of minutes.

Now the most abused substance throughout the state of Hawaii and slowly wending its way across the Pacific to the West Coast, "ice" shows some really extraordinary symptoms: lengthy and intense highs if enough is smoked, followed by comatose slumbers lasting up to 36 hours or more! The usual paranoia and hallucinations are also present to varying degrees as well. Since crystal meth or "ice" is beyond crack in its effects, treating users is much more difficult. *See the drug detoxification program outlined at the end of this section* for dealing with "ice."

Leonard's Story of Coming Off "Ice"

During my short research stay at Oscar's unusual clinic in San Francisco's Castro district, I met an accountant named Leonard L., who never gave me his exact age, but whom I judged to have been in his mid-to-late thirties. Friends had introduced him to "ice" while he was surfing off Makapuu Point on the extreme southeastern shore of Oahu in Hawaii. The stuff really sent his mental rockets soaring into the wild blue yonder, he claimed, but was "a real bummer . . . an awful and painful drag" afterward.

"Oscar here put me on a heavy dose of catnip tea sprinkled with some kind of sh-t," he loudly exclaimed. It actually was a small but equal combination of powdered and liquid spices: cardamom, cloves, and pure vanilla. "I used about an eighth of a teaspoon of each in a quart of the mint tea," he explained.

Leonard made catnip tea each day—3 Tbsp. of dried herb to a quart of boiling water; remove from heat, add spices, cover with lid, and steep 1 hour. Strain a cup and drink warm five times daily on an empty stomach. Leonard swore that this unusual brew worked. "I'll never touch that crap [meaning "ice"] again!" he concluded.

◆◆◆◆◆

MARIJUANA—ONE MAN'S POISON, ANOTHER MAN'S MEDICINE

In October, 1983 UCLA psychiatrist Ron Siegel informed a gathering of the American Psychological Association in Anaheim that man's inclination toward addictive substances began aeons ago when he was still part of the ape family. "*All* mammals, birds, insects, reptiles, and fish seek out ways to get high," he said. As man evolved into a higher creature of intelligence, this biological "need" for psychoactive substances remained an inherent part of him. Siegel also speculated that the great dinosaurs that roamed the earth during the Mesozoic era some 225 million years ago and feasted on giant flowering angiosperms were probably consuming up to a ton of marijuanalike plants each day; this "massive drug overdose" undoubtedly resulted in their extinction, he concluded.

Today over 20 million Americans smoke pot or marijuana. This is more usage than for any other illegal drug, with the majority of users being adults between 26 and 49. Pot is more lethal to the system than alcohol, morphine, heroin, or cocaine simply because it interacts with the body in *subtler* ways. Marijuana's most active ingredient is tetrahydrocannabinol (THC). Scientists acquainted with its peculiar properties and those of morphine's, have discovered certain specific binding sites for such plant hallucinogens deep within the brain itself. The body, in fact, produces natural opiates of its own, endorphins being a typical example.

Marijuana wreaks havoc with our front-line defenses against disease. According to the November 1987 issue of *Industrial Chemist* (p. 14), marijuana smoking "plays a crucial role in weakening the immune system by limiting the development of certain white blood cells."

A dangerous side to THC is that it isn't water soluble and can't be flushed out of the body as easily as, say, alcohol or caffeine could be. Instead, THC mixes with internal fat deposits and can linger in their plump pockets for as long as half a month. These fat deposits are found in some chemically sensitive areas—the brain, the hormone-producing adrenal glands, the ovaries or testes, and the placenta of a pregnant woman. Pilots who smoked a joint (one marijuana cigarette containing 19 mg. of THC) and then attempted a simple landing task on a computerized flight simulator 24 hours later, were unable to perform it correctly, noted the November 1985 *American Journal of Psychiatry*.

How Marijuana Causes Immune Blackouts

Marijuana use does not promote the effects—slurred speech, mood swings, staggering gait, and violence—typically associated with other intoxicating drugs. Its potential for harm to the immune system is also more insidious. Some scientists think that THC short-circuits the bioelectrical flow between different endocrine glands, resulting in "immune blackouts" of short duration. During this brief time, nasty viruses have a better chance of establishing themselves undetected deep within the body somewhere. The fact that marijuana users seem to be more prone to certain respiratory infections and lingering allergies is evidence of this.

The medical profession has lauded the therapeutic virtues of this illicit drug: reduction of some neurological complications inherent to multiple sclerosis, reduction of chemotherapy-induced nausea in cancer patients, and lowering of intraocular pressure common to glaucoma.

Three Ways to Overcome Marijuana Addiction

Various treatments have proven very useful in helping addicts to quit pot.

1. **NeuroElectric Therapy.** Margaret Patterson, M.D., developed a simple electrical device resembling a Sony Walkman in size that sends a weak electrical impulse through electrodes taped behind the ear that harmonize with natural brain rhythms and reduce drug craving and anxiety. The device has helped over 600 addicts in the last two decades, including Peter Townshend, the lead guitarist of and chief songwriter for the Who, a British rock group. Dr. Patterson claims a 98% success rate for her NeuroElectric Therapy (NET). (For more information on NET, write to Anthropological Research Center; see the appendix for address.)

2. **Nutrition.** Improved nutrition has also helped many addicts recover. Developed in part by the Tulane School of Public Health at Tulane University in New Orleans, the package consists of blended complex carbohydrates and fiber in powdered form, which is then mixed with fruit juice and taken whenever a drug craving occurs. Certain legume powders (soy protein isolate and chickpea) and fibers (rice bran, oat bran, guar gum, several seaweeds) generate more cholecystokinin (CCK), a gastrointestinal hormone, which then travels to the brain and shuts off drug and food cravings. According to James Carter, M.D., head of Tulane's nutrition department, Tulane's special nutrition package was given to 60 prisoners in the Atlanta, Georgia, jail with very good results. The pilot program resulted in all participants losing their desire for addictive substances including alcohol and tobacco!

3. **Catnip.** Several medical studies have shown that when high school or college kids switched from smoking pot to smoking catnip, they "experienced effects very similar to those produced by marijuana" (*Journal of The American Medical Association*, February 17, 1969; *Quarterly Journal of Crude Drug Research*, vol.

12, 1974, pp. 1846–1849; and W. A. Emboden's, *Narcotic Plants* [New York: Macmillan, 1979]). The cured, dried leaves were rolled in cigarette paper or else stuffed into pipes and leisurely smoked for the desired "high." (See the drug detox program at the end of this section for more data.)

Veronica's Desire for Marijuana Permanently Ended

As previously stated, Oscar is a one-of-a-kind drug rehab therapist. But the bottom line to the hundreds he's treated is that his remedies, however weird they may seem to some, get results! Without his help, many, in fact, would probably still be on drugs to this very day. But he's had to work "outside" the system in order to achieve what he has.

I asked him one day about his marijuana treatment, and he snapped back, "It's all in the diet, man . . . all in the diet!" I briefly cited the work being done at Tulane University, which didn't seem to interest him all that much. "My secret, if you can call it that, is in the pasta. I just have them [patients] eat as much as they want to their hearts' content.

"There was this chick Veronica. . . . Been a smoker of grass for some years. Couldn't seem to quit on her own. I told her to 'pig out on pasta' and eventually her cravin' for the stuff [marijuana] evaporated just like that (snapping his fingers together in midair for emphasis). Works every time!"

◆◆◆◆◆

PCP

In the same league as "ice" is phencyclidine (PCP or "angel dust"). Popular in veterinary medicine as an animal tranquilizer, it gives users feelings of invincibility alternating with paranoia, anxiety, rage, and depression. White blood cell counts plunge and leukopenia (abnormally low leukocytes in blood plasma) threatens the user's immune well-being.

The most common symptom, however, seems to be the rapid transformation of little Casper Milquetoast fellows into veritable supermen. A cop at the Los Angeles International Airport told me of an incident a while back in which "this little puny guy" successfully fought off four big, burly policemen with

Arnold Schwartzenegger builds, then plunged through a plate glass window, and kept running down a concourse until a hail of bullets dropped him in his tracks for good!

Radical treatment is needed here. Besides strong physical restraints for the patient, heavy doses of valerian root fluid extract (up to *60 drops* beneath the tongue every hour) and the Bach Flower Remedy of aspen are highly recommended by one Santa Monica, California, homeopathic drug counselor.

◆◆◆◆◆◆

R$_x$ AND OTC DRUG: A HIDDEN DRUG EPIDEMIC

In a series on "Drugging Our Elderly," *The Arizona Republic* (June 26, 1988) reported that "the extensive overmedication of older Americans" kills or seriously harms 2 million over the age of 65 every year. It is by far *the worst* drug epidemic that this nation currently faces, simply because it has been such a well-kept secret for so long, the Phoenix paper warned. It blamed institutions (hospitals and nursing homes) and individuals (doctors, nurses, and nursing home employees) for what it called the "calloused and utterly deplorable care of elderly subjects." This shameful treatment had resulted in a very different kind of addict—someone who receives drugs against his or her own will and better judgment, but can't seem to do anything about it. In its Tuesday, June 28 issue, the paper pointed out that "more elderly Americans die each year" from this type of "forced and legalized" addiction "than did the number of American servicemen killed during the entire Vietnam War."

A second side to this particular problem of drug abuse lays in the *voluntary* consumption of numerous over-the-counter (OTC) medications by tens of millions of other younger and middle-aged Americans. The March 12, 1990 issue of *Newsweek* magazine reported that pain pills, diet pills, sleeping pills, cough syrups, cold formulas, allergy medications, and laxatives "are being packaged, promoted and sold like toothpaste," when, in fact, "they're far more hazardous" than this. Extensive liver, kidney and stomach damage, not to mention hypertension, anxiety, restlessness, and hallucinations, have resulted from their careless and frequent use. Widespread advertising in magazines and newspapers and on radio and television by manufacturers have encouraged a sharp rise in public consumption of such OTC medicaments.

But advertising alone doesn't account for the enormous consumption of powerful prescription drugs in the state of Utah, which leads the nation in this type of substance abuse. Other factors are involved. Social scientists who've thoroughly examined the situation find that the majority of those addicted to such drugs are white, middle-class, well-educated, family-oriented, and staunchly Mormon as a rule. They note that the inordinate stresses and demanding sacrifices placed upon devout members of The Church of Jesus Christ of Latter-Day Saints in large part created a "need" in many of them for such potent pharmaceuticals. A variety of ingenious ways are employed by these people to persuade their doctors and pharmacists to prescribe and sell them those drugs which will alleviate some of their anxiety, depression, insomnia, loneliness, and nervousness.

Two of the most preferred prescription drugs in Utah, local sources say, are Novocain (procaine) and Xylocaine (lidocaine). According to *Scientific American* (March 1982), both "are structurally similar to cocaine and work by a similar mechanism. In fact, this journal noted, snorted lidocaine can't be distinguished from the same quantity of inhaled cocaine. Moreover, lab animals will work just as hard to get injections of procaine as they will for injections of cocaine. And this because the molecules of cocaine, lidocaine, and procaine are structurally similar.

Published research as well as data of my own obtained from interviews with many local Utahans, has repeatedly shown that those who constantly use prescription and OTC medications are *more* susceptible to respiratory infections, *more* susceptible to viral invasions, and take *longer* to get over bacterial problems than do those who aren't as frequently dependent on these substances. Allergies occur more often in the former than they do in the latter group. This kind of evidence points to a definite weakening of the immune systems in the young, middle-aged, and elderly victims of this type of coerced or voluntary addiction.

Nutritional Substitutes for R$_x$ and OTC Drugs

Besides some obvious social changes which have to be made, certain nutritional objectives also have to be met by those seeking treatment. Heading the list is *daily* consumption of vitamin C. *Non*acidic forms should be used in preference to those which contain straight ascorbic acid that can cause burning sensations inside the mouth, stomach, colon, and kidneys when frequently taken in large amounts. (Look for products listing calcium ascorbate and ascorbyl palmitate on the labels as sources for nonacidic C. See Great American Natural Products in the appendix.) Up to 10,000 mg. daily for youth and 15,000–20,000 mg. for adults of all ages. Also niacin (750 mg.) and pantothenic acid (100 mg.) each day helps as well. (See the detox program at the end of this section for additional suggestions.)

How Ethel C. Quit Her Prescription Drugs

My San Francisco informant told me of one patient visit in particular that he always enjoyed relating to others. "There comes in one day this lady dressed in mighty fancy threads. I'm talking about real upscale here. She had heard about some of my successes and wanted to know if I could help her mother. I said 'send her in.' A week later this retired English high school teacher came in to see me. Said her name was Ethel C. She had been taking a variety of over-the-counter and prescription medications for her, as she put it, 'many aches and pains.' She wanted to know how to quit taking them. I told her it was stupid to stop taking pills that her life might depend on.

"But I said I could help her cut out all those things which she was taking only for relief. I instructed her to make half of a coffee pot of mint tea each morning and to drink a number of cups of that warm throughout the day. I had her fill the top of a regular percolatin' pot with equal amounts of dried spearmint and peppermint, and the inside just half full of water."

"Did it help her?" I asked. "Must have," Oscar said, "because she sent me a short note some weeks later sayin' it did, and addin' that my grammar could stand some help, too."

◆◆◆◆◆
"SUGAR BLUES"/SALT SHAKEDOWN

A plethora of articles and books for the lay public or scientific community have been written in the last decade on the negative health consequences associated with intakes of white sugar and table salt. Basically all the authors have attempted to show through reasonable evidence the damaging effects of both. Rather than rehash what has already been written, it's my purpose here to show how an *acquired taste* for sugar and salt can interfere with normal immune functions and to demonstrate what can be done to control these impulsive *taste* habits.

The Dangers of Sugar and Salt to the Immune System

First, a crash course on the peculiar anatomy of the tongue. Taste sensations in humans arise from stimulation of specialized cells grouped in small clusters called taste buds. Taste buds exist in tiny bumps on the front of the tongue, in folds on the side of the tongue, and in circular grooves on the back of the tongue surface. Receptor cells on the top of each bud are constantly renewed about every ten days or so. Now three different cranial nerves furnish energy to these differently located taste buds; in turn, these three nerves are interconnected with the central nervous system itself, with the limbic system (the seat of the emotions in the brain), and with the hypothalamus gland (the main control console of the brain and site of hunger/fullness desires).

The work of Dr. Hugo O. Besedovsky, of the Swiss Research Institute in Davos-Platz, Switzerland, has demonstrated a feedback loop of communication between the immune system and the brain itself. Also the work of Dr. Elena A. Korneva of the Institute for Experimental Medicine in Leningrad, USSR, has proven that *sensation* stimulation to the front or back of the hypothalamus can determine whether the body's immune capabilities either *increase* or else are mildly to seriously *impaired*. And Dr. Viktor M. Klimenko, a colleague of Dr. Korneva's, has shown that immune responses in turn produce subtle but important chemical and electrical changes in the brain.

What all of this means in lay terms is essentially this: the *actual* tasting of sugary and salty substances *or* even the *craved* taste of them *immediately* dispatches electrical impulses through the nervous system to the limbic and hypothalamus portions of the brain via certain hormonelike agents called neuropeptides. In turn, these parts of the brain rapidly signal the gastrointestinal tract (where food is ultimately digested) *and* the immune system which then become cranked up to deal adequately with these sugary/salty substances. In the process, parts of the immune system start *over*producing certain cellular components in greater numbers than the body is then equipped to handle. The eventual results of such excessive stimulation can later spell trouble in the form of autoimmunity (adequately covered in Chapter Two). It would be fair to say then that not only does the frequent consumption of sugary and salty foods impair our health in obvious diseases like diabetes and hypertension, but also that the *initial* sensations of tasting them on the tongue combined with brain cravings for them tend to undermine immune defenses well before the actual problems themselves become apparent.

In another way, how we feel affects to some degree what we can or cannot taste. At the American Psychological Association's national conference which convened in New York City at the end of August 1987, a paper was read in which women suffering from depression could taste a harmless but bitter chemical called phenylthiocaramide (PTC), but happy and positive-minded women were *unable* to taste it. Hence, the emotions generated by the limbic areas of our brains can also exert an influence on our taste buds as well; this is an example of the "feedback loop of communication" that was discovered by Dr. Besedovsky in Switzerland.

Probably one of the real dangers to the introduction of sugar at an early age is that a human being develops a *gradual addiction* to it that can never be entirely eliminated. John Yudkin, M.D., a British nutritionist writing in *The Lancet* (June 22, 1963), observed that "our taste for sugar appears to be one that grows on what it feeds, so that we tend to like our food sweeter and sweeter." "People eat for palatability rather than for nutritional value," he concluded. His work and that of many other researchers since then has led to the assumption that *a taste* for sweet things eventually evolves into *a real addiction* similar in some ways to cravings for alcohol, caffeine, and nicotine. And the consumption of more and more sugary foods upsets the delicate communications balance between our nerves, brain, and immune system. Thus, it appears that the *taste for sugar* rather than the actual consumption of it, must be effectively dealt with in some rational way to stop the continual poisoning of our bodies.

How to Fight "Junk Food" Addiction

When nearly a thousand Minnesota high school kids were asked in 1985 what "the primary appeal of junk food" was to them, they overwhelmingly responded, "Because the stuff *tastes good!*" Where registered dieticians and licensed nutritionists were able to substitute fresh fruits, fruit juices, wholesome vegetable snacks, and vegetable juices such as carrot (which is naturally quite sweet anyway) for Twinkies, doughnuts, jelly rolls, soft drinks, and colas, they discovered that teenagers not only enjoyed these more nourishing replacements, but also seemed to have far fewer respiratory infections and less fatigue and moodiness. Thus, *substitution* of naturally sweet foods for items containing refined white sugar, fructose, sucrose, or NutraSweet seems to be one solution.

Another logical approach to the problem of sugar addiction is analyzing your own emotions. Two separate studies at the University of California, Berkeley (1975), and New York University, New York City (1986), investigated the food selections made by many different students dining in campus cafeterias and discovered that those who were moody and high-strung ate *more* sugary/salty foods than did others who were reasonably calm and felt good about themselves. The inevitable conclusion drawn from both reports, which appeared in two well respected nutrition journals, was this: insecurity breeds greater sugar addiction, while strong self-confidence seems to drastically reduce the *craving* for sweets.

A third factor is the simplicity of a meal itself. A psychiatrist from Johns Hopkins Hospital in Baltimore observed that there is a greater inclination toward sweet things when a variety of foods are served as opposed to a meal consisting of just one of those foods, even if it happens to be a favorite one. Not only is *less* eaten at a single entree meal, but also the desire for dessert sharply drops as well. Rodents given the choice of a three-course or one-course meal, will invariably choose the former and "overeat to the point of obesity."

The inclusion of strong tasting or smelling herbs in our meals more often will definitely curb our sugar/salt addiction. Professor Tim J. Roper of the University of Sussex in England, reported in *New Scientist* magazine (March 29, 1984) that the "flavour principles" of Mediterranean cuisine were a combination of olive oil, garlic, tomatoes, and herbs. Mexican cookery makes liberal use of ingredients that are by any objective standards unpleasant—hot chilies and cayenne pepper being prime examples. Then, too, many vegetarian dishes call for honey or molasses in place of sugar and kelp or dulse (powdered seaweeds) in place of table salt. The end result, Professor Roper says, is a considerable *decline* in the use of sugar and salt in these respective cuisines.

A fifth and final point to be made is an attitude readjustment to our present consumerism. When shopping in the supermarket, we're often inclined to purchase things that "look" good or "smell" good or even "taste" good (ever wonder why the free food samples given out are usually sweet or salty and very fattening?). We must especially monitor what our eyes behold, for whatever our gaze happens to fall upon that "looks" mighty tempting, an immediate signal flashes to the limbic "feel good" part of our brain and then is instantaneously dispatched through our nerves to the hypothalamus "hunger" center and on to our gut neuropeptides as well. In a matter of seconds we're experiencing a *hormonal* response that's almost subconscious to food our eyes have spotted which is tasty (sweet/salty) and appealing to our various senses. To turn the tide of such frequent autosuggestions *away* from junk food and toward healthier staples, we need to practice a certain amount of self-control and learn to discipline ourselves better when we're shopping for groceries.

Curbing the "Sugar Blues"

One of the most common addictions treated at Oscar's San Francisco drug rehab center is the craving for sweets. During the seven days one spring that I spent with him, I was surprised to discover just how many college students visited his place. "Word-of-mouth is always the best form of advertizin'," he wisecracked. Many of them were from across the Bay at the University of California campus in Berkeley.

Michelle P. and Roxanne J. were typical of this large college clientele. In the informal interviews that followed, both women revealed their addiction to sweets. The first thing Oscar did was to discuss their everyday social lives. It became apparent that each coed suffered from some form of insecurity and a certain amount of stress. Pointing to his right temple with a forefinger, he told them, "The first part of your problem begins up here." Then opening his mouth wide and sticking out his tongue he pointed to it. "The second part of your problem is here. Once we can adequately deal with both of these, you're on your way to recovery."

Oscar firmly believes that "sugarholics" (as he so aptly characterizes them) need to get their mental landscape in order before any dietary readjustments are made. He advised them to sort out their priorities and get rid of those things or people that were stress inducing. He also gave them a brief pep talk designed to make them feel better about themselves.

"Knowin' that you look great is very important to the therapy," he insisted. You gotta believe in yourself enough to say over and over again, 'Hey, man! I'm worth the effort to change the image of myself for the better." To get their minds off their problems for a while each day, Oscar recommended some biofeedback techniques, a few deep-breathing exercises or whatever else worked for them.

The next part was fairly simple. He "prescribed" certain foods that were naturally sweet, which would take care of the taste buds along either side of the tongue that stimulated sugar "blues." In emergency situations, he suggested sucking a Certs. While these obviously contain sugar, the amount released is very small and is measured out over a period of time. His preference, however, was for a short piece of licorice root bark from a local health food store chewed on throughout the day.

He also advised them to *sip* rather than drink or gulp down a mixture of half carrot and half pineapple juice. "The two really go great together," he said, "especially when you add a couple of ice cubes." Best taken through a *thin* straw in *measured* sips over the course of an hour, if possible, to really be effective.

By doing it *this way*, he thinks, "you're foolin' the brain into thinkin' it's gettin' its badly needed dose of sugar, but only not as much." Strawsipping grape juice is also possible, but doesn't seem to work as well as the former does. He also insists that *cold* prune juice works wonderfully well when slowly sipped.

And during meal times at the campus cafeteria, he suggested both girls chew on a *single* pitted date or fig while going through the line. "If you're brain is gettin' fed just a *little* bit of sugar, you won't be so inclined to load up your tray with a lot of desserts," he admonished. And *cold water* was the beverage rule for every meal. "If my advice is followed," he observed to me, "they'll have pretty much licked their sugar 'blues'."

◆◆◆◆◆

TOBACCO

What to Do About That Nicotine Fit

Times have really changed so far as the once popular habit of smoking is concerned. Common to many of the newsstand "big picture" magazines (*Look*, *Life*, etc.) that dominated the 1930s and 1940s were hundreds of cigarette ads, touting not only their glamorous aspects but also *with medical endorsements* as to their presumed health values of all things! ("Camels" and "Lucky Strikes" were typical of these.) Today, however, the recently retired U.S. Surgeon-General C. Everett Koop, M.D., has come out against cigarettes in the strongest terms imaginable, proclaiming those who still enjoy smoking to have as serious a drug addiction problem as those who use crack, cocaine, or heroin.

To paraphrase President Bush, there are "kinder, gentler" ways to quit the tobacco habit than going completely "cold turkey."

1. Avoid consumption of acid foods and instead opt for more alkaline staples. Research shows that smokers who eat junk food are apt to have more cigarettes in a day than those who supplement their diets with more fresh fruits and vegetables. Sugar and fat tend to flush nicotine out of the system more quickly, thereby creating more frequent cravings, whereas alkaline foods high in potassium cause a longer retention of nicotine in the system, which enables addicts to smoke *fewer* cigarettes.

2. Clinical testing has determined that heavy ex-smokers benefit from chewing a nicotine gum called Nicorette, made by Dow Chemical Company's Lakeside Pharmaceutical division. The medical journal *Lancet* reported in mid-February 1988 that one three-pack-a-day smoker quit his 21-year habit by this means. He then slowly weaned himself away from his 17 sticks of Nicorette a day by switching to bubble gum instead.

3. Reduce the stress of your surrounding environment or else remove yourself to one that is more conducive to peace. In the latter part of 1989, thousands of New England Telephone employees went on strike for several months. During that time until negotiations finally ended it, "there was some pretty heavy smoking going on around our offices here," said vice president of human resources, Peter Bertschmann. Normally a pack-a-day smoker himself, he jumped up three and four packs daily during those critical few months. Since the pressure abated in the early spring of 1990, he's dropped significantly to *less* than a pack a day. "Hopefully I can kick the habit soon altogether," he thoughtfully mused, "as I just don't see myself going down 17 flights of stairs to smoke outside" (the telephone company issued a total ban on inside smoking that went into effect July 1).

4. Judy H. works as an executive secretary for a prominent Indonesian company in Jakarta. Prior to her conversion to Mormonism, she was a two- or three-pack-a-day smoker. To help herself make the transition a lot easier into her new faith (which forbids smoking and drinking), she resorted to chewing carrots. As previously mentioned in my other book, *Heinerman's Encyclopedia of Fruits, Vegetables & Herbs* (Prentice Hall, 1988), she reported: "It took me about two weeks on this carrot program until I was able to quit smoking altogether. I would eat about 2–3 carrots a day. I found that the sweet taste of the carrots satisfied me enough so that I didn't crave a [Dunhill brand] cigarette [anymore]." Chewing celery sticks and radishes also seems to help, but not as well as carrots.

5. Acupuncture works pretty well for some people, too. I've had some heavy ex-smokers swear by the success of this therapy, when everything else seemed to fail. Consult only a qualified and competent expert though.

Nicotine, just like caffeine and other addictive substances, can negatively influence the immune system in a number of ways, the most drastic being to stop it from preventing cancer in the body. By kicking the habit *now*, smokers are assuring themselves of extra years of healthier living.

Smoking Addiction Cured with Diet and Secret Tibetan Herbs

A Korean chemist now residing in Chicago, Illinois, once heard me on a national radio program discussing what could be done about various addictions. He sent me a photocopied story about an amazing clinic in Tijuana, Mexico, which was featured in the July 10, 1990 issue of the Chicago *Korean Times*. Not only did he provide a translation of the article for my benefit, but included his own testimony about it as well.

Charles P. related in some detail how this clinic helped him overcome a terrible smoking problem. He mentioned that prior to going to East/West Wellness Center (also known as Agua Calente Val Paraiso), he went through nearly *five packs per day*! "I was a hopeless chain smoker!" he admitted.

But then he met Dr. Yun Hye-gu, one of just a handful of doctors in the world skilled enough to dispense the little known but very powerful herbal formulas from Tibet. Tibetan herbs, he learned from Dr. Yun, are far more potent than are regular Western or even Chinese herbs are. They need to be handled with great care and wisdom.

During the three some odd weeks he spent at Dr. Yun's clinic, he ate nothing but organic foods without white sugar, white flour, or salt in them. No red meat of any kind was allowed, just fresh cooked fish once a week. And no eggs or milk were permitted either, I might add.

The first thing he noticed on this diet after a week, was *a reduced inclination* to smoke. By the time a good week had passed, he said, his cigarette intake had dropped drastically to *less than a pack a day*! "I couldn't believe it myself, at first, until it dawned on me just how little I craved smoking. It was no longer a thing I desired to do."

The second part of the treatment was a daily administration of a particular Tibetan compound that "actually took away my taste for cigarettes," he claimed. He said that at first the effects of this formula were very subtle, but after a week or ten days, they become more pronounced and evident. So much so, in fact, that one day while he was in downtown Tijuana doing some shopping, and another smoker exhaled in his direction, "it actually made me sick to my stomach."

Mr. P. couldn't supply me with the list of secret herbs which made up the ingredients of this remarkable Tibetan formula. I contacted Dr. Yun to learn what they were, but he declined for obvious commercial reasons. "My competitors down here would love to know what it is," he replied by phone. However, he said any of my readers could contact him by phone or mail at the East/West Wellness Center (see the appendix), and he would be glad to help them as much as he could with some of the remedial aspects to his very successful recovery program for substance addictions such as tobacco, alcohol, and drugs.

◆◆◆◆◆

DRUG DETOX PROGRAM THAT WORKS

In the last twelve years or so, I've had the good fortune of meeting several dozen drug rehabilitation counselors, therapists, doctors, and holistic healers throughout the country and overseas, who've specialized in treating thousands of individuals addicted to the substances. From hundreds of hours of interviews and endless days spent with them, I've compiled what I believe to be a pretty good detoxification program that is an expansion of a more abbreviated version included in my last book (*Heinerman's Encyclopedia of Fruits, Vegetables & Herbs*; also see the Anthropological Research Center in the appendix).

1. Recognition of the problem. This is the first task confronting the addict. Denial of the addiction only exacerbates the problem. Many of those hooked on caffeine, nicotine, or sugar/salt will vehemently resist the idea that they are *just as much addicts* as alcoholics or dope users. But "truth is truth" as the familiar adage goes, and nothing will ever change this fact or make it easier to live with.

2. Desire for assistance. You can't help somebody unless they (a) want the help and (b) are willing to work with others who can help them overcome their problems. You may throw a sinking person any number of lifelines, but unless that individual grabs on to one of them and *hangs on*, no amount of effort will ever be able to keep the addict from eventually drowning anyway.

3. Recovery success is measured by degrees, never by leaps and bounds. An addiction is just like an old rheumatic back pain in some ways—it always seems to keep coming back when the weather becomes a little overcast and stormy. Life is constantly filled with all types of stress. Expect the unexpected and be prepared to handle crisis situations in a moment's notice—*sober* and without some familiar substance to give false hopes and empty escapes.

4. A completely revamped diet is absolutely essential to your physiological and sociological well-being. Certain foods are known to drive the engines of addiction. The body of a recovering addict *must be* properly fueled or else all other efforts will prove to be futile, sooner or later. In a few words here's some sound advice worth following to the letter:

- Replace sugar/salt with honey or molasses and powdered seaweeds.
- Eliminate vinegar and foods (condiments) containing it from the diet.
- Cook with olive or sunflower oils; avoid deep-fried fast foods.
- Replace poultry, pork, and most beef with fish, lamb, goat, and veal.
- Don't broil or fry foods; instead boil, bake, or steam them.
- Consume fresh fruits and fruit juices.
- Consume fresh vegetables and vegetable juices (except V-8).
- Drink more coffeelike beverages (Pero, Postum).
- Drink a lot of water (preferably distilled or mineral spring).
- Avoid alcohol, coffee, colas, and all soft drinks.

- Replace meat with legumes, nuts, and seeds for protein needs.
- Meal times should be pleasant occasions devoid of stressful moments.
- Eat five small meals daily instead of three large ones.
- Have *only* one or two entrees per meal, *never* any more than this.

5. Cleanse drug residues with liquids instead of solids. Herbal teas, tinctures, and fluid extracts seem to work more quickly and with less effort than do capsules or tablets of powdered plant materials. Three different types of herbal blends are suggested here for detoxification purposes. *They are to be taken on an empty stomach* for maximum effectiveness. They are each to be *consumed at different times* throughout the day, as indicated in the following discussion. When making an herbal tea, bring a pint or quart of water to a boil in a stainless steel, enamel, or glassware pot (*never* aluminum or Teflon®). Add coarse, tough materials (roots, stems, stalks, berries) first; then cover with lid and reduce heat to lower setting and allow to simmer for 5 minutes. Remove from stove, add more delicate materials (leaves, flowers), cover again, and allow to steep 30–45 minutes longer. Strain, flavor with honey or molasses, and drink as directed. If using only delicate materials, after water has boiled, remove pot from the heat and add the herbs desired. Then gently stir, cover and permit to steep for 40 minutes. Strain, sweeten, and drink according to directions.

6. Calm the nerves and brain centers with liquid concentrates. Unlike tinctures, which are simpler and can be made at home, fluid extracts are usually more complex in nature and require extra equipment and a greater amount of time and effort to make them as potent as they should be. Therefore, it's best to purchase them. They are generally administered sublingually (beneath the base of the tongue) in 15–20 drop amounts every couple of hours or as needs dictate. The following fluid extracts help curb renewed drug carvings: wild lettuce, valerian root, chamomile, rosemary. (See the appendix for Pure Herbs Ltd., which carries these several liquid concentrates.)

◆◆◆◆◆◆

A CAJUN RECIPE FOR CURING DRUG ADDICTION

In the last decade I've probably visited New Orleans, Louisiana, at least a dozen times. The mellow sounds of Dixie Land jazz, the eerie sensations of their nighttime Stephen King–type grave-yards, the hot and humid bayou marshes with their irresistible adventures keep bringing people like myself back time and time again. But the biggest attraction of all, perhaps, is that appe-tizing and mouth-watering Cajun cooking. Nothing so lip-smacking as this can be found anywhere else in the South.

The spicy elements that make each dish a gastronomical adventure are also the very same things that work miraculous recovery cures for drug addicts, believe it or not. Ida Lafitte-Ramirez is one of those unique individuals who has successfully bridged opposite talents into a real work of art. Her sidewalk cafe experiences were, at some point in time, translated into a down home medical expertise. The "Julia Child of jambalaya" turned into a kind of Dr. Lendon Smith somewhere along the way.

Ida's work with drug addicts hasn't been widely heralded in the press although it ought to be. The heart and core of Ida's recovery program consists of a few selected spices. That's right, s-p-i-c-e-s as in red-hot cayenne pepper, sharply penetrating horseradish, saliva-inducing mustard, tear-invoking garlic, and heart-warming ginger. Coriander, cumin, fenugreek, onion, oregano, and thyme are her second line of defense against the insidious addiction to drugs.

Ida believes that these strong and lusty spices somehow enable the body chemistry to "switch" from habit-forming and harmful drugs to irresistible and healthy culinary herbs such as these. "I guess it is because they are so . . . so . . . [searching for the right word] . . . so *piquant*, I suppose, that they work as well as they do in helping addicts reform their lives," she added with a certain finality.

Ida's remedies are really her recipes, and while most of her "food prescription" may be found in any cookbook specializing in Cajun and Creole dishes, yet it's from the jambalaya that most of her success comes. This throw-together mixture of rice cooked with smoked ham and sausage, skinned chicken, de-veined shrimp or shucked oysters and seasoned with pinches of the foregoing herbs is more of "an add what you please" dish than anything else. In other words, those not liking pork, poultry, or mollusks can opt for other kinds of meat ranging from exotic gator and wild deer meat to the more conventional beef or lamb.

The main point, however, is *most* of the aforementioned spices *need to be included* in small amounts in order to be effective in helping drug addicts quit their substance abuses once and for all. Ms. Lafitte-Ramirez told me that other kinds of ethnic cuisines could work just as well, but they need to be *spicy*! So it seems that the likes of Mexican, Thai, Indian, and Chinese foods, besides her own Cajun creations, have enormous therapeutic value in coping with general drug addiction problems.

◆◆◆◆◆

HYPOGLYCEMIA

The Great Disease Mimic

There are basically three types of hypoglycemia. Two of them involve tumors of the pancreas on the Islet of Langerhans. The third type of low blood sugar is called reactive or functional hyperinsulinism and is induced by a diet high in refined carbohydrates. They cause a dramatic rise in blood sugar, triggering an excess of insulin secretion from the pancreas. This drops the blood sugar quickly to an abnormally low level.

Dr. S. Gyland carefully followed the behavior of several hundred patients suffering from this last form of hypoglycemia. He cited the frequency of several symptoms with depression occurring in 77% of them and worrying and anxiety in 62% of the patients. Many of the illnesses complained about are thought to be "all in the mind" of the individual or psychosomatic disorders. These people are then led to believe that they need psychiatric counseling, when, in fact, all they require is a modification of their regular eating habits.

In a restudy of 115 patients who were referred for psychological treatment on the basis of diagnosis by exclusion, all 115 on competent, careful reexamination were discovered to have physical ailments that were actually the causes of their "emotional" symptoms. For one person in every ten, says a recent *Journal of Orthomolecular Medicine* (vol. 5, 1990, p. 8), sugar is a deadly food, paving the way toward a multitude of distressing physical symptoms, plus all the tortures of neurotic and even psychotic behavior.

How Hypoglycemia Adversely Affects Immune Functions

In addition to Dr. Gyland's own work, the research pioneered by the famous psychiatrist, Harry Salzer, M.D., also helped to prove that high intakes of refined carbohydrates can really foul up the mental and emotional states of people, which, in turn, throws a corresponding monkey wrench into the carefully tuned machinery of immune functions. Of the hundreds and hundreds of patients he treated over the years, Dr. Salzer discovered that about 40% or four out of ten of his patients experiencing some kind of neuropsychiatric illness, were, in fact, suffering from mild to acute hypoglycemia.

In several brilliant papers given by him on the subject during the early and mid-1950s, he concluded that for many of his patients horizontal on psychiatric couches, a simple change in diet could put most of them vertical at lunch counters instead. In one of his papers read before the Section of Nervous and Mental Diseases at the annual convention of the American Medical Association in June 1957, he listed the four most frequent symptoms discovered in more than 300 hypoglycemic patients who came under his immediate care and observation: depression, 60%; insomnia, 50%, anxiety, 50%; and irritability, 45%.

The recent work done by two Swiss researchers demonstrates that the neuroendocrine system in each of us is involved not only in the development of but in the *ongoing* regulation of the immune system. Dr. Walter Pierpaoli of the Institute for Biomedical Research in Quartino-Magadino and Dr. George J. M. Maestroni of the Laboratory for Experimental Pathology in Locarno have shown that *mental or emotional* interference with the cyclical release of the important hormone melatonin (released by the pineal gland) *profoundly* handicaps body immunity. Their work proves that any *socially* activated/*biologically* triggered disturbances in the brain, heart, and nerves can cause hidden but dangerous adverse effects within the neuroendocrine system which is immediately responsible for the smooth regulation of the immune system.

Thus, the four most common and obvious signs of hypoglycemia, namely, depression, insomnia, anxiety, and irritability, wreck havoc with our front line defenses. As a result, those with low blood sugar tend to get more colds and flus and take longer to recover from infections such as Candida, than others who don't have this particular problem.

How to Find the Sugar Hiding in the Food We Buy

According to the late nutritionist, Dr. Carlton Fredericks in his book, *Psycho-Nutrition* (New York: Macmillan, 1978), "the average American . . . swallows 1⅓ teaspoonfuls of sugar, every 35 minutes, 24 hours a day!" He declared "that most our sugar intake is invisible (until it surfaces on your hips)." Sugar is all around us in so many different things that most of the time we aren't even aware of it.

Of course, those who are more health conscious than some will certainly avoid the obvious foods already high in sugar content—candies, cakes, pies, ice cream, and so forth. But what about other *less* obvious foods *also* high in sugar? According to the March 1978 issue of *Consumer Reports* you'd better think twice about using French or Thousand Island dressing on your healthy salads if you're concerned about your sugar intake, because they contain between 23 and 30.2% of the stuff. Or if you're thinking about a healthier breakfast cereal such as granola instead of that other cardboard junk you already know is high in sugar, then you'd better think again because something like Quaker 100% Natural Cereal has a whopping 23.9% sugar in it.

In fact, foods you don't even suspect of containing sugar have more in them than may meet the eye. A jar of Coffee-mate nondairy creamer has about *8 times* as much sugar (65.4%) in it than does a can of Classic Coca-Cola (8.8%). Or how about a box of Shake 'n Bake Barbecue Mix for chicken with just about as much sugar (50.9%) in it as you'd find in a single bar of Hershey's Milk Chocolate (51.4%). Even something as innocuous as a can of Del Monte Whole Kernel Corn doesn't escape without its dose (10.7%) of sugar either.

The food companies have been getting more clever lately in hiding the fact that they put sugar in just about everything we consume. For instance, a recent trip to the supermarket told me that a 26-oz. can of Campbell's Tomato Soup had high fructose corn syrup in it as the *second* leading ingredient, but no where else did the label say anything about plain sugar being in it. This, of course, is their way of masking the facts, like slipping a knockout pill into someone's drink when they're not looking. Sugar is there all right, but just in another form. Sometimes consumers get a *double* dose of the same poison in one product. Take an 18-oz. jar of Skippy Creamy Peanut Butter for instance. Besides the obvious peanuts, the label also mentions dextrose as the second ingredient with vegetable oil, salt, and finally sugar bringing up the end. Dextrose, of course, is a naturally occurring sugar extracted from grapes and corn and widely utilized by the food industry these days to flavor hundreds of edible items.

An extensive listing of foods to avoid wouldn't be practical nor very effective here. An easy rule of thumb to follow is to just remember to read labels and look for *anything* ending in -ose, which indicates sugar is present in some form. The label doesn't have to spell out s-u-g-a-r in so many letters, but other words— corn syrup, fructose, dextrose, mannose, glucose, rhamnose, and so forth, can indicate that the same harmful ingredient is present. By looking at labels more carefully, you can curtail your sugar intake substantially.

Nonhypoglycemic Foods for Strong Immunity

Those adversely affected by low blood sugar can find great relief from this particular problem by frequently utilizing a variety of foods which will amply nourish them without creating biological havoc later on.

The following vegetables ought to be consumed fresh or semicooked in a 2-cup amount nearly every day. (Canned vegetables should be avoided due to their high sugar contents, but *some* frozen vegetables may be all right to use.)

Asparagus	Endive	Mushrooms
Avocado	Eggplant	Mustard greens
Beet greens	Escarole	Radishes
Broccoli	Green or wax	Sauerkraut
Brussels sprouts	beans	Spinach
Cabbage	Green bell	String beans
Celery	pepper	Summer
Chard	Kale	squash
Chicory	Kohlrabi	Tomatoes
Collards	Leeks	Tomato juice
Cucumbers	Lettuce (Romaine	Turnip greens
Dandelion	*not* iceberg)	Watercress

All canned, bottled and frozen fruits should pretty much be avoided as their sugar contents are extraordinarily high as a rule. Also many fresh fruits in season should either be entirely avoided (oranges, grapes) or else utilized *very sparingly* (apples, peaches, pears) by hypoglycemics. Also, nearly all fruit juices will tend to play havoc with existing blood sugar levels in those highly susceptible to such concentrated forms of sweet energy.

Legumes are highly recommended since they are complex carbohydrates and aren't assimilated as rapidly, as, say, mashed potatoes would be (a baked potato with the skin intact, however, is a complex carbohydrate). Complex carbohydrates serve as sort of a braking mechanism so that not too many carbohydrates are dumped into the body all at once. The following list should be resorted to often for light lunch and heavier dinner entrees:

Black beans	Lima beans
Black-eye peas	Mung beans
Chickpeas	Navy, white, and Great
Fava beans	Northern beans
Kidney beans	Split and whole peas
Lentils	Soybeans

Finally, certain grains should be consumed at least *twice* daily—once in the morning for a hearty breakfast and again in the evening as a late night snack before retiring. I've noticed that when hypoglycemics consume one or more of these grains several times a day, it seems to help regulate their blood sugar metabolisms.

Barley	Rice
Buckwheat	Rye
Bulghur	Triticale
Corn/popcorn (unsalted)	Wheat/shredded and cracked
Millet	Wild rice
Oats	

By merely making a few simple adjustments in the diet, someone suffering from hypoglycemia can avoid those constant "immune blackouts" that leave the body open to major infections. All it takes is a little knowledge, a greater amount of will power, and a lot of determination to make it work successfully.

A Zapotecan Indian Cure for Hypoglycemia

The Zapotecan, together with other interrelated Mexican Indian tribes like the Mazatecs and Mixtecs, occupy most of the state of Oaxaca and adjacent areas. Anthropologists like myself have studied the diets and folk medicines of such people in times past. Several important articles about one of their major health problems, namely, hypoglycemia, have been published in different scientific journals. Anthropologist C. W. O'Neill, for instance, explored the problems surrounding low blood sugar in the Zapotecan village of La Paz (also known as Escalerita) in a lengthy article published in *The Journal of Psychological Anthropology* (vol. 3, 1979, pp. 301–322). And just a couple of years later, Dr. Ralph Bolton of Pomona College in Pomona, California, covered the same topic in his own lengthy report, which appeared in the October 1981 issue of *Ethnology*. While mentioning the classic symptoms of *susto* or hypoglycemia among the Zapotecan (i.e., disturbed sleep, listlessness, loss of appetite, apathy, fatigue, depression and asociality), he also extended his research to some South American Indian tribes as well.

Much has been written about hypoglycemia by health and medical experts in this country and in Canada. But none of them, to my knowledge, has ever investigated other successful therapy programs practiced elsewhere in this hemisphere, probably because they were unaware that this problem existed in other societies. This is where my training as a medical anthropologist comes in handy and makes available to the average layperson valuable and important health information that might not otherwise ever be made public.

In 1977 and again in 1981, I spent considerable time in Mexico with various indigenous Indian cultures, collecting a great deal of helpful medical information relative to their remedies for sickness. As I went back into my files and poured over some of my bulky notebooks written in the field, I discovered to my happy surprise, a rather successful treatment for hypoglycemia furnished to me by one Zapotecan *curandera* or folk healer named Isabella Thipaak.

Her program, while amazingly simple, helps to reverse many of those symptoms common to low blood sugar. Here is an outline of the main points of her treatment:

1. Patient must avoid sweets, coffee, refined flour, aggravating spices, such as cayenne pepper (a difficult thing for Mexicans to do!), and garlic. [I might comment here that certain scientific evidence published in the *West Indian Medical Journal* (Vol. 31, 1982, pp. 194–197), *The American Journal of Clinical Nutrition* (Vol. 28, July 1975, pp. 684–685), and *Medikon* (Vol. 3, no. 3, 1977, pp. 15–17) prove that both spices are decidedly hypoglycemic and, therefore, ought to be avoided.]

2. The patient is to consume five to seven *small* meals spread out over the entire day, instead of just the two to three big ones most of us are accustomed to.

3. Breakfast should be before 8:30 A.M. and consist of nuts, eggs, cheese, corn tortillas, and half a citrus fruit, preferably sour (grapefruit, for instance). The second breakfast, as

Isabella called it, should take place around 10:30 A.M. and consist of more raw nuts or seeds (sunflower) and some simple vegetable soup (tomato). Then two lunches follow, one at noontime and the other at 3:30 P.M. Corn chips with guacamole, steamed corn or other lightly cooked vegetables, and some chicken is what she recommends to her hypoglycemic patients. The second lunch must also contain some other kind of animal protein, preferably a chunk of goat or lamb meat, if possible. A piece of fish can be easily substituted if neither of the others is readily available. Also a few nuts (Brazil) and a small serving of some type of cheese should be included as well. In between both lunches, a short 30-minute siesta is recommended to help relax the digestive processes for a while. Dinner for her hypoglycemic patients is around 6:30 P.M. and no later than 7 P.M. Here a larger selection of items is permitted: tacos, bean-filled tortillas, enchiladas, boiled corn, small roasted or baked potatoes, fresh mango or papaya, fresh or baked banana, baked pumpkin or squash, and so on. Not much, if any meat is served at this time; the emphasis is on complex carbohydrates and fruits and vegetables. (It's interesting to note here that most other meal guides for hypoglycemics published in the United States prohibit especially sweet fruits like bananas. However, Isabella has never found them to be a problem provided they are taken *only at night*.) A final "second dinner," as she likes to call it, just before retiring for the night usually includes a heated tortilla with a little cheese of some kind. She includes other foods native to the area, but they aren't included here because of their scarce availability in the United States. Her program can be readjusted to accommodate more finicky American tastes, if need be.

4. One of the most popular herbs used by Isabella in treating low blood sugar is manzanita berries and leaves. (Manzanita belongs to the same Arctostaphylos group that uva ursi does.) Her patients are encouraged to drink a cup of the tea every other day. They are taught to make the tea by boiling a pint of water and then adding one level teaspoonful of either the berries or leaves or half of each and simmering a few minutes. Then the container is removed from the fire and covered, and the contents allowed to set for a while before straining and drinking.

5. Proper rest is an absolute *must* for Isabella's patients. They are plainly told to take short siestas after the noon meal and another one, if necessary, after a hard day's work and just before eating the first dinner at 6:30 P.M. Also she insists upon a *full* night's sleep for them as well. (By her calculations, 8 to 10 hours constitutes a complete rest.)

6. Arguments need to be avoided as much as possible, as they tend to upset the emotions and bodily functions of a hypoglycemic patient. Spousal fights and neighborhood jealousies, common to the Zapotecs, are particularly troublesome for any treatment. She insists that her patients get along with their mates, other family members, friends, and neighbors.

◆◆◆◆◆

INSUFFICIENT SLEEP

A Sleep-Deprived State Leads to Serious Illness

What did the late television actor, Lorne Greene and master puppeteer, Jim Henson have in common with screen actress, Elizabeth Taylor, who in June 1990 was barely clinging to life? All three succumbed to deadly viral infections *due to a lack of adequate rest!*

Greene, best known for his roles as Ben Cartwright in "Bonanza" and Commander Adama in "Battlestar Galactica," died in a hospital quite suddenly a few years ago of pneumonia. Prior to his death, he had been trying to fulfill a heavy schedule of commitments, which kept him busy and with little opportunity for the rest his exhausted body needed. At some point along the way, he caught a simple cold, which quickly developed into a full case of pneumonia that required immediate hospitalization. His body's already weakened immune system never had a chance to recover fully, and he died unexpectedly. Greene, who had been in the best of health before this, was then in his late sixties.

Henson was the voice and inspiration behind many of the famous Muppet characters—Kermit the Frog, Miss Piggy, Gonzo and Big Bird. According to "Entertainment Tonight" on Tuesday, June 5, 1990, Henson had been working 15-hour shifts 7 days a week for many months without much let-up. He had been in the "peak of health," close friends and family members said, up until just a few days before his untimely demise. At that time, he complained of having a mild sore throat that just didn't seem to want to go away. One day he suddenly collapsed and was rushed to New York Hospital suffering from what one doctor disclosed as the worst "galloping pneumonia that I ever saw in my life." This combined with a strep throat infection was just too much for his system to handle and he quickly died at the age of 53.

Taylor was hospitalized April 9, 1990 at St. John's Hospital and Health Center in Santa Monica, California, with a terrible case of double pneumonia. According to various news releases, her confinement extended well into the summer, as she bravely fought the medical odds against her recovery. At one point she was just "a cat's whisker" from death, said one doctor. Again, as in the other two cases, she had been on a heavy schedule promoting her new line of perfumes and making commercials for them without much chance of resting as she should have.

The lesson to be learned from these three examples is that *proper rest* keeps the immune system strong and active! No matter how carefully you may eat or how many vitamin-mineral or herbal supplements you may take or how frequently you may exercise, the bottom line is that without *sufficient* sleep the body's front-line defenses are going to suffer terribly. And simply "catching" up on missed sleep on the weekend isn't going to help matters much either. A *consistent* program of adequate rest is necessary on a *daily* basis to keep our immune levels in tip-top shape; nothing less than this will do.

How to Have a Good Night's Rest

Tonight approximately 65 million American adults will crawl into bed somewhere, draw up the covers, lay their heads down on their pillows, and then, try as they might, won't be able to find restful sleep. You might very well be one of them. If you

- pass the entire night in the clutches of unremitting insomnia,

- take an hour or longer to fall asleep,
- do fall asleep but awaken at 4 A.M. and can't get back to sleep,
- are the victim of recurrent nightmares and sleepwalking,

then you probably suffer from some kind of sleep disorder. But whatever your particular sleep problem may be, help is available. The information presented here has been gleaned from a wide variety of medical and scientific journals reporting numerous studies made on the subject of sleep.

REM Sleep: The Stuff Dreams Are Made Of. There are five basic types of normal sleeping patterns: four stages of non-REM (no rapid eye movement) sleep and regular REM. Stages 3 and 4 of non-REM are known as Delta sleep, the most profound state of unconsciousness which the body can attain. Up to age 30, a person spends 20% of his or her total sleep time in Delta; after 30, however, Delta sleep time plummets dramatically to only 4% for men and 8% for women aged 70 to 80.

REM sleep is that level which the majority of us slumber at to varying degrees. Here brain waves resemble drowsiness more than deep sleep. Although mental activity occurs all night long, more than 80% will recall vivid dreams if awakened at this time. Face, limbs, and trunk muscles are slack, but there may be twitches due to bursts of activity in the central nervous system somewhere.

Dreams full of pleasant or interesting activities (as opposed to nightmares) constitute normal and uninterrupted REM sleep. To achieve such meaningful therapeutic dreams, one must understand something about what initiates sleep in the first place. J. Allan Hobson of Harvard Medical School and a world authority on the neurophysiology of sleep revealed in the 1960s and early 1970s that the brainstem and hypothalamus gland portion of the brain were implicated in sleep. Certain neurons, known as giant cells, increase their firing intensity before and after REM sleep. On the other hand, neurons known as locus coeruleus cells stop their electrical activity before and during REM sleep. So it appears that giant cells switch on REM and engage the dream machinery, while locus coeruleus cells switch everything off at the proper time.

Now there are certain substances which can either help or hinder the process of sleep initiation. Warm herbal teas like valerian root, catnip herb, or chamomile flowers all exert profound effects on both the brainstem and hypothalamus. This is due to certain naturally occurring sedative compounds such as valepotriates (in valerian), nepelactone (in catnip), and the amino acid tryptophan (in chamomile). In fact, as I reported in my second herb book over a decade ago, *Science of Herbal Medicine* (Provo, Utah, 1979, p. 52), "Chamomile has the amino acid tryptophan, which works like a sedative in the body, and will induce sleepiness much as warm milk [which contains the same ingredient] would." My discovery was later cited by two scientists from the Department of Medical Chemistry and Pharmacognosy, College of Pharmacy, University of Minnesota, Minneapolis in their extensive article on chamomile (p. 264), which appeared in Volume 1 of *Herbs, Spices, and Medicinal Plants: Recent Advances in Botany, Horticulture and Pharmacology* (Phoenix, 1986). Additionally, minute quantities of naturally occurring morphine, from the alfalfa and clover hay consumed by grazing milk cows, has also been reported in milk. When taken internally as warm liquids, they tend to encourage normal REM sleep and, thereby, help to induce the right kind of dreams which comprise a good night's rest.

The inclusion of certain foods high in tryptophan in a late dinner several hours before bedtime might also help to bring on dream-rich slumber. These include eggs, cheese (especially Parmesan and Swiss), yogurt, beef, ham, salmon, and almonds. Deer meat and other wild game are especially high in this sleep-inducing amino acid.

Conversely, other substances exert an antagonistic effect upon normal REM sleep and consequently should be avoided before bedtime. These include caffeinated beverages like coffee, black tea, chocolate, or colas; alcohol of any kind, nicotine from smoking cigarettes, and, oddly enough, prescription sleep medications, which can really wreck beautiful dreams. (This is because such drugs suppress dreaming for a while, and then when it finally does return, comes back with a vengeance in the form of terrible nightmares.)

Meditation to Ease the Troubled Mind of a Hopeless Insomniac. At their sleep laboratory at Hershey Medical Center of Pennsylvania State University, Drs. Joyce and Anthony Kales have studied hundreds of insomniacs. For those people whose sleeplessness starts with tension and anxiety, usually over some event of the day, after a night or two of troubled sleep, most resume their normal sleep patterns. The chronic insomniac, on the other hand, finds it hard to turn off his or her anxiety and tension. He or she is the person, they say, who doesn't let out anger or disappointment. Responding to the stress of the day, the chronic insomniac's racing thoughts activate his or her physical arousal system, making it more difficult to get to sleep. Chronic insomniacs, therefore, are physically more aroused just before bedtime. Their body temperatures and heart rates are higher, and they move around in a bed more than normal sleepers do.

The Kales maintain that four out of five of their insomniac patients have actual emotional problems (such as neurotic depression, obsessive-compulsive disorders or anxiety states.) A recent article ("OM at the Top") in the June 4, 1990 *San Diego Union* described the most effective way to mediate for helping to relax a tense mind and body.

1. First of all realize that "meditation is *not* the act of doing something" rather, "it's the act of *not doing* something." In effect, "meditation is something you have to relax *into*" by emptying the head of *all* thoughts!

2. This can be easily achieved through the simple dynamics of focusing, much as you might turn a camera lens different ways in order to get the sharpest, clearest image possible. Begin by concentrating on an idea or a word and pay absolutely no attention to other thoughts that may intrude.

3. The most helpful focusing of all is on slow, deep breathing. Breathing is the most essential ingredient to meaningful meditation that will help conquer your "hopeless" insomnia. It should be sort of a circular breathing that falls into your body and falls out of it again, until all you notice is that cycle of breathing and nothing else.

4. Occasionally, very soft and mellow music in the background can help induce a self-hypnosis type of meditation that's conducive to sound sleep. I've found that the recorded monotone and repetitive chants of a Navajo medicine man really

works quite well. As does personal prayer to Deity—whenever I can't get to sleep I commence a silent prayer to my Heavenly and Eternal Father and within minutes I'm in slumberland before ever finishing my final "Amen!"

Be Comfortable When Resting. A short list of various "do's and don'ts" will help to make your sleep more pleasant and enjoyable.

Don't wear tight or constricting clothing to bed. I was once a full-clad pajama fellow myself, but not anymore. I discovered some hears ago, while having to sleep in a hammock in a hot, isolated Maya village in the northern Guatemalan jungle, that I fared a lot better sleeping *completely naked.* To this day, I *never* wear a stitch of clothes to bed and I sleep like a baby as a result!

Don't sleep in the same bed with your mate or companion. Here again, I've discovered among primitive tribes that husband and wife nearly always sleep on *separate* floor mats, although still side-by-side each other. Lest some accuse me of becoming a marriage breaker by chance, let me suggest that husband and wife can occupy *two separate* beds which can still be pushed together for that romantic intimacy. But, at least, they'll each have plenty of room to stretch and move around without disturbing the other's REM dreams.

Do spend some money and get yourself a nice, down- or feather-filled pillow. Anything else is inferior and won't help you feel as comfortable as you'd like to. Its always nice to have a pillow you can punch and fluff to fit the shape of your head instead of cheap synthetic material that keeps popping back every time you hit it.

Do make sure that little annoyances are held in check so as to minimize possible sleep disturbances. Put heavy drapes across the windows of your bedroom if neighborhood street or business lights pose a problem. Use earplugs, which can usually be obtained from a sporting goods store that sells rifles, to cut out all unwanted noises.

Do your showering at night under fairly hot water just before retiring. The December 12, 1980 issue of *Science* reported that "the warmer you go to bed, the longer you'll sleep."

Researchers at the Laboratory of Human Chronophysiology at Montefiore Hospital in the Bronx, New York, found that adult males who took hot showers before going to bed had much better REM sleep than did a control group who took hot or cold showers upon arising the next morning.

Don't drink fluids before retiring or else your bladder and kidneys will frequently interfere with your sawing of logs.

The Myth of "Catching Up"—
How to Avoid Those Dreaded "Blue Mondays"

Let's get one thing straight here—there is no, repeat *no*, such a thing as catching up on your sleep. If you skip breakfast and even miss lunch, you can always make up for it somehow with a hearty dinner. Miss an important appointment, and it can usually be rescheduled for a later date. But miss out on your nightly sleep and you simply *cannot* call it back by sleeping in longer the next day. Ask any sleep study experts about this and they'll confirm the validity of it right away.

On weekends, most people are apt to go to bed later and sleep later the next morning, letting their inner body clocks take over. Between Friday night and Sunday morning, we could be out of step by up to four hours. On Sunday night, we return to our regular bedtime of, say, 11 P.M. By then, however, our bodies aren't ready for sleep until 3 A.M. So on Monday morning, when we are awakened by a 7 A.M. alarm clock, we are really in the middle of our sleep cycle. We feel sleepy and unalert. To avoid those dreaded "Blue Mondays," just try to get to bed and arise on weekends at the same time as during the week.

Shift work can be brutal on the sleeping patterns of factory, postal and hospital employees, bakers, long-haul truck drivers, police officers and firefighters. Dr. Charles Czeisler of Harvard Medical School devised a shift schedule for an Ogden, Utah, chemical company that closely followed nature's body clocks. He reported that complaints about sleep and digestive problems dropped dramatically and work production increased by 20-30%. He recommended that shift workers who have trouble sleeping should go to sleep at the same time every day and should eat a similar meal at the same time each day for the duration of the work shift. They should also stick with shifts that don't change too often. Also they should completely curtail their intake of coffee and colas in the last week before a new shift schedule goes into effect. Also, a person on, say, the 3–11 P.M. shift should try and switch to the 11 P.M.–7 A.M. shift on his next rotation period instead of attempting to move backward to the 7 A.M.–3 P.M. shift.

Overseas travel by airplane can be equally punishing on the system, unless certain precautions are taken *before* the trip begins. Avoid animal proteins, all sweets, and coffee at least 24 hours in advance. This will enable the body to nicely readjust itself to the new time zones one is entering. When I flew on Japan Airlines with nine other Americans to Tokyo the last part of May 1990, I avoided drinking coffee and cola beverages, which everyone else had. Some 15 hours later, upon arriving at Narita New Tokyo International Airport, everyone but me was still groggy and bleary-eyed, and I didn't even sleep a wink along the way!

Factor S, the Body Chemical That Puts Us to Sleep. Harvard Medical School researchers John Pappenheimer and Manfred Karnovsky spent 15 grueling years of painstaking work before finally isolating a natural human chemical called Factor S. This component, they reported in an early spring 1982 *Journal of Biological Chemistry,* is nature's own sleeping potion.

They gave this human Factor S to a variety of lab animals and found that it made rabbits sleep 50% longer than usual. They wrote that "it resembles the deep sleep that occurs when animals are allowed to sleep following prolonged sleep deprivation." The Factor S used in the animal experiments was laboriously extracted from 4½ tons of human urine collected in containers placed in public lavatories. From this amount, the scientists obtained 30 mcg. of Factor S, roughly the weight of a few grains of white sugar.

The substance is extremely potent and minuscule amounts can put animals to sleep. The researchers found that Factor S is composed of four basic materials: glutamic acid, alanine, diaminopimelic acid, and muramic acid. Glutamic acid is an essential neurotransmitter to help keep things running smoothly in the brain. Alanine is a nonessential amino acid produced within the body, but obtainable from certain food sources. And unlike glutamic acid, which excites brain reactions, alanine works just the opposite by inhibiting brain transmissions. Thus, a nice balance is struck between the former stimulant and the latter calmative. Diaminopimelic and muramic acids are very common in the cells walls of bacteria but not known to be produced in the human body. So both Harvard professors speculated that bacteria in the human intestinal tract may be essential for the production of Factor S.

Certain foods are high in glutamic acid and alanine and could, in fact, help to induce sleep in many people who can't readily fall asleep. For myself, I've discovered through personal experimentation with a number of volunteers, that occasional nighttime snacks of wheat germ, granola, cottage cheese, ham/ luncheon/sausage meat sandwiches, sliced turkey, duck, and wild game often helps to bring on slumber in an hour or less as a rule. Also, periodic nightly supplementation of pantothenic acid (100 mg.) seems to help as well.

While none of these things is an absolute guarantee toward producing more Factor S within the intestines, the process can be expedited a little more with the ingestion of *live* cultured yogurt or acidophilus. (Much of the foregoing information came from work done at the Brain Bio Center in Rocky Hill, New Jersey, and was reported in *The Healing Nutrients Within* (New Canaan, Conn.: Keats Publishing, 1987), by Drs. E. R. Braverman and C. C. Pfeiffer.)

To summarize briefly, nothing helps a weakened immune system more to bounce back to its full vitality and strength than consistent and uninterrupted sleep.

◆◆◆◆◆

SMOKING AND PASSIVE SMOKING

Once while looking through the stacks of old bound periodicals in the Marriott Library at the University of Utah in Salt Lake City, I came across a May 1, 1943 *Saturday Evening Post*. On page 66 was a Philip Morris ad entitled, "Why is America smoking more?" Further into the ad I discovered this: "You're *SAFER* smoking Philip Morris!" This was backed up by "reports from eminent doctors in medical journals" to this effect.

Cut now to May 18, 1988, some 45 years later and a quote from then U.S. Surgeon-General, C. Everett Koop, M.D., in *USA Today*: "Cigarettes and other forms of tobacco are addicting . . . in the same sense as are drugs such as heroin and cocaine!" My but how times change!

Not too long ago the Office of Technology Assessment (Congress's scientific advisory body) released a study estimating that the smoking costs the United States roughly $65 billion a year in disease and lost productivity through most of the 1980s.

Smoking is also becoming more a habit associated with the poorly educated, the economically disadvantaged and blue-collar workers. According to a report in the June 25, 1985 *Wall Street Journal*, those with college educations and higher-paying jobs were far less apt to smoke, than those with high school diplomas or dropouts doing blue-collar work. As the *Journal* noted in its article title, "Smoking of cigarettes seems to be becoming a lower-class habit."

In spite of this trend, however, many Americans still manage to smoke 1.32 billion cigarettes a day. Little wonder then that across the land every day, 408 of us will be diagnosed as having lung cancer, and 356 of us will die from it. In contrast to this, we chew 7.3 million sticks of gum every day.

One Addiction Feeds Another

The November 25, 1985 *New England Journal of Medicine* reported that smoking increases the tendency to drink more alcohol. In surveys taken across the country, "smokers were arrested for drunk driving three times as often as nonsmokers." Reports in other medical journals have also noted that smokers tend to drink twice or three times as much coffee or cola beverages as do nonsmokers. Smokers are also inclined to be more gluttonous at the dinner table than nonsmokers. All of which proves that one habit leads to another.

What's Bad About Cigarette Smoke?

The smoke curling up from a lit cigarette or billowing out of a smoker's mouth, contains a number of harmful ingredients, some of which may really surprise you. Things like carbon monoxide you probably already know about, but what about potential *radioactivity*? Both, in fact, are among the many hidden dangers lurking in tobacco smoke.

First, there's the nicotine problem. A two-year study with monkeys showed that oral nicotine consumption definitely induced hardening of the arteries, which raises questions about the supposed safety of chewing tobacco *and* nicotine gum. Japanese doctors at Kyoto School of Medicine discovered back in 1984 that nonsmokers whose family members puff more than two packs of cigarettes a day, actually inhale the equivalent of up to three cigarettes. The amount of cotinine remaining when nicotine is broken down inside the body was nearly identical in nonsmokers from heavy smoking families as it was in the lightest regular smokers—those who smoked less than three cigarettes a day.

Next is the tar content of cigarettes. A brief report in the January 8, 1982 issue of *Science* stated that nonsmokers are exposed to just as much tar emissions from secondhand smoke as are regular smokers who use low-tar cigarettes. In fact, the cloud of pollution around low-tar smokers really isn't that much different from the cloud surrounding high-tar smokers who don't inhale. Tar is a factor in lung cancer, and nonsmokers appear to be at nearly just as much risk as are smokers of low-tar brands.

Then, we have the carbon monoxide factor. This toxic gas increases the permeability of cells lining the inner artery walls, allowing the accumulation of cholesterol. This then helps to narrow and harden the arteries. Carbon monoxide also interferes with oxygen transfer at the cellular level, eventually poisoning the system. At the 60th Symposium of the American Heart Association in Anaheim in the latter part of November 1987, Dr. William Moskowitz of the Medical College of Virginia, presented compelling evidence to show that 11- and 12-year-old boys exposed to secondhand smoke in homes where one or both of their parents smoked had thicker heart walls and stiffer aortas than did another group of similar ages from nonsmoking homes. Clearly then, this toxic gas can be just as bad for nonsmokers as it obviously is for smokers.

The fourth bad constituent in cigarette smoke is an unidentified element now suspected of causing cataracts. According to a November 1989 issue of *Physician's Weekly*, doctors at Johns Hopkins Medical School discovered the formation of cataracts in *both* smokers *and* nonsmokers alike. This unnamed element affects the nucleus of the eye's lens in an adverse way by making it become opaque somehow.

After this come a host of nasty chemicals like acrolein, acetaldehyde, ammonia, and formaldehyde. All of them cause considerable damage of the olfactory receptor cells inside the nose, thereby impairing the ability to smell, not to mention injuring sensitive lung and brain tissue, too.

Finally, the *New England Journal of Medicine* of February 11, 1982 announced that certain alpha emitters of polonium-210 and lead-210 in cigarette smoke result in marked radiation exposure to the bronchial tubes of smokers *and nonsmokers* alike. In a person smoking 1½ packs per day the radiation exposure is equivalent to 300 chest X rays a year!

Passive Smoke Harmful to Nonsmokers

Many Americans have finally wised up to the dangers of smoking and voluntarily "kicked the habit." Yet for them and the rest of us who've never smoked, an ever-present danger remains: secondhand smoke. And the most recent research on the subject, said the June 11, 1990 issue of *Newsweek* magazine, a lot grimmer than many of us may have realized. Prominent San Francisco heart researcher Stanton Glantz has carefully calculated that "passive smoking causes 10 times as much heart disease as lung disease." Yale University epidemiologist Dwight Janerich also recently reported that the risk of lung cancer has doubled in people who've been exposed to a given quantity of secondhand smoke during their early lives. In other words, from the available evidence before us, one nonsmoker *now* dies for every eight smokers.

Pets are even adversely affected by their owners' addictive habits. The February 1990 issue of the University of California at Berkeley's *Wellness Letter* cited a Colorado study which showed that dogs of owners who smoked had a 50% greater risk of heart failure and lung congestion that did pets of nonsmoking owners.

An array of other evidence shows that passive smoke can significantly increase the levels of carcinogenic chemicals in the blood, produce frontal sinus headaches, induce peptic ulcers, foul up normal drug metabolism in the liver, and, worst of all, cause dramatic DNA changes in one's normal gene structure. Therefore, you should *avoid* secondhand smoke at all costs!

How to Increase Your Resistance to Harmful Effects of Tobacco Smoke

Whether you're a smoker who still indulges or one who's completely given up the habit or, like so many others, a nonsmoker sometimes exposed to cigarette fumes, there are a number of things which you can do to strengthen your body against tobacco smoke in general. Some of the things will help to cleanse the system of harmful impurities. Others will help repair tissue damaged by the smoke. And one or two may even help cut down personal addiction to nicotine. You can decide which ones might work the best for your particular situation.

1. Herbs, diet change, and acupuncture help you to "kick" the habit. Getting rid of the addiction is half or three-fourths of the problem. Certain things seem to help a smoker not want to smoke any more. And all of them are natural and safe to try.

James A. Duke, recently retired from the USDA Germplasm Resources Lab in Beltsville, Maryland, encourages smokers to try lobelia or Indian tobacco. Lobelia contains an alkaloid, lobeline, "which the Amerindians used to cut back on the smoking of tobacco," he says. The best way to use lobelia for this is in a fluid extract form. Pure Herbs of Madison Heights, Michigan (see the Appendix) has Indian tobacco available in the 1-fl.-oz. or 4-fl.-oz. size. Put 10–12 drops directly beneath the tongue on an empty stomach about twice daily or whenever the need to smoke occurs.

In India Ayurvedic doctors have used both a water decoction and an alcoholic fluid extract of common oats to help cure addicts of the opium habit. According to the October 15, 1971 issue of *Nature*, a clinical study was carried out with the alcohol fluid extract of fresh young oat shoots on a group of chronic smokers at Ruchill Hospital in Glasgow, Scotland. A control group of equivalent smokers received a placebo. In the oat extract group the total daily consumption by 13 patients was 254 cigarettes; at the end of the test it had dropped to 74. Five had stopped smoking altogether, 7 had reduced it to less than 50%, and in one no change had occurred.

In the placebo group the total daily consumption at the start was 215, at the end it was 217. Smoking had been stopped by none, reduced to above 50% by 6, and increased by 3; 4 reported no change. Clearly the oat extract "seems to reduce the number of cigarettes smoked per day, along with a diminished craving for smoking." A small Salt Lake City herb company makes this fluid extract of oats mainly for doctors who are trying to help their patients quit smoking, but sometimes they also fill requests from private consumers. Custom-Made Formulas (see the appendix) is the only U.S. firm I know of that presently carries this Ayurvedic antismoking extract.

A unique antismoking diet has been developed by A. James Fix, Ph.D., and David M. Daughton, a behavioral research team at the University of Nebraska College of Medicine. According to them, nicotine is an incredibly strong base substance. The more acid foods the body ingests, the more readily nicotine is flushed out of the system, and the more nicotine a smoker would need to take in to replace it. Whereas, the more basic or alkaline the foods are, the *less* nicotine is lost, and the less a smoker would need to take in from outside sources. In other words, the more alkaline the blood is, the less a smoker would need to puff so their theory goes,

They discovered that when sodium bicarbonate was used to increase the alkalinity of smokers' bodies, they seemed to have a much easier time quitting smoking. This lead them to their special alkalinizing diet for smokers. The best foods for this would be black strap molasses, lima beans, raisins, figs, beet greens, spinach, dandelion greens, brewer's yeast, almonds, carrots, celery, grapefruit, sweet potatoes, tomatoes, strawberries, peas, mushrooms, apples, onions, and summer squash. Foods to avoid because of their strong acidic effect on the blood are red meat, chicken, eggs, codfish, cheese (cheddar and cottage), bread, peanuts, honey, sugar, and anything fried or deep-fried in grease.

The *American Journal of Chinese Medicine* (vol. 10, p. 107) reported in 1982 that acupuncture has helped considerably in reducing tobacco addiction in chronic smokers. Consult a qualified, licensed acupuncturist with some years of skill and training behind him or her for this, preferably an Oriental if you can.

2. Certain herbs, vitamins and the *way* in which cigarettes are smoked can substantially reduce nicotine, carbon monoxide, and radioactivity levels in the blood. Wakunaga of America makes an odorless garlic (kyolic) and a garlic-ginseng combination, which are excellent for removing such harmful substances from the system. An average of three capsules daily of either product is recommended. You can obtain their aged garlic extract from any major health food store, but may need to contact the company in person for their garlic-ginseng combination (see the appendix). A Canadian company in Vancouver, Albi Imports, distributes Korean red ginseng in capsules, tablets, extract, tea, and powder throughout North America. Many U.S. consumers prefer to order direct from them (see the appendix). About 3 capsules/tablets or 12 drops of fluid extract or 1 cup of tea is suggested on a daily basis for flushing these things out of the body. (See the appendix.)

Vitamin C is also very good for this, but preferably in the liquid or fizzy powder which can be reconstituted in water or juice. Quest Vitamins U.S.A. of Foster City, California, makes an effervescent Electro-C Powder which has great cleansing action on internal tissues saturated with such harmful substances (see the appendix). One teaspoon in 8 oz. of liquid is suggested.

Also the manner in which cigarettes are smoked determines how much nicotine, carbon monoxide, and radioactivity may be present in the blood at any given time. According to the January 1983 issue of *Clinical Pharmacology & Therapeutics*, the *longer* a cigarette is puffed, the more apt the smoker is to get a greater increase of these things inside his or her body. The conventional wisdom here seems to be a shorter drag and not to smoke it down to the end as some do. A past issue of *Environmental Research* (vol. 11, 1976, p. 310) noted that those who get more exercise (dock workers) at their jobs, tend to have *far less* carbon monoxide levels in them when they light up, than sedentary smokers do (office workers and pregnant women). So, if you must smoke, be engaged in some physical activity while doing so, though it's still better to quit while you can.

3. Fortifying your immune system whether you smoke or are around those who do is absolutely essential to good health. Different medical journals have mentioned that vitamins A, B-6, and C in particular are essential for maintaining strong immune defenses when exposed to cigarette smoke. Various reports carried in them have recommended about 25,000 I.U. of A, about 10–12 mg. of B-6, and up to 3,500 mg. daily of C for this.

Finally, several other journals (*Archives of Environmental Health, November/December 1984,* and *New England Journal of Medicine, November 13, 1986*) have suggested that vitamin E (250 I.U.) and selenium (15 mcg.) be used together to reduce risks of incurring lung cancer. All of these things add up to an effective program for increasing your resistance to the hazards of smoking and secondhand smoke.

Clean Lungs with Coltsfoot Leaves

Ralph M. is what law enforcement officers might describe as a "career criminal." He is a hardened "lifer" (serving 20 to life) at Greenhaven Correctional Facility near Stormville, New York. A cop accidentally got in the way of one of Ralph's bullets, which put him behind bars at this fortresslike compound about a two-hour drive north of New York City.

Some years ago he read one of my herb columns in a national health magazine and decided to try my suggestion of drinking coltsfoot leaf tea for cleaning out his lungs. Nearly everybody in his prison block is a heavy smoker. Consequently, Ralph's respiratory system started showing signs of deterioration due to the strong secondhand smoke present throughout the facility.

Since prison rules are pretty tight about what visitors may or may not bring in, getting the coltsfoot leaves he needed for tea was something of a challenge. Four months later, after endless phone calls to his attorney, reams of paperwork, and a holistic-oriented medical doctor who regularly visits the inmates and can legally bring some of the herb in with him, Ralph finally acquired enough leaves to start making his tea.

A portion of one letter to me read:

> Doc—I've been faithfully taking that stuff you wrote about in your article. You wouldn't believe the hassling I got trying to obtain some of it through the proper channels. Dope gets in a helluva lot easier than some simple herb. Man! they [the guards] liked checked out every damned bit of leaf with tweezers and a magnifying glass the first time my medic friend brought some in. Now it isn't so bad, but they still like to look it over first before they let him bring anymore through.
>
> I've been drinking a cup a day for almost six months now. Recently, I got into the hospital infirmary to have another chest X ray done. You know what? My lungs are looking a lot cleaner than they did the first time round. Less shadows in the X rays the doc says. And I can breathe a whole lot better, too. And you know what? All of this damned smoke around here doesn't bother me as much as it used to. Your herb sure helped. Thanks a million!

My instructions in the article were: Bring 1 pint of water to a boil and add 1 level tsp. of dried, cut coltsfoot leaves. Cover, turn heat off, and simmer 40 minutes. Strain and drink 1 cup warm daily with honey added for taste. It's a great way to revitalize worn out lungs!

Summary

1. Boredom, stress, or depression usually bring on alcoholism, anxiety attacks, drug addiction, and smoking. Mental and emotional stress generally contributes to hypoglycemia and insomnia. Therefore, attention must be paid toward improving the attitude of the mind and the feelings of the heart.

2. The liver is the *primary* organ most affected by alcohol, drugs, and tobacco. Likewise, it also plays a major role in blood sugar metabolism. Vegetable beta-carotene (carrots, beets, dark leafy greens), tomato juice (with some lemon juice added), dandelion root (tea or capsules), B-complex vitamins (4 tablets daily

of the high-potency kind), and almonds are just some of the things to help it adequately recuperate.

3. Besides the agents that have been mentioned in this chapter, three other herbs stand out as doing a superior job of flushing harmful substances out of fatty tissue within the body. They are goldenseal root and prickly ash bark (equal parts of both powders in capsules, 3 daily) and red clover blossom tea (2 cups daily). They work best on an empty stomach.

4. Nothing quite compensates for preventing future short-circuiting of the immune system than a good night's rest!

5. To stop further "immune blackouts," the diet should consist more of fresh, wholesome lightly cooked or raw, live foods, instead of fried or deep-fried foods. Meat should be held to a minimum with preference toward lean beef, goat, lamb, and saltwater or freshwater fish, instead of chicken, turkey, or pork.

4

Managing Childhood/ Adolescent Health Problems

CHILDHOOD from ages 1 through 12 and the subsequent teenage years are fraught with myriad health problems ranging from zits and sniffles to earaches and sore throats. As young people grow up and become more sexually active, they become in time likely candidates for some very nasty and hard-to-shake venereal diseases.

This chapter concerns itself with about three dozen different ailments or conditions that a child or teenager is apt to encounter at some time or another in his or her young life. They include

Acne vulgaris	Gastroenteritis	Poliomyelitis/polio
Adenoid enlargement	Giardia	Reye syndrome
	Gingivitis	Rheumatic fever
Boils	Halitosis	Sexually transmissible diseases
Chicken pox	Infectious mononucleosis	
Constipation/ appendicitis		Strep throat
	Lactose intolerance	Tonsillitis
Cough	Lice	Toothache
Cradle cap	Malnutrition	Vaginal discharge
Diptheria	Measles	Warts
Ear infections	Mumps	Whooping cough
Eczema	Muscular dystrophy	Worms
Fever		

◆◆◆◆◆

WHAT TODD DID FOR HIS ACNE

The following letter was received by me September 11, 1988 from an 11th-grader in a small central Montana town high school:

"Dear Dr. Heinerman: Mom reminded me to write you about what we did for my acne problem. I had it real bad, all over my face and forehead and all. Well, sir, mom made me stop eating all junk food. No more candy, potato chips, fries, shakes, colas, soft drinks, and ice cream. I about died when she told me this. But I could see a change come over me right away. My acne seemed to stop getting worser [sic].

"Well, sir, the next thing I did was to start washing my face with this yicky-looking black soap mom called 'pinetar soap.' I washed first thing in the morning when I got up, when I came home from school, and before I went to bed. It seemed to help alot. Oh, I probably should mention that mom had me soak some cotton balls with tincture of witch hazel and wipe my face every night, which took off the excess oils from my skin.

"She also had me take some [Vitamin] C every day, but I forgot how much. [Author's note: It was 1,500 mg. daily in tablet form.] I also took a spoonful of some [Vitamin] E which she got from a local vet[erinary] store here in town. [Author's note: It was Rex's Wheat Germ Oil.]

"That's about all I done [sic]. But in a couple of weeks my acne was 90% cleared up. I'm 16 and hope this is of some help to you." /s/ Todd C.

◆◆◆◆◆

HOW DOROTHY CORRECTED HER CHILD'S SWOLLEN ADENOIDS

In the spring of 1988, I gave an herb lecture on the immune system in Lincoln, Nebraska. It was sponsored by The Golden Carrot health food store. A good-sized crowd attended. Among them was a 37-year-old mother named Dorothy M., whose 7-year-old child had suffered from enlarged adenoids. During a question-and-answer session, she raised her hand and freely shared with the audience what she had done to remedy this condition in her daughter.

Dorothy said that a local ear, nose, and throat specialist had told her that surgery wasn't really justified in this case. He simply recommended that her kid put up with the obstruction the best she could. Dorothy decided to try something on her own, which seemed to work well.

She made a strong solution of catnip and peppermint tea and then put the strained, hot fluid into a humidifier and had her child breathe the warm fumes in from this. As a result, the girl was able to rest better at night and not have to breathe through her mouth so much.

Dorothy kept this up for a couple of months until her daughter's adenoids had returned to the normal size and breathing became much easier. She claimed it would work for anyone else who's child may have a similar problem.

◆◆◆◆◆

A GRANDMOTHER'S REMEDIES FOR BOILS

A grandmother from Fargo, North Dakota, wrote a while back to tell me how she used to deal with boils in any of her children, grandchildren, friends, or neighbors.

First she scrubbed the area well with some strong soap and water. She preferred Irish Spring because "it cleans the skin the best." Then a thorough rising and drying followed. With most small boils, she insisted, it was then only necessary to keep them clean and dry, and they would usually clear up in a week or so.

However, for larger boils she would lance them with a large sewing needle that had been disinfected over a flame from a gas stove, lighter, or lit match. Then the boil would be gently squeezed between her thumb and forefinger until the pus ran out. This was wiped away with a cottonball soaked in hydrogen peroxide.

She would then swab the area with a little more cotton soaked in peroxide or even Clorox to make sure no outside bacteria got in. Then she would apply a little tincture of witch hazel, which somehow helped to "seal" or close the punctured skin.

She also had her "patients" drink plenty of red clover blossom tea "to keep the blood pure." She made the tea by adding 1½ Tbsp. of dried flowers to a pint of boiling water. She covered the mixture and let it steep for 30 minutes before straining and serving warm with honey.

◆◆◆◆◆◆

GRANDMA'S REMEDIES FOR CHICKEN POX

This same Fargo, North Dakota, correspondent also shared with me some of her methods for dealing with chicken pox, which she proudly proclaimed in her letter as being "mighty effective."

First thing was dealing with the fever and headache, she said. She would have the sick child drink some *cool* peppermint tea *and* bathe in a tub of *cold* peppermint tea water but *without* using any soap! She would get out her large porcelain pot used for canning fruit in the summer and fill it with about 3 gallons of water. This would be placed on the stove and brought to a rapid boil, after which about 4 *cups* of *dried* peppermint leaves would be added (dried leaves are stronger than fresh ones, she swore). The heat would be turned off and the pot covered with a lid. Everything would steep for several hours until cool, and then it would be placed into her refrigerator overnight. If there isn't sufficient room for such a large pot, then strain the contents into several gallon jugs and place in your fridge that way. Next day when it's cold, give some to the youngster to drink every couple of hours and pour the rest of it into a tub already filled with about 5 gallons of regular water. Have the kid lay down and soak in this for a while. It should help stop the itching and reduce the fever.

Next have the youngster wear some light cotton gloves while sick so as not to scratch himself or herself. The gloves can be lightly rubbed over those areas that itch like crazy to bring some degree of comfort without having to actually scratch the red spots. Also, rubbing the face, scalp, arms, and legs with calamine lotions helps to reduce this itchiness. Another method to control the urge to scratch is by *lightly* rubbing on some tincture of witch hazel and then exposing these body parts to a blowing circular fan for about 10 minutes.

Then she would see to it that the youngster got plenty of rest and was well entertained with good books, puzzles, games, and so forth to take his or her mind off of the illness itself. The child would also be given about 3,000 mg. of vitamin C, usually crushed up if it was a tablet and stirred into some fruit juice. (A powdered fizzy kind is available from Quest Vitamins U.S.A.; see the appendix for details.)

◆◆◆◆◆

HOW MY DAD CURED AN APPENDICITIS ATTACK AND HOW TO KEEP THE BOWELS REGULAR

Children and adolescents generally don't pay much attention to something like bowel movements. Consequently, they can become constipated and in some cases eventually suffer from appendicitis.

When I was about 7 years of age, we lived in the small farming community of Salem, Utah. It was here that I came down with an attack of appendicitis, which my father successfully treated without the aid of a doctor. First, he had me lay on my left side and flex my knee which helped to ease the pain a little.

Next he prepared a combination of bayberry bark and slippery elm bark tea (equal parts of each steeped in 1 quart of boiling water for 1 hour). I drank a warm cup of this about every 2 hours. My dad also gave me several warm enemas of spearmint and catnip tea, which relieved my pain even more.

At night he would apply poultices to the tender area just to the right of my navel and below it. In a pint of boiling water, he would add 1 Tbsp. of crushed mullein leaves and some grated, raw ginger root. He would let the mixture simmer on low heat for 3 minutes before adding just enough cornmeal to make a thick paste. He would then ladle some of this onto a double-thick 8-inch by 8-inch piece of gauze and then apply to the right side of my abdomen. A folded towel would be placed over it to retain the heat as long as possible. The procedure was repeated several more times when the application became cold.

During this spell of sickness, I was kept on a liquid diet pretty much, drinking mostly papaya or mango juice, besides the aforementioned tea. My recovery about four or five days later was without incident and I returned to school the following week as normal and healthy as were any of the other kids my age then.

Two of the best things to clear up constipation are prune juice (three glasses daily) and FarmLax, a product made by old Doc Yoder in the Amish community near St. Petersburg, Florida (see Old Amish Herbs in the appendix).

◆◆◆◆◆

AMISH REMEDIES FOR EVERYTHING FROM COUGHS TO HALITOSIS

In the last decade, I've had the good fortunate of lecturing in a number of old-order Amish communities scattered throughout the eastern and southern United States. These plain living folks, remembered mostly for their horses and buggies than anything else, had to devise simple remedies over the years to treat different childhood maladies when doctors weren't always readily available. I've collected together on the next several pages the *most effective* ones, which my family, friends, or staff members have tried to themselves and discovered to work. Certainly, these treatments are *not* meant to be used instead of visiting a pediatrician, but *in addition* to consulting with a qualified physician.

Cough Remedy (Smicksburg, Pennsylvania). In a teapot bring to boil 1 quart of well water. Add half a handful of dried horehound herb, quarter handful of dried coltsfoot leaves, and just a pinch of wild cherry bark. Let simmer on back part of coal-and-wood stove for a few minutes; then set aside and allow to steep for an hour. Strain through cheese cloth and give half cup of *warm* brew to sick child to slowly *sip*. Flavor with sugar if you like. (Note: I recommend honey instead.)

Cradle Cap (Napannee, Indiana). Wash infant's head with warm water and Johnson's Baby Shampoo *twice daily* (morning and night). If buildup of thick scales in hair becomes excessive, olive oil can be applied to the scalp and left there for 10 hours. Sometimes a soft lanolin lotion works just as well. If infection sets in, wash scalp with pine tar soap.

Diptheria (Butler, Ohio). Of course, youngsters today are immunized against diptheria, and so this very serious disease is rare in the United States. Whatever the illness, this nutritious broth serves as both food and medicine when nothing else can be given to a sick child. In 1 quart of water, boil up some beef liver and heart until thoroughly cooked; remove the pieces of organ meats and put broth back on stove. Add 1 Tbsp. of dried hops and 2 Tbsp. of dried, coarse slippery elm bark. Cover and simmer toward back of stove for about 10 minutes. Then remove and let it steep another 10 minutes. While still very warm, uncover and add 1 Tbsp. of fluid extract of Indian tobacco or lobelia (see Pure Herbs in the appendix) and 1 Tbsp. fresh squeezed lime juice. Stir good and cover again. A few minutes later, uncover and strain the liquid off. Give half a cup to the child every couple of hours.

Ear Infection (Sugar Creek, Ohio). Take a quarter chunk of a small, peeled onion and crush good with heavy flat iron. Then peel and do the same thing with one garlic clove. (Be sure bottom of flat iron is clean and not dirty from sitting on top of your wood range.) Take both these mashed objects and put them in half a pint of Southern Comfort, Blue Thunder, or comparable cheap whiskey. Cover and let soak for two days. Strain through muslin and put a few drops of this stuff into child's ear with an eye dropper. Best to have child lay on his side so liquid won't run out of the ear that's bothering him and can clear up the infection. May have to do this several times a day. At night drops can be held in ear with a piece of clean cotton while child sleeps. (Note: You can use a hammer or other blunt instrument for crushing the onion and garlic in the event you don't have an old flat iron laying around handy somewhere.)

Eczema (Walnut Creek, Ohio). Combine together equal parts of the following herbs: burdock root, chickweed herb, plantain herb, mullein leaves, and white oak bark. (In this case equal parts would be about 5 Tbsp. of each ingredient.) Place them in the bottom of a large porcelain pot (stainless steel can also be used) and add 2 quarts of distilled water (Perrier water may be used too). Cover with lid and set toward the back of the stove where the firebox isn't so hot (low heat) and slowly simmer for 3 or 4 hours until just half of the liquid remains. Then strain this carefully through muslin. One cup of the cool liquid is taken internally whenever a fomentation (soaked cloth) is to be applied. Soak a sterile piece of cotton or flannel material, gently wring out, and cover those parts of the skin with eczema. Then wrap some waxed paper (or plastic sandwich wrap) around the cloth and hold in place with small strips of tape. Leave on overnight. Repeat this procedure for a week or until condition shows signs of clearing up. Most effective for other skin problems, too, such as psoriasis.

Fever (Wooster, Ohio). Make a tea of two handfuls each of mullein leaves and catnip herb; soak in boiling water for an hour, covered with a lid, and away from the stove. Strain and give a 1 cup of warm tea to sick child every couple of hours to sip as needed. Sweeten with molasses. Best thing for holding any fever in check. In case of glandular swelling, apply fomentation of tea to sides of neck and throat as needed.

Gastroenteritis (Lancaster, Pennsylvania). Put a small handful each of barley and brown rice in a medium-sized pot. Cover with 2½ inches of water, put lid on and cook for 30 minutes on back of stove or until grains are done. Be sure that there is plenty of water to make for a very runny porridge in the end. Strain the juice off and let it cool. Sweeten with a little molasses or honey. Put in a clean glass bottle with a nipple and give to the sick toddler or young child to drink. Do this couple of times each day. It should stop the diarrhea pretty quickly.

Giardia (Lancaster, Pennsylvania). Kill an old setting hen, plunge it into boiling water to remove all the pin feathers, and clean out the innards. Then chop half of it up with a meat cleaver and throw into pot filled with a quart or so of water. (An already butchered chicken from your local supermarket will do just as nicely for those not acquainted with how things are usually done "down on the farm.") Next chop up a small white onion and a clove of garlic (presumably peeled) and add, along with three or four strips of green onion. Boil in middle of stove where firebox is hottest for 30 minutes, then shove to back of stove where fire isn't so hot. (Translation for novice folks: Cook on high heat for half an hour, then reduce to low heat and simmer for same length of time.) In last few minutes (about 10) of cooking, uncover and throw in a chopped whole lemon and a pinch of black pepper. Cool, strain and give some of this herbal broth in bottle with nipple to sick child to help kill parasites causing its runs.

Gingivitis (Dover, Delaware). To stop this gum bleeding, mix together a pinch each of salt, and powdered kelp, and black walnut in a small dish. Then moisten with water a *soft* bristle toothbrush and dip it into these powders until bristles are well covered. Gently brush the gums with this morning and evening. Rinse mouth with half a cup of *cool* peppermint tea or witch hazel tea. A little powdered oak bark may also be added to the other herbs if bleeding is very severe.

Halitosis (Dover, Delaware). First try to determine the origins of the youngster's bad breath. Could be due to indigestion, sore throat, bad cavity, or persistent runny nose. Then have the child rinse his mouth with half a cup of kyo-green powdered drink (see Wakunaga in the appendix). Or just chop up a bunch of parsley real fine and a couple of fresh mint leaves (or 1 Tbsp. of dried leaves), add to a pint of boiling water, cover pot with lid, and simmer for 20 minutes. Cool and strain; rinse mouth with quarter cup of tea. A quicker way to get rid of bad breath is just to chew a wad made of two sprigs of parsley wrapped up inside a fresh mint leaf. Place this wad on back molar and grind away, letting the juice get all over your mouth and tongue and slowly trickle down your throat.

◆◆◆◆◆

HERBAL EXTRACTS AND VITAMINS FOR TREATING INFECTIOUS MONONUCLEOSIS

A Canadian naturopathic doctor prescribes certain herbal fluid extracts to his teenage and college-age patients who suffer from Epstein Barr virus (EBV). He has them take 8 to 10 drops goldenseal root beneath the tongue in the morning, 8 to 10 drops of echinacea in the afternoon, 5 to 6 drops of chaparral in the evening, and 10 drops of garlic just before retiring.

In addition to this he has them take 4,000 mg. of vitamin C and 50,000 to 100,000 I.U. of vitamin A every other week until the EBV becomes dormant. To get rid of the sore throat and enlarged tonsils that usually accompany more aggravated cases of mono or "kissing disease," this naturopath suggests gargling with 2 fl. oz. of brandy in which has been stirred 1 tsp. of lemon juice and a pinch of table salt.

◆◆◆◆◆

GOAT MILK FOR LACTOSE INTOLERANCE

This same Canadian doctor recommends that fresh or canned goat's milk be fed to all young children unable to handle regular cow's milk. For very young infants, he advises their mothers to breast feed them instead, since cow's milk contains the alpha S-1 protein to which many people are so allergic. (Also see the chapter on allergies for further information about such food intolerances. However, it should be noted that lactose intolerance is considerably different than allergy to milk. Lactose-intolerant individuals don't have the enzyme lactase necessary to digest the lactose. Those who are allergic to the *casein* component of milk won't be any better off by switching to goat's milk.)

◆◆◆◆◆

FIVE STEP METHOD FOR GETTING RID OF LICE

A registered nurse of Cajun background in New Orleans listed the steps needed to get rid of lice:

1. Child or young adult should bathe each day. Scalp especially should be washed with pine tar soap and rinsed thoroughly. After which a tablespoonful of straight apple cider vinegar should be applied to the hair and thoroughly rubbed into the scalp before combing or brushing is done.

2. Fresh clothes, both undergarments and outer wear, must be changed every day. They should be laundered with a good, strong detergent (such as Wisk) and a cup of apple cider vinegar should be added to every load of clothes.

3. Sheets and pillow slips should be changed daily. And the mattress and bedroom should be sprayed with some Listerine antiseptic from a squirt bottle with a fine mist adjustment to it.

4. Internally, the individual should take liquid kyolic garlic (2 capsules for child under age 12, and 3 capsules for teenagers) or black walnut (2 capsules for child or teenager).

5. Attention should also be paid to the colon. Regular daily bowel movements are important in helping to rid the body of lice.

◆◆◆◆◆◆

HOW TO PREVENT MALNUTRITION

Generally associated with many Third World countries, malnutrition is actually widespread throughout America. Poverty, insufficient food supplies, psychological disturbance (such as that suffered in child abuse), anorexia nervosa, recurrent vomiting, and any chronic illness leading to a "wasting away" of body flesh and weight all contribute to malnutrition.

Ironically, however, gluttony and consumption of "junk foods" low in fiber and loaded with sugar and fat lead to *over*nutrition, the principle cause of *mal*nutrition found in all industrialized nations of the Western world. Both forms of malnutrition affect tens of millions of America's youth today whether they live in inner-city ghettos or swanky upper-class suburbs.

While much obviously could be written on ways to cope with this problem in the young, several important solutions are presented here to help remedy the situation. First, *a good breakfast* for growing kids is absolutely essential! Inexpensive but nourishing foods for such a meal would include cooked oatmeal, shredded wheat/granola combined, milk, whole wheat toast with butter, scrambled or poached eggs (*not* fried), cottage cheese, fruit-flavored yogurt, honey, and fruit juice (citrus) or fresh fruit (melons). Even a peanut butter-and-jelly (low sugar) sandwich on whole wheat bread with a glass of milk is better than a doughnut or nothing at all.

Those who are able to afford a wider variety of foods should visit their local health food store or nutrition center where organic foods are sold. Fresh goat's milk, bottled organic fruit juices (apple, mango, papaya, for instance), cooked millet, buckwheat pancakes, fresh or frozen berries (blackberry, boysenberry, raspberry, strawberry), assorted cheeses (Edam, Gouda, Monterey), organic fresh fruits (grapes, plums, and melons like crenshaw and cantaloupe), and exotic whole-grain breads are just some of the things that upper-income folks should consider feeding their children for breakfast each morning. Also having their children drink different kinds of herbal tea blends (such as what Celestial Seasonings makes) for breakfast helps to improve their overall health. Such teas can be made the night before, refrigerated, and served chilled with ice the next morning. Kids seem to like cold drinks a lot better than hot ones.

Second, a light lunch that's quick but nutritious works well for impatient youth always on the go. Inexpensive choices include whole wheat sandwiches (peanut butter-and-jelly, grilled cheese, fried egg *without* mayonnaise), assorted bowls of canned soup (chicken, potato, tomato), and suitable beverages (milk, citrus juice replacements, cranberry/raspberry, but *no* soft drinks or colas). More expensive selections would include seven-grain sandwiches (avocado and tomato, tuna and tomato, sprouts and tomato), freshly made soups (cheddar cheese, lentil, golden mushroom), fresh salads, and health soft drinks (ginseng soda, *real* cherry cola).

Third, substantial dinners for growing, active kids should be centered more on *single* entrees rather than complete meal courses. Low-cost, tasty but nutritious items are vegetarian pizza, simple stews (with potatoes, carrots, and inexpensive meat or fish cuts), casseroles (with macaroni, cheese, rice, tomatoes, and the like), meat loaf, spaghetti and meat sauce, tacos, burritos, and so on. More expensive choices include roast lamb, roast beef, steak, prime rib, freshwater/saltwater fish (salmon, trout, halibut, sturgeon), steamed vegetables (artichoke hearts, brussels sprouts, snow peas), salads (coleslaw, papaya and kiwi), fresh fruits in season (blackberry, cherry, currant, date, elderberry, fig, guava, kumquat, mango, nectarine, orange, peach, pear, pineapple, watermelon).

Regardless of a family's economic situation, malnutrition *can be prevented.* Parents should encourage their kids to *avoid* as much as possible those things which *rob* the body of important nutrients: candy, soft drinks and colas, potato chips, French fries and hamburgers, doughnuts, Twinkies, hot dogs, pies, ice cream, and so on. Additional and affordable supplementation can come from vitamins A (10,000 I.U.), B-complex (one tablet), C (500 mg.), E (50 I.U.), and occasionally a powdered multi-mineral mix (see Quest Vitamins in the appendix).

♦♦♦♦♦♦

HELP FOR MEASLES AND MUMPS

The late Utah herbalist Dr. John R. Christopher recommended the use of different herbs in various forms for treating measles (both red and German kinds) and mumps in his book *Childhood Diseases* (Springville, Utah: Christopher Publications, 1978). Common to both ailments are the warm catnip enemas for proper bowel evacuations, yarrow and valerian tea for reducing fevers, and raspberry yellow dock tea made with apple cider vinegar instead of water for bathing itching skin. The only two herbs not shared by both are chamomile tea for kids with measles and mullein tea for those with mumps.

To make a tea out of any of these herbs, just bring a pint of water to a boil and add 1 Tbsp. of dried, coarsely cut herb; then cover with a lid, remove from heat and steep 30 minutes. Strain and use as indicated while still warm. In the case of chamomile, the sick child should drink half a cup every few hours. And with mullein, a fomentation should be made using a clean cotton cloth soaked in the hot tea and placed around the neck and throat and covered with plastic and also a towel to retain the heat longer.

♦♦♦♦♦♦

NUTRITION TO THE RESCUE FOR MUSCULAR DYSTROPHY

Muscular dystrophy (MD) is a serious muscle-wasting disease passed by mothers to their offspring, usually sons. It is caused by a lack of or a genetic defect in the important muscle protein called dystrophin. This is the disease which comedian Jerry Lewis has made famous with his yearly telethons. In all there are some 40-plus such muscular disorders, including amyotrophic lateral sclerosis or Lou Gehrig's disease, which claimed not only the famous baseball player, but also British film star, David Niven. Besides the evident wasting and atrophying of body muscles, varying degrees of mental retardation occurs in about 30% of those thus afflicted.

The journal, *Acta Medica Scandinavica* (Vol. 219, pp. 407–414) for 1986 reported on the success that some Swedish doctors have had with certain health food supplements in treating muscular dystrophy at the Ostra Hospital in Göteborg. Five patients with this disorder were given selenium (0.2–0.3 mg.) and vitamin E (10–100 mg.) for the first 12 months, and then increases of each (selenium, 1–1.3 mg., and vitamin E, 500–600 mg.) for the remaining two years. All patients improved subjectively and objectively. Grip strength and ability to perform physical tasks improved in all five. Most had fewer symptoms and two even experienced increased capacity for exercising.

Several doctors from the Department of Internal Medicine at Ostra Hospital with whom I later communicated further informed me that as yet unpublished data from more extensive research showed that a high-potency B-complex vitamin (3 tablets daily), a good calcium-magnesium blend (400 mg. calcium and 800 mg. magnesium), potassium (2,000 mg.), and foods rich in copper (oysters, nuts, and blackstrap molasses) and manganese (pineapple juice, cooked oatmeal, spinach, and Müeslix, a European nut-seed-grain blend dry cereal now sold in the United States, were all exceptionally good for treating most varieties of MD (An added health note by way of interest: Jeanne Freeland-Graves, a professor of nutrition at the University of Texas at Austin, has found that women who drink a glass of pineapple juice don't develop osteoporosis so fast; those who do are generally very low in manganese as a rule.)

◆◆◆◆◆

HERBS FOR RESISTING POLIO

According to *Antibiotics Annual, 1958–1959* (pp. 106–107), St. Johnswort (fluid extract and tea) reduced the incidence of poliomyelitis in infected mice to 66% versus a 92% occurrence in untreated mice. Nearly similar results were achieved with a tea made from raw garlic clove (only 64% in treated groups versus a whopping 90% in untreated mice).

Suggested dosage for the alcoholic extract is about ½ drops twice daily beneath the tongue or half a cup twice daily on an empty stomach. Greater amounts of liquid kyolic garlic can be used, however, with very minimal side effects. About 3 capsules twice daily on an empty stomach with juice or water is suggested. (See the appendix for Pure Herbs in regard to the hard-to-find St. Johnswort fluid extract and Wakunaga of America for the readily available kyolic garlic.)

◆◆◆◆◆

REYE SNYDROME—RARE BUT FATAL
IF NOT TREATED QUICKLY

In recent times this has become a rare condition among young children and adolescents. However, cases still occur and occasionally make the headlines when uninformed parents give their kids aspirin to reduce the pain that accompanies influenza, chicken pox, and other viral illnesses.

When Reye syndrome occurs, it is always marked by extreme vomiting, raging fever, mental confusion, and convulsions. Your first order of business is to elevate blood glucose levels by giving the child orange or some other kind of fruit juice. Next is the management of liver failure and the prevention of blood clots. This can be accomplished by giving the child or teenager a glass of tomato juice into which has been stirred half a teaspoon of powdered ginger root. Getting the individual some fresh air quickly is important, and mouth-to-mouth resuscitation may be necessary. *Reye syndrome victims require hospital emergency treatment right away!*

◆◆◆◆◆

SUCCESSFULLY BEATING RHEUMATIC FEVER
WITH HERBAL TEAS

The same *Streptococcus* bacteria that causes scarlet fever, bacterial tonsillitis (this chapter), and sore throat (allergy chapter) brings on rheumatic fever as well. This dangerous disease occurs mainly in schoolchildren and can cause arthritis, fever, abnormal movements, and/or inflammation of the heart. In the last instance, by damaging the heart valves themselves, it can have the unwelcome long-term effect of coronary heart disease.

Treatment should be chiefly aimed at reducing the inflammation as much as possible. Herbs high on my list of natural recommendations would be chamomile, mullein, plantain, and yarrow. A tea made of equal parts (1 Tbsp. each) steeped in a quart of hot water for half an hour, strained, sweetened with honey or blackstrap molasses, and given to the child a cup at a time every 4 to 6 hours is one of the best things I know of to bring the inflammation under control.

This tea should be alternated with another one for bringing down the fever. In a pint of boiling water, add 1 tsp. *each* of dried catnip herb and dried, coarsely cut white willow bark. Cover and simmer 2 minutes on low heat, then remove and steep for 20 minutes. Give half a cup to the sick child twice a day on an empty stomach. Oh, and be sure to sweeten with honey or molasses to mask the strong taste.

Once the child has recovered, he or she should be put on a fairly steady supplementation of vitamin C (500 mg. daily) and kyolic garlic (1 liquid-filled capsule every other day). Also an occasional (once a week) fish oil-derived vitamin· A capsule (10,000 I.U.) as well.

◆◆◆◆◆

WHAT TO DO ABOUT SEXUALLY TRANSMISSIBLE DISEASES

From the mid-1940s until the mid-1970s, gonorrhea and syphilis were the two main types of venereal disease afflicting the majority of those suffering from such infections. However with today's increased sexual activity among America's youth, there has been a dramatic rise in the incidence of three other venereal diseases, namely, chancroid, chlamydia, and genital herpes (otherwise known as herpes simplex II). Today these three constitute the majority of sexually transmitted diseases (STDs) so prevalent throughout the country.

Most STDs remain with their human hosts for life and are

virtually impossible to get rid of. Take the herpes simplex virus, for instance. Researchers at the University of Minnesota in Minneapolis now report that prolonged contact with herpes-infected cells disarms key compounds of the immune system, preventing them from attacking this virus or several other related infectious agents that they would ordinarily destroy. It seems that the herpes-infected cells generate a unique glycoprotein on their surfaces which temporarily disarms natural kill (NK) cells and interleukin-2-activated killer (LAK) cells. With both NK and LAK cells briefly paralyzed, the herpes simplex II virus can scoot away and lie dormant in different body tissues for long periods of time until reactivated later on. The best approach then to the problem of such STDs is to make sure they remain inactive for as long as possible.

"Fever Treatments" Control STDS

Two Seale, Alabama, Seventh-Day Adventist physicians have utilized an interesting method for managing STDs. In their 1981 book, *Home Remedies,* Agatha M. Thrash, M.D., a pathologist, and Calvin L. Thrash, Jr., M.D., an internal medicine specialist, describe their use of "fever treatments" to bring such venereal diseases under stricter control. These can be administered in a number of ways: whirlpool bath, Russian steam cabinet, blanket pack, and bathtub.

The easiest and most convenient of these for in-home use would be the last one. The afflicted young person should sit in a reclined position *in* the bathtub with the feet *toward* the tap. The body is snugly wrapped in a clean sheet and several wool blankets or old quilts. A couple of folded bath towels may be used as a comfort support for the shoulders, neck and head. An additional cushion may also be necessary for the buttocks as well, since the knees will be drawn up during this reclining position. Both feet should be placed a pan of hot water that reaches above the ankles; when additional hot water is needed just turn on the tap and let enough run in until the pan water again becomes as hot as the person can tolerate.

On a chair or stool by the tub side should be a basin of ice water and, if necessary, a small electric fan. Also a glass and straw for ice water as well as an oral thermometer. Everything but the person's head is wrapped beneath the sheet and blankets. Every few minutes the face should be lightly sponged off with ice water and the young adult given a sip of something cold to drink (preferably cold water). The idea here is to elevate the body temperature to 102° or 103° F. By so doing, these various STD viruses are substantially weakened and seek to become dormant somewhere within the body.

Both doctors counsel that any person trying this should drink in advance several 8-fl.-oz. glasses of salt water (2 Tbsp. of regular table salt to each quart of water) to prevent dehydration. Also taking a good mineral supplement (about 4 tablets) may be a good idea. Each treatment lasts for about 1 hour, followed by a 1-minute cold shower rinse and brisk rubdown with a large, heavy towel. Figure doing this about three times a week for several months or until the particular STD viruses have become dormant enough for the outward symptoms to disappear.

The doctors also warn that other existing health conditions may contra-indicate a treatment like this. If the youth has juvenile-onset diabetes, low blood pressure, rheumatic heart disease, anemia or tuberculosis, then fever treatment should *not* be applied!

Natural Remedies for STDs

Internally, the best natural remedies to administer are as follows: goldenseal root capsules (2 to 4 daily), kyolic garlic (3 capsules daily), and chaparral (2 capsules daily). If the young person has hypoglycemia, drop the first two herbs, double the chaparral, and add 6 capsules of sarsaparilla root instead. Vitamins A (50,000 I.U.) and C (15,000 mg.) should also be included as well. All these dosages are for young people 16 years of age and up.

Probably the toughest part of this program for youngsters with STDs to follow, will be abstaining from certain kinds of junk food. Anything deep-fried (french fries, chicken, doughnuts, potato chips), fried (hamburgers), sweet (candy, soft drinks, colas, pastries), and spicey (catsup, mustard, pickles, and mayonnaise) *must be avoided* in order to keep such viruses from becoming active again, for they tend to thrive in biological systems that are especially acidic; conversely, they don't do very well in blood that is made alkaline by consuming lots of raw fruits, vegetables, grains, seeds, nuts, legumes, and so forth.

Finally, consider this advice from the late Rabbi Wolfe Kelman, a major leader of Conservative Judaism. His counsel was intended not only for those of the Jewish faith but for young people of other religious beliefs as well. The good rabbi believed that young people had an obligation to themselves if no one else to take better care of their bodies than what they often do. He often likened the human body at conception to a brand new car. By the time a boy or girl reached adolescent, their cars were in top shape and ready for rapid use if need be. But he always admonished young people to "drive" themselves sensibly rather than to always "race their engines" in the full heat of passion. He was forever gently suggesting that they get a good, firm grip on their sexual impulses and learn to abide by the simple rules of good moral conduct so that their respective vehicles would give them many wonderful years of excellent service. Otherwise, they might find themselves frequently in need of medical repairs to take care of this or that problem, which could easily have been avoided if they had just learned to apply the brakes a little more often when their engines of passion tended to overheat and wanted to go into overdrive.

Admittedly, STDs are some of today's toughest medical challenges facing health care providers. And while various remedial measures like those cited within these pages definitely help to correct the problems, it is more in the realm of *safe* (sexual) driving practices that the most good can be done in avoiding them. Obeying the speed limits of life and taking things slow and easy will keep young people fitter and healthier for their best years yet to come, Rabbi Kelman was fond of noting.

♦♦♦♦♦♦

TREATING STREP THROAT AND TONSILLITIS

An elderly Cajun healer residing in the outskirts of New Orleans shared with me her most effective remedy for treating both kinds of throat infection some years ago. Warm a little brandy (about 3 Tbsp.) over a gas range flame in a tin flour cup for a couple of minutes until it's quite warm but not so hot as to injure the mouth or throat. Then add about 10 drops of fluid extracts of mullein and 5 drops of Indian tobacco or lobelia (see Pure Herbs in the Appendix). Then add a pinch of table salt, stir with your finger, and give to the sick child to slowly gargle with. After each gargling, he or she then expectorates and repeats the process again. Have the child do this two or three times daily.

◆◆◆◆◆

HOW TO STOP TOOTHACHE PAIN

There are several things which I've employed from time to time to stop a nagging toothache in myself, other adult friends or their children. Each of these methods works and has been tested enough through the years to vouch for its effectiveness.

Method One. Peel a single clove of garlic. Then mash it thoroughly with a hammer, large glass ashtray, clean brick or rock, or similar heavy object. Then apply mashed garlic directly to the site of the pain itself. Repeat every four hours as necessary.

Method Two. Thoroughly saturate a small cotton ball with fluid extracts of Indian tobacco (lobelia) *and* valerian root. Then position inside the mouth against the aching tooth. Replace every hour or so as needed to keep pain down until you can get to a dentist.

A nifty way of holding the garlic pulp or cotton wad in place better is to put each of these items on a small piece of white bread which has been covered with a light spread of peanut butter. As everyone knows who has eaten the stuff, peanut butter will stick anywhere in your mouth for quite a while, in spite of the presence of saliva.

Sometimes a hot or cold pack placed against the outside of the jaw also helps to reduce the pain. A second dry cloth or hand towel is then placed over the wet one to retain the heat or cold longer.

◆◆◆◆◆◆

HOW TO TREAT VAGINAL DISCHARGES

Many schoolage girls develop a white discharge from the vagina from time to time. It may cause itching and occasionally is bloodstained. Factors that prompt this include candidiasis infections or dermatitis induced by bubble-bath soaps, bath oils, or nylon underpants; or it may be a sign of an STD in adolescence or an indication of sexual abuse.

One of the simplest treatments is to make a vaginal douche that can then be slowly inserted to cleanse the infected area. In a small tin cup put almost a pint of Pierce's tincture of witch hazel, which can be obtained from any drugstore. Then add 4 Tbsp. of hydrogen peroxide and 2 Tbsp. of apple cider vinegar. These should complete a full pint of liquids. Stir in ½ tsp. of powdered goldenseal and then pour everything into a clean douche bag.

Have the young lady then apply this either in the bathtub or on the toilet. The bag should never be more than 2 feet above the hips. Insert this douche gradually and retain for about 10 minutes if possible. Pregnant women should *never* attempt such a douche.

The young lady should also be given 3,500 mg. of vitamin C and 50,000 I.U. of vitamin A daily as well. Consult the first chapter under candidiasis for dietary suggestions. Two capsules daily of goldenseal root or kyolic garlic can also be given along with the vitamins.

◆◆◆◆◆◆

HOW ONE PHYSICIAN REMOVES WARTS NATURALLY

Those common, small and brownish warts many people seem to get, occur mostly on the hands, neck, and back. Those occurring on the soles of the feet, however, are called plantar warts, while those in and around the sexual organs are termed genital warts. All of them are caused by viruses known as human pipilloma viruses. They are caught from other people with warts. The types of papilloma viruses causing skin warts are different from those that usually cause genital warts.

In my earlier book, *Heinerman's Encyclopedia of Fruits, Vegetables & Herbs* (p. 18), I gave an account of one doctor in Morganstown, West Virginia, who has successfully treated over 400 cases of warts all over the country using nothing but ripe banana peels! Matthew Midcap, M.D., instructs all his wart patients to cut a square piece of ripe banana skin and apply the inside white mushy part against their warts, holding it in place with adhesive tape. This rather odd dressing should be changed every 6 or 8 hours with a fresh section of peel.

To help expedite things, I recommend an additional ingredient. Crush one aspirin tablet to powder. With an eyedropper, put no more than 2 or 3 drops of water on the inside of the ripe banana skin; then sprinkle on the crushed aspirin. Now apply this preparation to the wart and tape in place. For genital warts, substitute powdered mayapple for the aspirin.

◆◆◆◆◆

WHAT TO DO ABOUT WHOOPING COUGH (PERTUSSIS)

This is a highly infectious disease caused by bacteria and spread through exhaled and coughed droplets. It is quite common in unimmunized preschoolers and most serious in infants under six months of age. Symptoms occur in three phases, each lasting about two weeks. In the first phase, sneezing, a runny nose, and slight fever develop, with the cough coming later. During this time the child is most infectious, but because the symptoms often mimic those of a common cold, a correct diagnosis is unlikely to be made. It is in the first phase that the most vigorous treatment needs to be given.

Follow many of the recommendations already given in the first chapter under the common cold, and also give the child or infant some warm lemon balm tea to drink. Of all the mint family, this particular plant seems to be the strongest for killing viruses. According to a Polish report in the *Journal of Pharmacy and Pharmacology* (Vol. 38, pp. 791–794) for 1986, certain identifiable components within lemon balm attach themselves to certain harmful viruses (herpes, influenza, and cancer) and thereby prevent their absorption to host cell receptors.

Tea, however, is by far the most effective way to utilize lemon balm for research has shown that the gelatin in capsules render this antiviral activity inert. Bring a pint of water to a boil and add 1½ Tbsp. of dried lemon balm. Remove from the heat, cover, and steep 20 minutes. Strain, sweeten with honey, and serve warm to sick child in feeding bottle or cup.

In the second phase of this disease, the cough worsens and occurs in spasms lasting half a minute or more. The child's face turns red and he or she becomes blue. Intake of breath after the cough produces the characteristic whoop, hence the name "whooping cough." The cough may be triggered by the slightest movement, crying or even eating. Vomiting often occurs after coughing and the child may even have nosebleeds and small hemorrhages in the eyes. The appetite is poor, and this coupled with vomiting can produce dehydration and weight loss. Convulsions may also occur, especially in infants. This second phase can last for nearly a month. The sick child runs the likely risks of getting pneumonia or other chronic lung infections at this point in time. If you suspect your child has whooping cough, *consult proper medical attention at once!*

My folks, who never believed in immunization or trusted the medical profession, elected to treat my own case of whooping cough on their own when I was about 4 years old. My dad's mother had been an experienced herbalist from Temesvar, Hungary (now part of Romania), and was still alive at the time of my sickness to treat me. However, treating very serious problems such as whooping cough on your own is *not* recommended. My grandmother's remedy might be used to augment a physician's treatment.

My grandmother, Barbara Liebhardt Heinerman, put 1 quart of water to boil on the stove. To it she added about 6 heaping Tbsp. of dried, coarsely cut wild cherry bark. Covering the pot with a lid, she allowed this mixture to boil down slowly to just about half of its original volume (slightly less than a pint). With the bark and pint of liquid still in the pot, she next added 2 Tbsp. of dried horehound herb and covered again; the heat was then turned off and the brew permitted to steep for 30 minutes.

Then she would strain off the dark, bitter liquid and return the same to the stove in a smaller pot. After getting it hot again, she then added 3 or 4 Tbsp. of dark honey and stirred it thoroughly. After removing from the stove, she added 1 tsp. each of lemon juice and brandy. This she kept bottled in the refrigerator and would give to me *warm* in half cup amounts throughout the day. This helped to clear up my whooping cough eventually. A gruel made of boiled barley and millet with some powdered slippery elm bark added sustained me through my lengthy ordeal of sickness and kept me from wasting away.

◆◆◆◆◆

ELIMINATING THE WORMS IN YOUR LIFE

Occasionally in some of my herb lectures, when time and mood permit, I will work in certain tongue-in-cheek humor for the benefit of my captive audiences. One of these is a rather droll description on how to get rid of the worms in a person's life. "Take garlic, for instance," I remember telling a standing-room-only crowd in a plush Vancouver, B.C., hotel recently. "It's highly effective as a worm remover." A deliberate twenty-second or half-minute pause elicited the question I expected from someone in the audience—"How do you use it?" My simple reply was merely to chew a clove of the stuff and *any* worms around you would surely be apt to stay a good distance away. As always, the large assembled group roared their approval with rings of hearty laughter.

On a more serious side, though, garlic is, indeed, an effective agent to use in getting rid of intestinal parasites, particularly in children. I've discovered that a steady supplementation of 2 capsules of kyolic garlic swallowed with some juice or water into which has been stirred 1 level tsp. of ground pumpkin seeds will help to eliminate even the worst case of tapeworm!

Another way this can be done is to take ¼ tsp. each of powdered pumpkin, watermelon, and cucumber seeds that have been crushed to a powder and add them to 3–4 Tbsp. each of honey and distilled water. Then add ¾ tsp. of liquid kyolic garlic. Cap the bottle with a lid and shake thoroughly until well emulsified. Give the child 1–2 Tbsp. of this every 4 hours each day for a week or until expelled worms are no longer evident in the stool.

A favorite treatment of the late Utah herbalist Dr. John R. Christopher was to make a paste out of a single garlic clove that has been finely minced or grated and ¼ tsp. of Vaseline. To this could be added a few drops of fluid extract of Indian tobacco or lobelia (see Pure Herbs in the appendix). This paste is then applied to those body parts afflicted with ringworm, covered with gauze and left overnight. During the daytime, the child's skin or scalp can be rubbed with a good garlic oil several times. (Consult the Great American Natural Products in the appendix for an excellent garlic oil. Or just mince a few cloves of peeled garlic and a few strands of green onion and immerse them in a pint of olive oil for a week, before straining and refrigerating to use.)

Summary

1. For many external problems, cleanliness is an absolute must. Pine tar soap is highly recommended for this.

2. For both internal and external problems, certain herbals seem to work very well. Among them are garlic, goldenseal, and chaparral.

3. The mints are particularly useful to allay inflammation in most childhood/adolescent occurrences.

4. Tincture of witch hazel works well in relieving the itching sensation induced by a number of them. Also herbal fluid extracts and teas work better with children than does swallowing a lot of capsules/tablets would.

5. Nourishing broths (beef, chicken, fish) made with cooked grains (barley and millet) and added herbs (slippery elm bark) are good to feed sick children.

6. Proper bowel movements, adequate rest, and good food are essential for a child's physical well-being.

7. Plenty of fluids (juices, water) must be given to sick kids.

8. Teenagers need education regarding the limits their bodies can go.

5

Holding the Line Against "Infectious" Heart Disease With Spices

◆◆◆◆◆

WHAT YOU DON'T KNOW ABOUT HEART DISEASE

Recently at a weekend health workshop held in Seattle on June 24, 1990, I asked regional members of the Northwest National Nutritional Food Association (NNFA) to tell me what they thought were the most likely factors contributing to coronary heart disease, currently our nation's number one killer! Typical responses were pretty much what I expected: elevated cholesterol levels, "bad" cholesterol, fatty foods, salty foods, sweets, smoking, obesity, lack of exercise, and so on.

Now the majority of those in attendance were what one might describe as pretty well read in health matters in general. After all, since health and nutrition happen to be their main business, it behooved them to be more knowledgeable than the average person in these things. Imagine then their astonishment when I introduced evidence to show that some of these factors weren't as important in causing coronary heart disease (CHD) as were certain other things they hadn't even mentioned.

As examples I cited the factors of smoking and salty foods in the one instance and the herpes simplex virus for the other. According to *The American Journal of Medicine* (February 27, 1984), the Japanese consume extraordinary amounts of salty foods and smoke like crazy, yet episodes of heart disease continue to be very rare in that country as a whole. More to the crowd's amazement were the excerpts I read to them from an article in the Friday, June 15, 1990 *New York Times*. According to Dr. David P. Hajjar, a professor of biochemistry and pathology at

170

Cornell Medical College in New York, 80 to 90% of all Americans have been infected with herpes simplex I virus, which he and other scientists now believe is the *major* cause of hardening of the arteries in many adults.

"If we can nail down the connection between herpes and atherosclerosis, then this discovery will have major, major ramifications," he informed *Times* reporter, Natalie Angier. After reading this, I asked for a show of hands as to how many present ever had cold sores at some time in their lives. With the exception of half-a-dozen souls, everyone else in that grand ballroom timidly raised their hands.

Looking over my glasses at them from behind the elevated lectern where I stood, I soberly stated: "Not only does this then make all of you more likely candidates for the process of atherosclerosis within, but it also tells me just how little the average American really knows about heart disease. *Immune*-induced atherosclerosis is more prevalent than the diet-induced kind," I concluded.

◆◆◆◆◆

THE FIVE ENDPOINTS OF CHD

No discussion about coronary heart disease would be complete without mentioning its initial five endpoints in passing. Briefly put, they are as follows:

1. Angina pectoris is defined by doctors as short-duration chest discomfort as a result of exertion or excitement and relieved in 5 to 15 minutes by rest and confirmed by two separate physician interviewers.

2. Coronary insufficiency is defined as prolonged chest pain (greater than 15 minutes) associated with transient non-specific ST-T wave changes and normal blood enzymes.

3. Myocardial infarction is diagnosed as prolonged chest pain associated with appropriate Q wave changes and/or serum enzyme changes.

4. Sudden death is defined as having occurred within 1 hour in a person for whom there was no other explanation for death.

5. Nonsudden coronary heart disease is death occurring after 1 hour in a person in whom an acute myocardial process was already in progress.

What's so amazing about some of these five endpoints, however, is the incredible influence that the body's own immune system has upon them.

◆◆◆◆◆◆

HOW IMMUNITY AFFECTS HEART DISEASE

The medical thinking used to be that CHD was prompted by bad diets (greasy food), bad social habits (smoking and drinking), and bad stress (anger or depression). Only in special cases, such as rheumatic fever in early childhood, were doctors even willing to consider some kind of an immune connection to heart disease developing later on in adult life. But a growing body of evidence within the last couple of decades has begun to change the minds of many physicians about how they now view CHD. More and more, they're discovering that the present state of a person's own immune health has *a lot* to do with how well or poorly the heart itself is performing. In other words, *strong* immune defenses pretty much guarantee a sound heart, while *weakened* defenses spell disastrous results, often in the form of atherosclerosis.

There are a number of different factors that have a significant bearing on the way our immune systems behave. For instance, did you know that loneliness can really send otherwise first-rate immune performances plummeting like crazy? Said Mother Teresa of this problem in the March 1980 issue of *McCall's* magazine,

> The biggest disease today is not leprosy or cancer. It's the the feeling of being uncared for, unwanted—of being deserted and alone. . .

One recent study from the *American Journal of Psychiatry* (April 1987) showed how true her words are. Women who had undergone major life changes such as bereavement had "significantly lower" natural killer (NK) cell activity than did subjects who were similar in age and sociodemographic characteristics but who had *few* such dramatic life changes.

Other studies have demonstrated similar things. Those who mourn the loss of a loved one for any length of time not only have suppressed immunity, but also *higher* incidence of coronary heart disease. It seems here the atherosclerotic process is fed two different ways: one, by negatively felt emotions from within the heart which, in turn, lower immune resistance to disease, and the other, by certain mischievous viruses being able to penetrate the valves of the heart successfully and initiate hardening of the arteries.

Another bizarre way by which the immune system can be flattened just enough to create heart disease is in the *continual* listening to country-western music of all things! In an appropriately entitled article, "Lookin' for Science in All the Wrong Places" in the March 1989 *Discover* magazine, the highly provocative work of University of Minnesota anthropologist James M. Schaefer was cited at great length. Dr. Schaefer discovered that tear-jerk lonesome blues, songs about the sad and often abusive aspects of life among certain working-class people, tended to increase the consumption of alcohol. "Hard drinkers," he noted, "were more likely to choose slower paced, wailing, self-pitying music." Follow-up work conducted by various medical doctors on such hard drinkers has definitely shown heart impairments in the majority of them. Interestingly, these same hard drinkers have considerably higher rates of infectious diseases than do nondrinkers or moderate drinkers.

Besides the alcohol which obviously wrecks the immune system and the heart in different ways, there is also the matter of the *sounds* themselves. A musicologist friend of mine with a background in medicine conducted a little experiment a few years back in which he examined the activity of certain immune cells in hard rock musicians. During the playing of their "heavy metal" music, each one's natural kill (NK) cell activity was way down, but within an hour after such racket had subsided the entire band's NK cell activity rose again to normally strong levels. Thus, certain sounds like country-western, jazz blues, or hard rock can open the way for nasty viruses like herpes simplex I to penetrate the arteries.

A third common factor in the development of heart disease

is hostility. Two prominent San Francisco cardiologists, Meyer Friedman, M.D., and Ray Rosenman, M.D., elaborated on this in their best-seller, *Type A Behavior and Your Heart* (New York: Alfred Knopf, 1974). The classic Type A person, they reported, exhibits three distinct characteristics: he or she is likely competitive and ambitious, speaks rapidly and interrupts others frequently, and is seized by hostility and anger with uncommon frequency. In common parlance, "Type A" refers to anyone who is chronically on edge.

An analysis of such individuals by both cardiologists revealed a strong link between their hostility, as measured by Type A interviews, and the severity of their diagnosed atherosclerosis. Moreover, when hostility and Type A traits disappeared in others of the same age and sex who were similarly interviewed, the severity of atherosclerosis drastically declined to almost unbelievable proportions! The consensus here then is that hostility somehow triggers the internal release of substances such as hormones which negatively affect immune levels and heart activity when an overabundance of them are produced. As mentioned in the *Journal of Chronic Diseases* (vol. 18, p. 758) for 1965, "gonadal, adrenal, thyroid and pituitary hormones have all been studied in relation to atherogenesis in experimental animals" so far as anger and hostility go. Hormones interact with blood lipids (fat molecules) in a much more dramatic fashion when immune defenses are *down* than when they're active, alert, and up

By now you have gotten the point that *it just isn't a diet of rich foods* which contributes to heart disease. More often than not, it's other factors we seldom ever consider. A fourth factor, coming into vogue as doctors' knowledge about CHD continues expanding, is the vital role played by "social stress' in the atherosclerotic process.

Back in the very early part of the 1980s, scientists at the Bowman Gray School of Medicine in Winston-Salem, North Carolina, fed 30 macaque monkeys a low-fat diet based on recommendations of the American Heart Association. Fifteen of the animals were also subjected to "social stress." They periodically introduced newcomers into established groups, including a sexually attractive female whose role was to "enhance competition and social uncertainty."

When the monkeys were killed 21 months later and autopsies were performed upon them, the researchers discovered an amazing thing. The 15 macaques who had lived in the tense environment were found to have *far more* atherosclerosis—fat deposits in the coronary arteries if you will—than the others. Yet periodic checkups had revealed no noticeable differences between the two groups in blood pressure or serum cholesterol, usually two very good indicators for the absence or presence of CHD. The team leader, Jay Kaplan, explained that brief, repeated surges in blood pressure and hormonal secretion during moments of turmoil—fighting over the female, for example— probably caused damage to the arteries, which then accelerated the formation of fat deposits. Such findings help us to better understand how people with normal blood pressure and cholesterol readings can still develop CHD.

When I briefly spoke long distance by telephone with Dr. Hajjar of Cornell Medical College in New York on Friday, June 29, 1990 about some of these very things, he concluded that "any or all of them could precipitate dormant herpes simplex I viruses into quick action." And once they've managed to infect normal cells by way of an ingenious "piggyback" method within the arterial walls themselves, these herpes viruses could begin altering how cholesterol is metabolized in the body. This class of viruses tends to suppress the activity of enzymes that normally break down stored cholesterol within arterial cells. That inhibition, he maintains, soon leads to the accumulation of cholesterol plaques. In time, plaques can cut off the flow of blood to the heart, resulting in a major heart attack.

◆◆◆◆◆

HOW MODEL IMPROVED HER CHANCES AGAINST CHD WITH MASSAGE

A lengthy article about some of my research appeared in a Summer 1986 edition of *New York Newsday*, the widely read and often controversial New York City/Long Island newspaper. A leading model from Manhattan, who is well known in fashion circles, contacted me about what she did to reduce her risks of ever getting heart disease. Honoring her request for anonymity, I'll just refer to her as Chancel.

Because modeling is so competitive and highly stressful, she was always under a great deal of pressure she said. Added to this were those occasional golden opportunities lost to someone else and the ensuing depression which accompanied them. "My life was like a roller coaster in those days," she admitted, "trying to stay on top and avoiding downfalls as much as possible." She became more snappish and irritable with others as well.

One week, while modeling a new line of designer spring wear for photographers, she experienced a peculiar sensation never felt before. "It was almost as if my heart were missing some of its beats," she said. When they increased, she promptly sought the advice of a prominent cardiologist. He ran a series of tests and discovered that she suffered from a reciprocal rhythm or echo beat. While this cardiac dysrhythmia wasn't all that serious, he reassured her, at her continued pace of anxiety and excitement, it could portend something a lot worse if left unattended.

She decided to try massage as a way of helping her to relax, after a friend who danced with the Joffrey Ballet told her how much it had helped him. She purchased a good vibrator which easily slipped over her hand. With this machine, she was able to work on her head, neck, face, throat, arms, chest, abdomen, thighs, and legs for about 20 minutes every evening. Another friend came by to do her back three times a week for another 20 minutes or so.

"This really seems to have helped me," she concluded. "In a couple of weeks my heartbeat was back to normal and I've been a lot more relaxed ever since." Massage not only improved circulation, but also greatly reduced her risks of cardiac failure as well. So, whether done mechanically or the old-fashioned way by an expert, massage is very good for those suffering from major or minor heart problems.

◆◆◆◆◆

ATHEROSCLEROSIS: A MULTIFACTOR PROBLEM

Several intriguing pieces of evidence emerge from the medical literature to demonstrate just how much a variety of factors can play in the development of immune-induced hardening of the arteries. The first two reports clearly illustrate that the process begins well in childhood, while the latter shows how an *entire* community once *completely free* of heart attacks eventually developed the same high rate as found in neighboring cities.

Two reports published about 18 years apart appeared in the *Journal of The American Medical Association* on July 18, 1953 and May 17, 1971. Both dealt with the incidence of coronary heart disease in U.S. soldiers killed in action during the Korean and Vietnam wars. In autopsies performed on 200 corpses with an average age of 22.1 years, M.A.S.H. surgeons discovered "some gross evidence of coronary arteriosclerosis" in 77.3% of the hearts they closely examined. And in the later Vietnam conflict, doctors there noticed that out of 105 autopsied cadavers with an average age of 22.1 years also, "forty-seven patients exhibited some degree of atherosclerosis in one or more of their coronary vessels; twenty-seven patients had involvement of two or more vessels; and five patients had severe (3 plus) disease in one vessel (and in four of these, all three coronaries were severely involved)."

The team of surgeons in Vietnam concluded "that some degree of coronary atherosclerosis is present in 45% of young, healthy American males." Some 19 years have passed since they made this observation, but that figure hasn't changed much even though older American males have begun to take high-fiber, low-fat diets more seriously. What's involved in both groups of young men are a variety of factors, some dietary and others social in nature, which started the atherosclerotic process early in their lives.

As Peter Libby, a cardiologist with Tufts University-New England Medical Center in Boston told me by phone, Thursday, July 5, 1990:

> Coronary heart disease is a multi-factorial health problem. Many things are involved. The herpes virus induces a great output of macrophages [scavenger cells] and T [thymus] cells from the immune system. And macrophages are notorious for producing strong chemical oxidizing agents which can oxidize LDL [low-density lipoprotein] cholesterol. This "bad" cholesterol, in turn, promotes atherosclerosis.

I asked Dr. Libby if other factors such as anger, hostility, competetive stress, loud rock music, childhood checkenpox, consumption of alcohol, and a fairly steady diet of junk food could also be involved in CHD as well. He admitted that "most of these things are probably interrelated with the development of atherosclerosis in young people," but couldn't say for certain just to what extents. I reminded him that all of the aforementioned things figured prominently in the lives of most of those soldier boys from the Korean and Vietnam wars, and surely contributed to early beginnings of heart disease found in so many of them by Army surgeons during routine postmortem examinations.

The other example involves a somewhat different but closely related set of social circumstances which kept an entire town free of coronary heart disease for many years. The town in particular is Roseto, Pennsylvania, a small Italian-American village surrounded by the four neighboring communities of Nazareth, Bangor, Stroudsburg, and East Stroudsburg. Until the 1960s, CHD was virtually unheard of there. Stewart Wolf, a professor of medicine at Temple University in Philadelphia and John G. Bruhn, a medical sociologist, received a generous endowment from the National Heart, Lung and Blood Institute to research this amazing medical phenomenon.

The results of their intensive study were eventually published by the University of Oklahoma Press under the auspicious title of *The Roseto Story: An Anatomy of Health*. Here's what they found that kept native Rosetoans so heart disease-free:

- Rosetoans adhered to a tenaciously held life-style reflecting Old World values and customs and characterized by predictability and stability.
- Family relationships were extremely close and mutually supportive.
- This quality extended to neighbors and the community as a whole.
- There was a well-defined man-woman relationship where the man was the uncontested head of the family.
- The elderly were cherished and respected, and they retained their authority throughout life.

- The atmosphere was friendly, and residents had an optimistic attitude.
- Most striking, there was no "keeping up with the Jones's."

In summary, the cornerstone of Rosetoan life was the family, and families were tied to each other through intermarriage to form "clans." Drs. Wolf and Bruhn explained that personal and family problems were usually worked out within the clan or with the local Catholic priest. Family celebrations were frequent and social life evolved around the town's 22 civic organizations.

For five consecutive summers both doctors held clinics in three of the neighboring cities to gather medical histories, do physical exams and blood workups, take urine samples, check blood pressures, and perform electrocardiograms on most of the populations over 25. When compared to similar data previously gathered in Roseto, the other results clearly "showed that Rosetoans seemed to be incredibly immune to myocardial infarction." But once they moved from their village, their resistance to heart disease vanished, and they became just as vulnerable as other Americans.

Then in the mid-1960s, Roseto began changing, but unfortunately for the worst in terms of community health.

- The number of first-generation Rosetoans diminished through death.
- Young Rosetoans went away to college, sometimes never to return.
- Interethnic and interdenominational marriages became increasingly frequent.
- The birth rate began to decline.
- Church attendance decreased.

At the same time, social restraints against displays of wealth and vanity started to crumble. In a word, the newer generation of younger residents became more worldly and materialistic than the previous one had been. Women started giving more attention to their personal appearances, joining weight-reducing programs, getting face-lifts, buying sexier-looking clothing, getting new hair-dos, and so forth. Men joined country clubs and initiated golf tournaments. Between 1966 and 1976, Cadillacs, Mercedes-Benzes, and even a couple of Rolls Royces appeared in town. Several very expensive (over $100,000) homes went up.

"Their egalitarian standards broke down," Dr. Wolf noted. "We predicted that Rosetoans would pay for this. And the price would be that the town's relative immunity to death from myocardial infarction would gradually come to an end."

The prediction indeed came true. Beginning in 1966, there was a striking increase in death rates from heart attack. In 1971, death from myocardial infarction occurred for the very first time in Roseto in men under 55, a group previously always immune. By 1975, Roseto's heart attack rate matched that of their metropolitan neighbors.

Clearly then, as Dr. Libby, the cardiologist from Tuft's University-New England Medical Center in Boston, told me in our phone conversation, "Coronary heart disease is a multifactorial health problem" with "many things [being] involved" in the process. And as crazy as it may seem to some, things *other than* alcohol, junk food, stress, bad moods, and viruses are usually implicated somewhere along the way. As the Wolf-Bruhn study clearly demonstrated, the breakdown of established traditions and long-term relationships and their replacements with personal self-centeredness, greed, and materialism contributed *a lot* to the development of atherosclerosis in a younger generation of Rosetoans.

It's almost as if the stresses created by these different factors somehow weakened their immune systems just enough to permit viruses like the herpes simplex kind to become reactivated and combine with fat molecules to form deadly plaques inside the main arteries of the heart.

The Virus Link to Atherosclerosis

In the previous pages we've looked at different factors which seem to activate certain viruses that initiate hardening of the arteries. Here we examine this virus connection itself. Over a nine-year period, half-a-dozen significant papers were published in various medical journals specifically relating to this unusual link. A quick look at each of them should prove beyond a shadow of a doubt that coronary heart disease *is,* indeed, an infectious malady just as much as cancer or diabetes might be. The *Journal of Experimental Medicine* (vol. 148, 1928, p. 335) reported an interesting study conducted with 130 chickens. Two groups of these fowls were infected with a special type of herpes virus common to poultry (Marek's disease), while two other groups remained virus-free. An infected and an uninfected group were then fed cholesterol-supplemented diets, while the other infected and uninfected groups were given diets very low in fat.

Both groups with Marek's disease showed "striking grossly visible atherosclerotic lesions . . . in large coronary arteries, aortas, and major aortic branches"; this even applied to one of the infected groups with *normal* cholesterol levels recorded *before* the experiment began. On the other hand, both uninfected poultry groups showed *absolutely none* of the evident signs of atherosclerosis, even when one of them registered *elevated* cholesterol levels prior to the study. The team of scientists conducting this research concluded that "the atherosclerosis in these [infected] chickens closely resembles chronic atherosclerosis in human arteries."

The same team from the Department of Pathology, New York Hospital-Cornell Medical Center and the Departments of Microbiology and Avian & Aquatic Animal Medicine, New York State College of Veterinary Medicine, Cornell University (both in Ithaca, N.Y.), duplicated their work a year later with another 290 white Leghorn chickens and the same kind of poultry herpes virus. Their concluding remarks in the September 1979 *American Journal of Pathology* are worth taking note of, especially in light of the fact that the same results were again achieved as in their former experiment:

> This change closely resembled chronic atherosclerosis in humans. These results may be important to our understanding of human arteriosclerosis, since there is a widespread and persistent infection of human populations with as many as five herpes virus.

Three of the original team members continued their investigations of this peculiar phenomenon, but were joined this time by Dr. David P. Hajjar (cited earlier in this chapter). In their paper that appeared in the *American Journal of Pathology* (vol. 105, 1981, pp. 176–184), they mentioned two of the principal lipids or fats which accumulate in both human and chicken atherosclerotic arteries, namely, cholesterol (CH) and cholesteryl esters (CEs). The scientists soon discovered that in herpes-infected poultry there were "significantly *different*" types of CH and CEs than were found in uninfected or healthy chickens. They suggested this evidence proved that at least one kind (Marke's disease) of herpes virus severely "altered lipid metabolism," leading to hardening of the arteries.

A fourth paper, which appeared in the May 15, 1983 *Federation Proceedings*, clearly stated that all of this previous research "established a *direct* relationship between [herpes virus] infection and atherosclerosis!" In all the testing done up to that point, *only* infected poultry developed humanlike hardening of the arteries, whether they registered normal or elevated cholesterol levels. On the other hand, uninfected birds, even those with really high serum cholesterol levels, "did not develop this arterial disease." Based on their findings they even speculated that "other animal models of atherosclerosis (nonhuman primates, pigeons, pigs, rabbits, horses, etc.)" could very well be infected with different kinds of herpes viruses. And since "humans are widely and persistently infected with up to five herpes viruses," they concluded, coronary heart disease in humans could very well be attributed to this class of infections in most cases.

In the October 1983 issue of the *Proceedings of the National Academy of Sciences,* three Seattle, Washington, researchers investigated the likelihood of either cytomegalovirus (CMV) or Epstein-Barr virus (EBV) possibly inducing atherosclerosis in human beings. Their preliminary findings, while far from conclusive, did indicate, however, that both types of viruses are "widely distributed in human and can remain latent indefinitely." Their singular conclusion was that "herpes viruses and *other* viruses" are "possible etiologic factors in the development of atherosclerosis" in people.

The final paper published in the January 1986 issue of *American Journal of Pathology* by Hajjar and colleagues merely underscored what the other five previous reports had already confirmed with additional experimentation. Their abstract summary best describes what all these findings indicate but which the greater majority of Americans still don't realize: *Coronary heart disease in humans is due to "specific herpes virus infection" that significantly alters cholesterol metabolism and leads to heavy accumulations of fat deposits within artery walls of the heart!*

In my recent phone conversation with Dr. Hajjar, he said that this ongoing research right now is "some of the hottest around" and that three other major medical centers around the country are now heavily involved in pursuing the link between herpes and hardened arteries. Besides Cornell, they are Dr. Henry Jacobs group at the University of Minnesota School of Medicine in Minneapolis, Dr. Joseph Melnick's team at Baylor School of Medicine in Waco, Texas, and Dr. Earl Benditt's people at the University of Washington in Seattle.

"I think you'll see later in this decade," he said, "more information coming out supporting the idea that atherosclerosis is largely caused by herpes viruses and *other* viruses." With that data in hand, he thinks, doctors will then be able to treat coronary heart disease for what *it really is,* an "infectious" malady— no more, no less.

How an Army Staff Sergeant Stopped His Hardening of the Arteries

Throughout the 1980s, I gave dozens of health lectures throughout the Lone Star State of Texas. At one of those in late 1983 in the town of Killeen, a staff sergeant and his wife attended from nearby Fort Hood, the largest army land base in the entire United States. We'll call him Joseph M., a big, burly fellow nearing the midcentury mark in his life. His wife had talked him into coming, feeling that the theme of my speech that night—"Health Care for Your Heart"—might be useful to her husband.

"Nagged is more what she did," he growled in typical military fashion. Then pointing to the stripes on his uniform, he added somewhat sarcastically: "I didn't get these from taking orders but by giving them!"

He'd been experiencing chest pains for several months, Mrs. M. mentioned, and had had recent breathing difficulties as well. Clearly, this big guy with the beer belly you could almost push in a wheel barrow, was definitely "cruising for a coronary" somewhere along the way. How do you reason with a man who insists on meat every day with a meal and who prefers to be called by his old Army nickname of "G.I." (as in "G.I. Joe") instead of his given name of Joseph?

Standing there in front of me with his legs astride and his hands placed authoritatively on his hips, "G.I." presented more of a picture of defiance than an image of cooperation. But I wasn't discouraged by any of this, seeing how determined his wife was to have him mend his ways and get well. The first question I posed was where he took most of his meals each day. Before his wife could speak, he snarled in a low voice, "The mess hall!" She added, however, that he ate dinner at their home on the base most of the time. This important fact helped me direct my advice to them.

I expressed a familiarity with the eating habits of our men in uniform. To which the sergeant asked in mild surprise: "Oh, did you ever work in a chow hall?" "No," I said, my knowledge comes from an article entitled "Food Preferences of Enlisted Personnel in the Armed Forces," which appeared in the December 1978, *Journal of The American Dietetic Association.* "Your typical breakfast of o.j., bacon and eggs, and a doughnut needs to change," I soberly pointed out, "or else you'll probably be dead in a year or less." After this, his attitude became less hostile and he listened a little more carefully to what was being said.

Since diet was the crucial thing here, I made the following recommendations that would, if followed, I added, "bring your cholesterol way down, sir, and dramatically reverse your progressive hardening of the arteries."

Breakfast: A bowl of cooked oatmeal, two slices of unbuttered whole wheat toast, and 1 to 2 cups of hot Postum (a cereal grain-based coffee substitute beverage) on Mondays, Wednesdays, and Fridays at the base dining hall. His choice of packaged cold cereal, two slices of wheat toast, and some more Postum each Tuesday at the chow hall. But on Thursdays, I advised his wife to make some bran muffins and told him to eat about three or four of these before he went on duty. And when he was at home on the weekend, I suggested that she fix him a big stack of buckwheat pancakes flavored with pure maple or dark honey.

Lunch: I advised "G.I." to stick with salads at least four times a week. "They're for sissy recruits," he mumbled, but his wife quickly brushed this complaint aside with, "He's always like that when he has to do something he doesn't like." Sgt. M. informed me that a variety of salads were available in the chow line: cole slaw, macaroni salad, celery and carrot sticks, cucumber and onion salad, frijole salad, pickled beet and onion salad, carrot-raisin-celery salad, and kidney bean salad, among others. I told him to make generous use of these, but to avoid cottage cheese, jello salads, and tossed green salads with mayonnaise-based or oil-and-vinegar dressings on them. I also reminded him to not eat any breads with this meal and to drink either black or green tea, since the natural occurring tannins are known to reduce serum cholesterol and triglyceride levels.

Dinner: Since he ate this meal at home, the couple would have greater control over this menu. Knowing I couldn't do much to change his "meat-and-potatoes" mentality, I opted for the best of both worlds instead, giving him what he wanted and, at the same time, what I believed would be good for his heart. Wednesdays, Thursdays, and Fridays were always to be devoted to some kind of fish, either fresh- or saltwater, steamed or baked in a little lemon-lime juice. The fish of choice was to be served with two different vegetables, one raw (as in carrot, tomato or V-8 juice) and one lightly cooked (brussels sprouts, artichoke hearts, or broccoli, for instance). Preferred breads with this meal were to be one of several dark grains, like pumpernickel or rye perhaps. Dessert was to be in the form of some type of fresh *citrus* fruit such as half an orange, tangerine, or grapefruit. Saturdays and Sundays would find lamb being served with mint jelly, cooked brown rice, and a vegetable salad. Finally, Mondays and Tuesdays would be beef anyway he liked it, so long as fried onions or a small garlic clove were included with the meat. Along with this would be potatoes, either boiled or baked, and with a little plain yogurt seasoned with some powdered kelp and a dash of lemon juice. Except for the fish days in which vegetable juice was to be served, "G.I." was encouraged to drink just *plain cold water* with his other meals.

Staff Sergeant M. took no supplements of any kind because of an aversion (mostly psychological) to them. But I was pleased to hear from his wife about four months later. In a short letter she said: "My husband's cholesterol level has dropped 27 points, his chest pains have virtually ceased, and his breathing has improved. Your diet seems to have worked!"

◆◆◆◆◆◆

SPICES TO STOP "INFECTIOUS" CHD

The following list of spices used to improve the flavors of many dishes from different lands, have been selected because of their therapeutic importance to the heart. In most cases they accomplish two things at the same time to help prevent virus-induced coronary heart disease:

1. They reduce elevated serum cholesterol and triglyceride levels which have been implicated in the process of atherosclerosis.
2. They destroy certain harmful microorganisms known to alter the way in which cholesterol is safely metabolized by the body.

This alteration is believed to lead to hardening of the arteries. Some of these spices include more traditional healing herbs such as ginseng. But they can be incorporated with the preparation of meals or just taken separately in the forms of either a tea, tincture, tablet, or capsule on an empty stomach. Sometimes a combination of several together help to enhance the medical efficacy of both (garlic and ginseng, for instance). Most of these are readily available from any local supermarket, health food store, or nutrition center. In some instances, a food or herb emporium specializing in Oriental products may be the only source available for something not commonly found elsewhere (moer is such an example). Finally, consult the appendix for places to obtain some of the commercial products mentioned in passing: Wakunaga for garlic and Albi Imports for varieties of ginseng.

Black Tree Fungus

Black Tree Fungus (Moer) *(Auricularia auricula-judae; Exida auricula judae)*, a common mushroom or black lichen, is found growing in damp moist forests, usually on tree stumps and logged timber. The Chinese prefer those growing upon five types of trees—the mulberry, the sophera, the paper mulberry, the elm, and the willow (that of the mulberry is considered to be poisonous). The remaining four fungi are used as a texture food in many Szechwanese and Mandarin dishes due to their reputed longevity properties.

The spores are shaped somewhat like a human ear, are sticky and smooth when moist and damp, but leathery when dried out. They vary in size and are dull-brown inside and light brown on the outside. They yield a neutral but pleasant taste and function best in a medicinal sense when steamed first before being consumed.

An analysis of moer's therapeutic benefits was outlined in an interesting report that appeared in the May 22, 1980 *New England Journal of Medicine.* The highly popular Szechwanese dish, hot bean curd, which calls for generous amounts of black tree fungus, was found to inhibit normal blood platelet aggregation. An ingestion of 70 grams of moer severely blunted the usual clustering or clumping of those irregularly shaped disks called blood platelets in as little as 3 hours and lasting for up to 24 hours.

The report concluded by observing "that chronic consumption of antiplatelet foods" like moer, onion, and garlic, "may contribute to the low incidence of arteriosclerotic disease observed in certain ethnic and geographic groups." For instance, recent clinical evidence shows that mainland China in general and particular its southern provinces are virtually free of coronary-artery disease.

In the September 25, 1980 *New England Journal of Medicine,* a student from the University of Washington School of Medicine in Seattle mentioned her own experience with these "wood ears" while residing in rural Taiwan in 1972. She said that on two separate occasions she experienced unexplained severe bruising. However, when she consumed a lot of Suan-la tang or sour-hot soup, which contains quite a bit of this particular fungus, she noticed that she didn't bruise so badly. Also those Taiwanese who frequently eat a lot of Suan-la tang *didn't* have heart disease!

Another report from a group of doctors at Cornell University Medical College in New York City observed a similar transitory antiplatelet effect induced by the pungent rootstock of the tropical plant, ginger, also a common ingredient in many Oriental recipes. (See discussion of ginger root in this section for complete details.)

The best place to purchase moer (also called muerh) is from a reputable Chinese grocery store usually located in any major metropolitan area. For those not acquainted with the headlines that this fungus recently made, a quick review may be in good order. The former mayor of New York City, Ed Koch, suffered a mild stroke while in office during August 1987. Dr. J. P. Mohr, head of the Stroke Center at Columbia-Presbyterian Medical Center, prescribed a daily aspirin for the mayor and also put him on a low-fat, low-salt diet with lots of fresh fruits and vegetables. The doctor, however, encouraged the mayor to keep eating a modified form of Chinese cuisine, particularly dishes with black tree fungus, which he recommended along with garlic as potential blood thinners. All this was disclosed at a press conference and later reported in the November 1987 *University of California, Berkeley, Wellness Letter.* In effect, then, moer exhibits wonderful anticlotting effects and can certainly help prevent the onset of atherosclerosis.

Garlic Bulb

Garlic Bulb *(Allium sativum).* The Chinese and Japanese have probably done more research into the medicinal effects of garlic than anyone else has. Little wonder since garlic figures so prominently in the cuisines of both cultures. One scientist who has devoted a great deal of time and energy to the study of this spice is Benjamin Lau, M.D., Ph.D., a professor and chairman of the Department of Microbiology at California's Loma Linda University School of Medicine. In his small book *Garlic (for Health)* [Wilmot, Wisconsin: Lotus Light Publications, 1988] he shows how garlic can help reduce the risks of certain contributing factors to coronary heart disease.

Elevated serum cholesterol and triglyceride levels promote atherosclerosis. Lau and two associates gave a group of 32 subjects with high cholesterol (220–440 mg./dl.) 4 capsules of liquid kyolic garlic extract daily for up to six months. Their early findings were quite the opposite of what they expected and quite discouraging: instead of lowering cholesterol, the garlic was, in fact, raising it even higher! Yet they persisted in their experiment and "beginning in the third month, we saw a significant drop in serum lipids." By the end of half a year, lipid levels were at the low levels his team desired to see. He postulated that garlic causes fat deposits to shift from the liver and heart into the bloodstream, thereby producing initially higher serum lipid levels. But with the continued use of odor-modified garlic, these excess lipids are broken down and excreted through the intestinal tract. A review of all pertinent research done with garlic and atherosclerosis was authored by Lau and his colleagues and appeared in *Nutrition Research* (vol. 3, 1983, p. 119)

A second blood factor contributing to heart attacks and strokes is the amount of clotting material and the time it takes to clot. Blood cells called thrombocytes or platelets ordinarily cluster to help prevent blood loss in case of injury. Fibrinogen in the blood works with the platelet clumping through a complex process to help stop bleeding and to facilitate healing. Without this process, a simple cut could result in fatal blood loss. A third blood component, plasmin or fibrinolysin, dissolves the fibrin clots when they are no longer needed. Research shows that those subject to heart attacks and strokes have excessive fibrinogen (which causes clots) and not enough fibrinolysin (which breaks up clots). Citing evidence from Indian researchers, Dr. Lau shows how the sulphur compounds in this spice can lower fibrinogen, extend clotting time, and increase the ability to break up clots in those regularly consuming garlic. On the other hand, those not using this spice frequently suffer just the opposite effects.

Hypertension is a third cause of of strokes and heart attacks. In his book, Dr. Lau presents data to show the value of garlic in reducing high blood pressure. In the 1940s, one scientist tested 100 hypertensive patients by prescribing large amounts of garlic, gradually tapering it off as the experiment progressed. He discovered that after just a week's treatment, 40 patients had a drop of 20 mm Hg or more in their blood pressure. A more recent study of the Chinese Cooperative Group involved seventy hypertensive patients who were given the equivalent of 50 grams of raw garlic a day. Thirty-three of them showed a marked lowering of blood pressure; 14 showed moderate reductions in blood pressure, for an overall success rate of 61.7%.

Dr. Lau also cites diabetes as an additional "risk factor in the development of atherosclerotic disease." Garlic happens to have strong hypoglycemic properties to it. Indian scientists have shown that blood sugar levels plunged when volunteers consumed garlic in 1958. Almost two decades later, other Indian researchers demonstrated rabbits made diabetic by injections of alloxan, experienced dramatic reductions in their blood sugar levels when given extracts of garlic. And Japanese scientists working for Wakunaga Pharmaceutical Co., makers of kyolic garlic, proved that liquid garlic extract prevented the rise of blood sugar after oral loading of glucose in a standard glucose tolerance test.

Finally, viral infections can contribute to CHD as well. A study co-authored by Lau and two others and published in the September 1986 issue of *Antimicrobial Agents & Chemotherapy* showed that garlic extract inhibits the production of lipid or fat by the yeast, Candida albicans. And Japanese scientists from Kyoto Perfectural University of Medicine in Kyoto and the Wakunga Pharmaceutical Co. Research Center outside of Hiroshima, reported in the journal *Oncology* (vol. 46, 1989, pp. 277–280) that kyolic garlic extract manifested strong antitumor activity. These and similar studies prove that garlic is an excellent antibiotic agent and can certainly kill or inactivate those viruses that tend to promote atherosclerosis.

When I was in Japan in May 1990, I visited Yoshio Kato's Oyama Garlic Lab in Amagasaki. Patients who come to this clinic receive nothing but a variety of garlic remedies for an assortment of ailments. Garlic is sprayed from a showerlike apparatus onto people suffering everything from cancer and heart disease to hepatitis, herpes, and frostbite. It's quite an amazing thing to see!

Two Japanese News Reports Save Their Hearts With Kyolic. One of the more remarkable uses for garlic that I've just recently discovered has to do with its positive stimulation of weak hearts. A Scandinavian researcher with whom I spoke at the First World Garlic Congress held in Washington, D.C., at the Willard Hotel in late August 1990 pointed this out to me in some detail. Actually, it only reconfirmed what I already suspected from an incident that had taken place in Japan in the very last week of May of the same year.

In the busy and bustling downtown Ginza shopping district, I was fortunate enough to meet two reporters from one of the country's largest daily newspapers, *The Yomiuri Shimbun*. Yoshi-yuki and Junichi are typical of the thirty something Japanese men on their way up the ladder. But during the course of their arduous climb, both experienced mild fibrillations that soon sent them scurrying to cardiologists.

They each decided to try a liquid product consisting of fluid garlic extract, B-complex vitamins, and liver extract. In Japan it goes by the name of Leopin Liquid, but is sold here in the United States under the name of kyolic. They took an average of three liquid-filled gelatin capsules daily. Within just a few weeks their heart functions returned to normal. (See the appendix.)

Ginger Root

Ginger Root *(Zingiber officinale)*. In the ancient Sanskrit texts, as well as in the later classical literature of the Sangam, Buddhist, Arabic, Greek, and Roman periods, and even in the records of the famous European navigators Marco Polo and Vasco da Gama, does ginger appear, usually in concert with galangal and turmeric, two other relatives of the Zingiberaceae family. But sringavera, as ginger was known in ancient India, was used not only to improve the flavor of many foods and beverages, but also to make them more digestible as well to the system. Hence, this particular food item also served as an effective medicament.

The British, who once occupied India for more than a century, made some interesting uses of the root. King Henry the VIII incorporated ginger in his own special recipe for a remedy against the bubonic plague. In "merry olde" England of the seventeenth century, patrons of local pubs liked to sprinkle ground ginger on top of their ale, then stir it with a red-hot poker before downing the stuff; this was recognized as a beneficial cordial for inclement weather.

A retired Indian scientist, Dr. L. D. Kapoor, speaks of ginger's stimulating value in his book *CRC Handbook of Ayurvedic Medicinal Plants* (Boca Raton: CRC Press, 1990). Powdered ginger is extremely useful, he says, to rub on the extremities of the limbs to check cold perspiration and improves blood circulation in the collapse stage of cholera. The same application may also be used to ward off early paralysis from sudden attacks or strokes when liberally applied and vigorously massaged into critical acupuncture points located on the wrists, in the bend of each arm, on the sides of the neck, along the temples, at the top and base of the spinal column, on the inside folds behind each knee, on the ankles, and center bottoms of the feet. This works best by making a paste of some freshly ground root (half a root) and a little (¼ pint) alcohol. Or simply soak some shredded root (4 Tbsp.) in a little alcohol (2 cups of vodka preferably) for about five days, shaking the glass jar in which this mixture is twice a day. The strained fluid extract can then be applied externally on these vital body points and also administered sublingually (beneath the tongue) in 10-drop amounts twice daily until the paralysis dissipates.

Ginger's real value, however, in preventing hardening of the arteries is somewhat similar to the actions of moer. A group of Cornell Medical School researchers commented on these benefits in the September 25, 1980 *New England Journal of Medicine.* They noticed that when one of their members consumed "an excellent marmalade" consisting of 15% ginger and lesser amounts of grapefruit and crabapple the night before, his blood platelets failed to group together as usual. It seems that the gingerol in the root suppressed the arachidonic acid ability to inspire platelet aggregation. Furthermore, the molecular structure similarity between gingerol and aspirin, another recognized blood thinner, is uncanny to say the least. Two ginger capsules daily with meals may help to prevent CHD.

Ginger also manifests certain antioxidant properties as well. In an earlier chapter, the harmful effects of free radicals on the body was discussed. In a nutshell, these scavenger molecules run amok within the system, causing a breakdown of vital organs like the heart, liver, and lungs. Some scientists think that free radicals, in fact, could be another factor in the complicated process of artery hardening within the heart. Certainly the use of ginger seems to make sense in those easily susceptible to atherosclerosis.

Ginseng Root

Ginseng Root (Korean: *Phanax ginseng;* **Siberian:** *Eleuthorococcus senticosus)*. Retired USDA scientist, Dr. James A. Duke and his co-author, Dr. Edward S. Ayensu, former chairman of the Department of Botany at the Smithsonian Institution, discuss at considerable lengths the virtues of both types of ginseng in their in their two-volume work, *Medicine Plants of China* (Algonac, Michigan: Reference Publications, 1985). The panaxin in Korean ginseng, they say, acts as a potent stimulant for the midbrain, the heart, and the blood vessels. The powdered Korean root has been administered to patients experiencing arrhythmia with shock-like conditions, hypotension, and general shock. In all instances, 3.12 grams of the powder or several cups of the root tea appeared to have substantially strengthened myocardial contraction and elevated the blood pressure. They and other scientists conclude that Korean ginseng root should be regularly prescribed "to persons past the midyears" for healthier hearts.

Doctors from several major hospitals in Japan published a report on Korean ginseng's cholesterol-reducing properties in the *American Journal of Chinese Medicine* (vol. 11, 1983, pp. 96–101). The key principles within the root called saponins were responsible for lowering the high levels of blood cholesterol and triglycerides in normal rats fed extremely large amounts of fat.

Siberian ginseng has also been used for various heart conditions as well with excellent results. Duke and Ayensu cite a report which appeared in *BioScience* (vol. 29, 1979, p. 324) to the effect that this spiny ginseng brought about 90% improvement in neurasthenia cases, 60–90% improvement in hypertension cases, and 75% lowering of lipids in hypercholesterolemia cases. Furthermore, they say, studies conducted between the 1972–74 period showed that Siberian ginseng roots were highly effective against bronchitis as well as heart disease and produced no noticeable side effect.

The very best grades of both ginsengs are obviously sold in Chinese herb shops rather than health food stores. Four of the most popular brands preferred by Oriental men and women are: Heavenly Grade Korean Red Ginseng (extract, powder, and tea), Li Chung Yun Siberian Ginseng (capsules and liquid extract), Jin Sam Jung (a strong Oriental herbal tonic with ginseng as one of its main components), and Antler Horn Tonic (consisting of ginseng, antler horns, and other Oriental herbs). (See the appendix and Albi Imports, Burnaby, B.C., Canada, for obtaining these.)

As several scientific studies have shown, the combination of garlic and ginseng *together* work much better in the system than if either are taken alone. The Soviet journal, *Antibiotiki Ministerstro Zdravookhraneniia* for January 1982 contained a report of 250 children from infancy to 14 years of age being treated with for acute dysentery caused by Shigella sonnei. Those treated with just antibiotics alone didn't do as well as those treated with antibiotics *and* Siberian ginseng. The *Hiroshima Journal of Medical Science* for September 1985 also reported on garlic and ginseng working better together at preventing liver damage induced by carbon tetrachloride than if they were administered separately. Thus, an individual could take 2 capsules of the liquid kyolic garlic extract along with 1 of the Albi Imports ginseng products and probably achieve *greater* success in preventing "infectious" CHD than by taking them at separate times or just using one or the other instead.

A Canadian "Mountie" Benefits From Ginseng Tonic. Lt. H. F. of the Royal Canadian Mounted Police (RCMP) reported the following to me after I had spoken at the Canadian Health Food Association convention in Toronto in November 1988.

H. F. said he had never been one for taking "pills and such" (as he put it). But about a year before we met, he noticed his legs and arms started to get colder than usual. His doctor pronounced the problem as bad circulation coupled with a weak heart that could "use a kick or two" to get it going faster. The medicine prescribed "only made me sicker, so I quit taking it altogether," Henry added.

Then he heard from one of his Chinese friends about a product called Jin Sam Jung distributed by Albi Imports (see the appendix). He bought a bottle and began taking 1 level Tbsp. every morning before breakfast. Within about six weeks, he noticed a definite improvement in his circulation. While they may not always get their man, at least this Mountie got his herb, ginseng, in a tonic he liked.

Onion Bulb

Onion Bulb *(Allium cepa).* The ancient Egyptians made use of the onion in ancient times. The Bible (Numbers 11:5) tells us that the Hebrews were fed "fish, cucumbers, melons, leeks, onions, and garlic." And *An X-Ray Atlas of the Royal Mummies* (Chicago: University of Chicago Press, 1980) notes that every pharoah's corpse was liberally packed with onions.

Ironically, though, the kings of ancient Egypt seldom ever ate garlic or onions, esteeming them as "stinking weeds" fit only for their slaves. Had they utilized them more often in their diets, they probably wouldn't have suffered so much from arteriosclerosis. An intriguing story concerning the unraveling of this medical mystery may be found in the anonymously written *Medicine & Pharmacy (An Informal History): I. Ancient Egypt.* It seems an English chap named Sir Marc Armand Buffer, who was a noted pathologist, contracted diptheria in the 1890s and had to travel to Egypt for rest and recovery.

While there, he discovered that mummy tissue could be softened in a solution of alcohol and sodium bicarbonate, thereby permitting pathological examination which had heretofore been impossible on account of their extremely brittle conditions. In a lab room in Cairo, Dr. Ruffer used his scalpel on the mummy of the Pharoah believed to have lived during the time Moses and Aaron were in Egypt demanding that their people be set free.

The eighth and ninth chapters of Exodus repeatedly refer to "the heart of Pharoah [being] hardened." His embalmers had removed his heart upon his later demise, but had left just enough of an aorta for Ruffer to study. There, lo and behold, under the microscope was evidence of typical senile calcification of the aorta, with the interlamellar material thickly coated with calcium phosphate and presumably old lipid deposits. It seems then that this Pharoah's "heart had indeed been hard!"

Onions prevent arteriosclerosis several different ways. For one thing, said *Science News* on April 21, 1979, they contain an important prostaglandin (A-1), a compound known to reduce hypertension. Also this same component, notes *Prostaglandins, Leukotrienes & Medicine* (vol. 24, pp. 43–50) in 1986 prevents the grouping of blood platelets by simply altering arachidonic acid metabolism in them; this, in effect, keeps blood clots out of the body.

The May 23, 1990 *Journal of The American Chemical Society* points out that onion contains a fascinating brew of *over* 100 sulphur-containing compounds, which account for all of this spice's remarkable therapeutic effects in one way or another. Earlier in this section under garlic, it was mentioned that fibrinolysin dissolves blood (fibrin) clots when they are no longer needed to check hemorrhaging. Well, according to the January 1966 *Indian Journal of Medicinal Research*, onion not only reduces serum cholesterol levels, but also *increases* the production of more fibrinolysin to help reduce the incidence of thromboembolism (an obstruction by a clot in one of the blood vessels or heart cavities).

Another definite benefit to the heart is onion's strong hypoglycemic activity, noted the September 11, 1976 issue of *Lancet*. According to the late Dr. John Yudkin, formerly of Queen Elizabeth College in London, excessive sugar intake correlated very well with ischemic heart disease. In the *British Medical Journal* (vol. 20, p. 810) for 1966, Dr. Yudkin reported that heart patients who refused to "reduce their sugar consumption after one or more myocardial infarcts" could be counted on to die much earlier than others who completely eliminated sugary foods from their diets altogether. Several other studies in past issues of the *American Journal of Clinical Nutrition* (vol. 17, 1965, p. 334, and vol. 18, 1966, p. 237) have clearly demonstrated that men and women consuming 220 grams of sugar daily in their diets for almost a month had higher triglyceride and serum cholesterol levels in their blood than did others who were on low sugar diets

In light of this evidence, the wonderful hypoglycemic property of onion can certainly be appreciated in preventing arteriosclerosis. I might add my own personal testimony to what has already been given in this regard. This author as of 1990 is a 43-year-old white male with an average weight of around 190 and a height of 6 feet 4 inches. He sits for upwards of 10 hours a day at his word processor writing books and articles on all kinds of subjects. And when he lectures or teaches classes, he usually sits on a stool most of the time before his captive audiences. The only real exercise he gets is a little walking each day. His diet is heavy in beef, showing preference mostly for steaks and prime rib. When he consumes them, he *does not* trim away the fat but eats *everything* except the bone. However, he seldom ever eats carbohydrates (bread, potatoes, etc.) in the same meal with his meat, but has them at a later meal devoid of animal protein. He also unfortunately indulges himself in too many pastries.

In a word, then, he engages in those things which doctors have found to promote arteriosclerosis like crazy! And yet, every year he undergoes a complete blood workup and every two years a thorough heart scan. His serum cholesterol generally hovers around 176–180 mg/dl and his triglyceride count is minimal. The last time he had an angiogram, his heart was nearly "squeaky clean" of plaque deposits or, as his physician put it, "John, your heart vessels are as clean as a hound's tooth" (however clean that's supposed to be).

And what is my little secret to all of this? Why nothing more than onions *and lots of them* whenever I eat meat or any meal for that matter. I like to slice a large yellow onion and lightly sauté that next to my medium-rare steak. I also have an insatiable craving for green onions, which I generally eat with my lunch every day. In fact, if anything, I usually get a number of complaints from those around me—my fiancée, my office staff, my students, and fellow colleagues—about the terrible onion odor frequently present in my breath. To this day, I can thank onions more than anything else for keeping me virtually free of arteriosclerosis.

Like garlic, the many disulfides in onion also exhibit strong antioxidant properties as well. Not only does an onion kill harmful bacteria like *E. coli* and *S. cerevisiae*, but it also helps to curb the activity of those nasty free radicals. Staph, salmonella, and other scavenger molecules just don't stand a chance of infecting the heart with atherosclerotic lesions so long as onion is in the diet *often! Food Research* (vol. 23, 1958, pp. 274–279) once reported that the antibiotic and antioxidant properties are greatest in yellow onion that is uncooked or *lightly* cooked. (Note: Hypoglycemics can't tolerate garlic or onion very well.)

A French Chef's Recipe for Remedying the Heart. Marcel Le Cler is a chef at a little French bistro on the outskirts of Montreal. He has an established clientele of older folks, many of whom curiously enough, had been former patients of a leading Quebec cardiologist.

"He fixes zem up first and zen sends zem to me to do ze rest," he proudly proclaimed with a classic accent. What Marcel does, in fact, is to serve each of these recovered cardiac patients a special "Heart Tonic Soup" (as he calls it). The soup is a consommé usually made from boiled veal, and includes not one but *three* different kinds of onions—Bermuda (white), leeks, and green onion. All are finely chopped and added, then the soup is simmered for a while to draw out their full flavors.

Those who've stayed with the soup on a fairly regular basis, that is, having a couple of large bowls each week, have had fewer recurrences of heart problems than have those who've consumed it only intermittently. Marcel swore by the stuff and claimed that it really *did* extend the years of many of his doctors referrals.

Sage Root

Sage Root *(Salvia miltiorrhiza).* Several centuries ago when the Dutch enjoyed did a brisk business in spices, they frequently acquired sage from the French and then shipped it on to China, where they received in return four pounds of tea for every pound of sage. The dried, whole, rubbed, or ground leaves are extremely aromatic, herbaceous, and spicy with a unique balsamic bitter taste, fragrant, warm, and astringent. The flavorful properties help to add zest to pork sausage products, fried chicken, meat loaf, meat balls, hamburger mixes, condiments, pickles, confections, chewing gums, nonalcoholic beverages, and some specialty baked goods. In the home kitchen, sage has an affinity for poultry stuffings, pork dishes, roasts, gravies, casseroles, or soups. It's also good with baked fish, cheese dishes, Spanish omelets, pasta, and hamburgers. It adds zest to such vegetables as tomatoes, eggplant, lima beans, and onions. One sage leaf or a pinch of rubbed sage is enough for one portion of meat, fish, or omelet.

In mainland China a particular species known as red-rooted or purple sage is widely employed as a popular and highly effective medicine for treating everything from drug-resistant staph infections to myocardial infarctions. The root part is always used; it yields a slightly bitter taste that momentarily numbs the mouth with a tingling sensation. But in the body the oleoresins present in this root are strongly invigorating to the heart and liver, blood circulation, kidney and bladder functions, and so forth.

Drs. Duke and Ayensu refer to it in their *Medicinal Plants of China* as being useful for dispersing accumulated blood and swelling in the vessels or around the heart, for reducing coronary hypertension, and for calming myocardial disturbances. Back in 1975 when China was just opening up to the West, a delegation from the national Academy of Sciences visited there. One of the Americans, a parasitologist, suffered a major heart attack. A physician with the group properly diagnosed his condition with the aid of an ECG as myocardial infarction. The patient's chest pains became excruciating and so treatment was immediately started. Five hours later, he suffered another major heart attack and so emergency measures were quickly instituted, including cardiac massage.

A group of Chinese heart experts arrived at the hospital located in the provincial center west of Shanghai and reviewed all the evidence. The leading cardiologist recommended that an herbal medicine be used at that point, since the patient's situation looked grave enough that he might not make it if another setback occurred. Consent was readily given and an intravenous injection of an extract of this particular sage root was soon given to the strickened parasitologist. In a short time circulation commenced around the small blood vessels of the man's heart, and over the next two weeks the American regained his health. From there he was taken by plane to Tokyo for a further checkup and within five weeks he was back home in the United States actively engaged in his usual routine of things.

In the event that readers are unable to procure this particular species of sage from any major metropolitan Chinese herb shop (ask for it by the Chinese names of pinyin or dan shen or tan-shen), then ordinary rubbed sage *(Salvia officinalis)* leaves can be substituted. It's best though to go for either the Greek or Spanish varieties instead of the English kind if possible. Ideally, if one is able to obtain the extracted oleoresin from the Dalmatian kind of sage that's used in sausage seasonings, then by all means use this if you're unable to get the Chinese sage root.

Several licensed and practicing British medical herbalists I know of in London make a nifty fluid extract out of the Dalmatian oleoresin (10 drops), a little raw grated ginger root (2 Tbsp.), and a pinch of cayenne pepper (1/16th or tip of a teaspoon) put into a pint of brandy, shaken twice daily and allowed to set in a cool, dark place for approximately two weeks. The liquid is then strained through double cheese-cloth and put into a small, clean, well-stoppered bottle. They prescribe this to many of their angina patients, recommending 7 drops under the tongue three times in between meals.

On the other hand, if one can find the Chinese sage root, then just make a simple tea out of it. Bring a pint of water to a boil; add 1 level Tbsp. of the dried root. Cover and reduce heat to simmer for *no longer than 3 minutes.* Remove from stove and permit to steep for half an hour. Strain and drink 1 cup *warm* on an empty stomach twice daily where myocardial and angina problems are likely to occur.

A report by Japanese scientists on Chinese sage root was published in *Chemical & Pharmaceutical Bulletin* (vol. 31, pp. 1670–1675) for 1983. Blood platelet aggregations were induced into rabbits and rats by means of collagen. Sage root was then administered. Several tanshinone compounds within the root halted this clotting action rather nicely. This may help to explain a little why Chinese sage root is so wonderful for treating infarction and coronary pains.

Finally, the carnosic and labiatic acids in sage exhibit strong antioxidant and bactericidal properties against free radicals, staphylococcus, and other bacteria which are notorious for injuring the heart different ways. It may also be well to point out here that Chinese sage root exhibits a marvelous tranquilizing effect upon the central nervous system. According to a report in the May 1979 *Acta Pharmaceutica Sinica*, nervous lab animals "became calm and tame" after an extract tan-shen was administered to them. And when combined with phenobarbital practically all restless animals in two different (all of 20, and 9 of 10) fell asleep. This demonstrates the remarkable sedative action of the root upon the heart and nerves.

Slippery Elm Bark

Slippery Elm Bark *(Ulmus fulva)*. The late popular plant forager and herbal lore writer, Euell Gibbons described how he made chilled slippery elm junket and slippery elm breading for fish in his *Stalking the Healthful Herbs*. Gibbons raved about its wonderful nutritional value, which contain nineteenth-century Native Americans tribes and frontier doctors in the eastern United States knew all about as well. In his electric blender, Gibbons added 1 heaping Tbsp. each of powdered Irish moss and slippery elm bark and mixed them together on the grind cycle for a few seconds. Then he put a pint of milk in the top of a double boiler and cooked it until scalding hot. After which he stirred in 2 tsp. of the powdered herb mixture into enough cold water to make a paste; this he next added to the hot milk. He continued cooking and stirring for another 10 minutes, before straining everything through a double layer of cheese cloth. He then sweetened it with a little honey and added a pinch of nutmeg for flavor. When he poured this mixture into a dessert dish and chilled it in the refrigerator a while, it became a firm junket that was a delight to eat. "Here was a medicine to my liking," he quipped—"filet of elm deluxe."

After gutting and cleaning a string of nice freshwater fish, he prepared his breading material this way. In a brown paper bag he put several heaping tablespoonfuls of powdered slippery elm, along with ½ tsp. of salt (I recommend the equivalent of kelp instead), and 4–7 heaping Tbsp. of a good fish garni (storebought spice mixture for flavoring seafoods). Then he dropped in each of his several fish filets, shook them until they were thoroughly coated, and then lightly fried them in safflower or sunflower seed oil. He discovered that his slippery elm breading didn't come off as the fish fried like so many other coatings usually do. "The fish browned very nicely," he concluded, "and those who ate them pronounced them delicious.

Slippery elm is extremely mucilaginous, meaning that it turns into somewhat of a slick, slimy, gelatinous liquid when cooked in water. This is due to a rather remarkable amino acid-carbohydrate complex high in calcium and potassium, with moderate amounts of phosphorus and magnesium, and trace amounts of silicon, zinc, and manganese. The early frontierman, John. D. Hunter described its nutrition this way in the 1823 edition of his *Manners and Customs of Several Indian Tribes Located West of The Mississippi:* "I have subsisted for days on it, while traveling through the country of unfriendly tribes. The elm bark will support life for a great length of time." His only gripe was that without meat of some sort, it produced indigestion and considerable passing of gas worse than that produced by eating beans! One of the early migrating Mormon groups leaving Winter Quarters, Nebraska, and heading out to Utah, also survived on this as well. In Andrew Jenson's *L.D.S. Biographical Encyclopedia*, mention is made of Bishop David Evans's Company who "ran out of provisions and had to . . . live three weeks on quarter rations, consisting of [powdered] slippery elm bark and flour."

In light of very recent research, the vegetable protein content of this particular tree bark could be very helpful in treating heart attacks and a whole range of inflammatory diseases. Researchers at Johns Hopkins University Medical School in Baltimore, Maryland, and T Cell Sciences, Inc., in Cambridge, Massachusetts, have used a genetically shortened version of a natural human protein called complement receptor one (CR1) to limit the damage from heart attacks suffered in rats.

According to an initial report delivered at the 1989 annual meeting of the American Heart Association, certain proteins can block the action of a part of the immune system known as the "complement system." This is a collection of other proteins that are activated when the body is invaded by bacteria, fungi, viruses, or other foreign substances. Among other actions, the complement proteins activate certain special blood cells to rush to an injured area to clean up the debris left from an assault on a bacterium, for example.

But one unpleasant side effect of activating these specialized blood cells is that the cells can inadvertently trigger an inflammation of normal tissues. This is believed to be the cause of some inflammatory diseases like arthritis, vasculitis (inflammation of the blood vessels), glomerulonephritis (inflammation of the kidneys), and myasthenia gravis (inflammation of the muscles).

Now in a heart attack, the initial damage to the heart muscle is produced by a sudden blockage of blood flow by a blood clot. Additional damage to the heart muscle occurs when blood flow is restored through clot-dissolving agents. This additional damage is caused by complement-activated blood cells that rush into the damaged area with the restored flow.

In experiments with rats, blood flow to part of the heart muscle was temporarily stopped to mimic a real heart attack and then restored. In rodents treated with CR1, the area of damage in the heart muscle was more than 30% smaller than in animals that had "heart attacks" but were not treated with this altered protein. In a follow-up study, far fewer complement-activated cells were found in the damaged area of the hearts of CR1-treated rats than in untreated rats, indicating the protein was, indeed, limiting heart damage by blocking the complement system.

It seems the Almighty in His infinite wisdom already put such abbreviated versions of the human CR1 protein in two particular herbs, namely, slippery elm and yarrow. In almost two decades of extensively lecturing and writing on the subject of herbs throughout North America, I've probably encountered a little over two dozen heart attack cases wherein both of these herbs have been enthusiastically recommended by me. In about two-thirds or some 17 instances, the recovered individuals have written back to me indicating just how much both herbs helped them.

Now I had always suspected that it was the protein-carbohydrate complexes in both that helped them overcome their initial heart attacks a lot sooner than would normally be expected. But my proof so far as slippery elm went rested mainly with the testimony given by R. E. Griffith in his 1847 edition of *Medical Botany. With the Uses of Important Species in Medicine, the Arts, etc.*, in which he attributes recovery from heart pains to this bark. More solid evidence, though, came from the August 1969 *Journal of Pharmaceutical Sciences*, which described in detail how the proteins and carbohydrates in dried yarrow flowers affixed themselves to sites of inflammation where tissue repair work could commence.

In light of the Johns Hopkins-T Cell Sciences discovery, I think slippery elm and yarrow work along similar lines for minimizing further damage to the heart after a heart attack has occurred. My suggestion then as now is to take 4 capsules of each powdered herb daily on an empty stomach for at least six months or more.

Tarragon

Tarragon Leaves & Flowering Tops *(Artemisia dracunculus)*. Our last spice in this chapter for improving "infectious" heart disease happens to be an aromatic little number that is the very special ingredient in the world-famous Dijon mustard from France. Dried tarragon leaves evoke a flavor and aroma quite similar to that of anise in some ways. The spice is necessary for making béarnaise sauce, which is used with eggs and asparagus. Tarragon also works wonders in green salads and in pea, chicken, mushroom, tomato, and vegetable soups. It definitely adds an interesting flavor to beets, carrots, celery, green beans, onions, summer squash, and zucchini. Not too mention complementing poultry, veal, cheese, stuffed shellfish, baked fish, and a host of other meat dishes. Tarragon is a favorite in both French and Armenian cuisines.

In fact, the famous French herbalist from Provence, Maurice Mességué frequently used tarragon to treat the likes of the Ali Khan, King Farouk of Egypt, and the "Pope of the People" the late John XXIII. He discovered in his healing practice that tarragon was good for sluggish livers, hearts, stomachs, and kidneys and bladders. Also he noticed that those convalescing from recent heart attacks or suffering from acute stress and anxiety (personality type As), benefited more when they took tarragon on a regular basis.

However, this is one herb you simply *cannot* take just any old way to help your heart. Of all the different preparations that seem to have worked the best both for treatment as well as for prevention, the alcohol fluid extract is by far the best! And since no one sells it, you'll either have to have it specially made for you (see Custom-Made Formulas in the appendix) or else make it yourself.

To a quart of good-quality red wine (*not* white because of the trace amounts of arsenic for clarity and sulphur dioxide for preservation), add 7 to 10 sprigs of tarragon that have been snipped into small pieces with a pair of scissors. Cork or cap the bottle and set in a cool, dry place for 21 days, shaking the container a couple of times each day (once in the morning and again at night). Leave the tarragon in if you wish and store in a cool, dark place or refrigerate on a lower shelf or inside the bottom door rack and use as needed. Recommended dosage is between 10–15 drops beneath the tongue each day.

A report in the November 2, 1979 *Journal of the American Medical Association* explained how moderate intake of a little wine or hard liquor each day helped to lower the risks of coronary heart disease. And just a year before this, the November 1978 issue of *Human Nature* reported that a jigger of whiskey or a glass of red wine elevated the amount of "good" HDL (high-density lipoprotein) cholesterol known to prevent heart attacks from occurring. A later review of the existing medical evidence to this effect was published in the August 1985 *American Journal of Medicine* with similar conclusions. Finally, the Spring 1985 *Journal of Nutrition for the Elderly* and the September 1985 *Journal of the American Dietetic Association* both pointed out that a little wine (½ glass daily or full glass every two days) definitely improved the overall health and morale of elderly folks confined to geriatric units, nursing homes, and private residences.

Thus, we can see that when an addictive substance such as alcohol is used in moderation and with common sense, it can be a boon rather than a bane to good health. And when an incredible spice like tarragon is combined with something such as red wine, then only positive results can be forthcoming in the prevention and treatment of virus-induced arteriosclerosis. It's interesting to note in closing that throughout mainland China, folk practitioners with minimum medical training called "barefoot doctors" have often utilized a Chinese species of this particular spice to treat "acute and chronic convulsive attacks" of the brain, heart, liver, and stomach; so claims the English version of *A Barefoot Doctor's Manual* anyway.

How Tarragon Elixir Prevents Classic Heartburn. Marcel LeCler, my chef friend from Montreal, also had a great remedy for heartburn and acid indigestion which included the use of fresh tarragon. He swore it would "cure" the worst intestinal miseries that anyone might ever have the unpleasant misfortune of experiencing.

Begin with about a pint of naturally carbonated water. Next snip two sprigs of fresh tarragon into fine pieces. Add them to the container of carbonated water. Cover with a lid and shake vigorously for 15 seconds or so. Let it stand this way for a couple of days in a cool, shady spot somewhere, remembering to shake the contents the same way every day.

At this point it can be refrigerated. When classic heartburn or the symptoms of a hiatal hernia occur—sour feeling in the throat and an urge to regurgitate—just sip a few tablespoonfuls of this elixir through a straw and watch these problems vanish in a matter of minutes.

Summary

1. Other factors besides salt, sugar, fat, stress, and obesity cause CHD.

2. The herpes virus, loneliness, certain types of music, hostility and anger, and competition also manifest negative influences upon the heart as well.

3. Mischievous viruses produce more macrophages and T cells that can then interfere with normal cholesterol metabolism; this interference usually leads to hardening of the arteries.

4. The breakdown of close family ties and neighborly relations and the increased emphasis on materialism also seem to promote greater CHD.

5. Studies with poultry infected with a herpes virus yielded an atherosclerosis very similar to that found in human arteries as well.

6. Certain spices and herbs seem to help prevent and treat "infectious" coronary heart disease. They are black tree fungus, garlic, ginger, two kinds of ginseng, onion, sage, slippery elm and yarrow, and tarragon.

·~~~~ 6 ~~~~·

Recurrent Allergies: Doing Something About "Bad News" Bacteria

MENTION THE SUBJECT of allergies to a layperson, and he or she is apt to think of things which either make you sneeze or itch or both. But allergies are more than just a lot of unnecessary wheezing or breaking out all over in hives due to pollen or substance hypersensitivity. In fact, they can be as diverse as continual lack of physical energy to more deadly manifestations of ill health like pneumonia. This is because of the vicious bacteria responsible for their presence.

In this chapter, we'll examine not only the biochemical but also the social and environmental reasons behind many of the following allergy-related problems:

Asthma, bronchitis, and emphysema

Chronic fatigue syndrome

Conjunctivitis

Ecological illness

Food allergies

Hay fever

Lyme disease

Pneumonia

Sinusitis

Skin rash

Sore throat

◆◆◆◆◆

ALLERGIES: WHAT YOU NEED TO KNOW

The Prerequisites for Unfriendly Bacteria

Forget what you may have heard or thought causes allergies, because I'm about to show you some factors that you've probably never even heard of before or thought could possibly be linked to them. This business about pollen, house dust, strange perfume, cat hair, auto exhaust smog, and the like producing most of our allergies is yesterday's medical news. While they still play an obvious role as mechanisms by which many allergies are triggered, they aren't the main causes by any means.

The real culprits are "bad news" bacteria—sort of a 1990s-style neighborhood gang of microbial thugs that beat up poor, unsuspecting immune systems for the most unlikely of reasons. Like *shyness*, for instance. That's right, s-h-y-n-e-s-s of all things! These days the bashful and timid are more apt to suffer from hay fever than are those who are bold and aggressive.

According to the September/October 1990 issue of *Psychosomatic Medicine*, it isn't just President George Bush who is adversely affected by the so-called "wimp factor." It takes its heavy toll on shy adults as well. At the University of Arizona in Tucson, some 375 college undergraduates were divided into four basic groups based on the degree of shyness that each student had reported on a questionnaire that focused on shyness with strangers, fondness for large parties, and recollections of childhood shyness and fear of going to school. The research team led by Iris R. Bell, also administered questionnaires assessing mood disturbances and allergies, including hay fever, asthma, eczema, hives, and drug allergies leading to anaphylactic shock.

And guess what they found? Why that there were *more* reports of depression, fearfulness, chronic fatigue, and hay fever emerging from the 72 students in the most-shy group than from any other single participant group. Nearly 40% of students in the two groups ranking highest for shyness suffered terribly from hay fever, as compared to just about one-fifth of the remaining students.

But wait a second! If you think this is weird, then consider another follow-up statistic in the same study. Hay fever afflicted close to half of the 18 students reporting the most shyness, but struck *none* of the 19 students ranked as the most outgoing and personable in the 375-person sample.

Dr. Jerome Kagan of Harvard University presented other evidence in 1988 to support this very thing. Kagan noted that there is a *greater* frequency of hay fever among close relatives of extremely shy children than among relatives of outgoing children. It's believed by scientists studying this new link between emotional states and allergies that the hay fever-shyness connection may originate from alterations of neurochemical receptors deep within the brain that regulate mood, smell, and, most of all, immune functions.

A recent article in *The Wall Street Journal* (November 6, 1990, p. B-1) discussed the health repercussions of fear and stress in the office place and work station. These days with mounting economic uncertainties everywhere, workers from all kinds of jobs—from corporate boss to lowly mailroom dispatcher—are becoming more fearful of layoffs and outright dismissals.

And this is making for sicker employees with an alarming increase in allergy-related problems, according to Leon J. Warshaw, an executive director of the New York Business Group on Health, a coalition of businesses concerned about health care. In fact, a poll taken earlier in 1990 among employees at various New Jersey businesses, showed that a whopping 25% of them suffered from fear-induced allergies of some kind.

A second prerequisite necessary for "bad news" bacteria to thrive within the human body is a lifetime ingestion of various antibiotic substances. These need not always be the daily consumption of something potent in a pill form to ward off serious infection, but can start as early as childhood with all of those inoculations given to children. My colleague and friend, Laurence Badgley, M.D., of Foster City, California, has repeatedly stated, for more than a decade now, that most of the AIDS cases one hears, sees, or reads about these days can be traced to all of those immunizations received at infancy, particularly the smallpox vaccination. And Lendon Smith, M.D., another colleague and good friend, wonders now if all of those shots he administered to thousands of youngsters when he was a practicing Oregon pediatrician years ago, haven't caught up with them in their adult years in the form of allergies. Certainly, doctors are loathe to discuss this likely connection, but the evidence is all around us, especially in the dramatic surge of substance hypersensitivity cases seen these days by more and more physicians.

"The bugs are very clever," said Alexander Tomasz, a biochemist at Rockefeller University in New York City. He was referring, of course, to "bad news" bacteria that somehow can develop an uncanny resistance to 99% of our modern antibiotics. Now scientists have known for more than half-a-century that these bacteria have developed resistance to drugs, but they had erroneously imagined that such resistance developed through mutation in the bacteria's genes that was passed on to new colonies of bacteria. However, as it turns out, Tomasz says, these bacteria can import foreign genetic material that enable them to construct entire new defenses against antibiotics. When scientists examine DNA from such drug-resistant bacteria, it seems that "they call in blocks of material that must have come from somewhere else within the body," he noted. His comments were voiced at the annual New Horizons science writers' seminar at the University of Pennsylvania in Philadelphia, which this author attended, during the first weekend in November 1990.

A third prerequisite, required for nasty bacteria to set up permanent households within a person, is a high lead and other heavy metals content in the system. Such poisonous metals often come from the foods we eat. Commercially grown grapes, bottled or canned grape juice, and iceberg lettuce all rank high in lead content due to the excessive spraying of vineyards and fields in which they grow. That's why I've declared such items (unless they're organically grown, of course) to be "junk foods." Furthermore, such widespread exposure to heavy metals makes these "bad news" bugs more drug resistant.

Consider the case reported by a Canadian microbiologist from the University of Alberta Hospitals in Edmonton. According to reports in *Science News*, November 12, 1988, and *National Geographic*, September 1990 she and some of her colleagues traveled to Beechey Island in the Northwest Territory and removed tissue specimens from the frozen remains of two Arctic explorers who had been dead and well preserved since 1846. The tissue samples were kept frozen for transport and then cultured in the laboratory. The researchers grew six strains of a common intestinal bacterium, subjecting it to the antibiotics clindamycin and cefoxitin. The bacteria showed an amazing resistance to both drugs, an unexpected finding since both men died before the development of antibiotics. This led scientists to examine the food both explorers consumed. What they discovered was a high lead content in the bones of each man, due to having eaten food stored in tin cans soldered with lead. Today this isn't a problem in the canning industry, but now lead is more pervasive than it was 142 years ago due to excessive spraying of crops. A final reason why obnoxious and allergic-inducing bacteria may prefer to linger in places they're not welcomed, can be traced back to what our moms ate *before* we were born. According to *The New York Times* of August 30, 1990, certain foods consumed during pregnancy can initiate allergies in the baby that show up in the first months of life. This discovery challenges the popular assumption that breast milk is always the best food for an infant. Not anymore, unless the nursing mother refrains from eating certain allergy-provoking foods. Thus, my advice to an expectant mother would be this: "Be careful of what you consume, because you may be setting your unborn child up for a lifetime of allergies." Among those foods a pregnant woman should avoid or use with extreme caution during pregnancy are *all* dairy products (especially pasteurized milk), eggs, and any kind of red meat (except for pink salmon).

Dr. Ranjit K. Chandra, a pediatric immunologist at the Memorial University of Newfoundland, has found that proteins derived from an expectant mother's diet can turn up in the amniotic fluid, which the developing fetus continually swallows. These proteins can, in turn, sensitize allergy-prone babies to certain foods before they're ever born.

An 18-week-old fetus could form specific antibodies to allergenic proteins that are consumed by the mother, he noted. Then when the infant is born and later encounters the same proteins in childhood, teenage years, or adulthood, again either directly from solid foods or else indirectly through breast milk from foods the nursing mother ate, allergic symptoms may suddenly show up without a logical explanation.

Dr. Chandra tested a restricted diet in 121 women who had already given birth to at least one child with allergies. In a subsequent pregnancy, half the women were placed on a diet that entirely did away with cow's milk and other dairy products like ice cream, cottage cheese, and yogurt, eggs, beef, and peanuts throughout their pregnancy and until they finished nursing. The remaining women continued on their typical diets throughout the study. Among 55 women on the restricted program who completed the study, just 17 infants developed eczema. But among the 54 women with no dietary restrictions, nearly twice (30) the infants developed eczema. His findings suggest that babies are least likely to develop allergies when their moms adhere to a strict diet during both pregnancy and nursing.

How Four People Conquered Their Allergies Without Pills or Potions

In the following brief case studies, I'm going to show you how four different individuals conquered their own allergies. But none of them did it with any vitamin-mineral or herbal supplements.

How Gaining Self-confidence Helped Lick Respiratory Problems. Raymond P., age 24, is one of those fellows with a heart as large as the outdoors. But the kid also has some rather awkward traits that put him into the "nerd" category with many of his peers. He's tall and gangly and seems to have two left feet. Furthermore, he sometimes talks with a slight lisp, and his thick glasses and buck teeth also make him stand out at times as the hayseed hick from the country farm.

One day in the fall of 1990, he came into my office and asked what I would recommend for his shortness of breath. He said a local allergist had told him he was hypersensitive to the box elder trees surrounding the University of Utah campus. I just happened to be reading an article in the August 1990 issue of *Demographics* that showed that children from broken homes run a 35% greater risk of developing allergies than those from stable domestic environments.

We chatted amiably for a while on his past. Seems his parents had become separated when he was a small kid, and subsequently both had used him as a kind of short rope in their tug-of-war vendettas. He was constantly caught in the middle of all this. As a result, he developed a terrible inferiority complex, which went a lot deeper than even his physical appearance or ways belied.

I gave him a pep talk about the fact that looks don't count as much as what you've got in your head and heart. Beginning with my own unhappy childhood as a physically (not sexually) abused youngster to my disturbed mother's own suicide in January 1960, when I discovered her body in one bedroom of our home, I traced for him my own early life of shattered dreams, broken promises, and seemingly insurmountable obstacles. I told him how, during those troublesome years, my own hay fever about drove me crazy, especially in the summer. "I wore thick glasses just like you do, was called 'four-eyes' and other cruel things too shameful to mention, stuttered like a broken record, and was voted least likely to succeed in life by some of my classmates," I added. "And yet look at me now in the prime of my life. I still wear thick glasses, but I look better with them on than off. I am lauded in the media for my work with herbs and health, have delivered over a thousand *extemporaneous* lectures throughout North America, and was recently given an entire page writeup biography in Vol. 128 of *Contemporary Authors*. Not bad for a Neanderthal," I concluded. "And, by the way, my hay fever is history!"

I told Raymond he needed to take some Dale Carnegie courses or other classes that emphasized self-image enhancement. "You need to get past how you look and what others think of you," I emphasized, "and concern yourself more with just how Raymond perceives Raymond. He promised he'd do this, shook my hand, and left.

About a month later, he dropped by my research center. He said a personal motivation class he had been taking three times a week had really given him "a new lease on life" (as he put it). "Thanks to your advice, I now see things a lot differently with this course. It's helped me to see just how special a person I really am inside. It's given me more self-worth than I've probably had in years." He said that for the first time, "I began to feel comfortable with myself. I stopped being ashamed of who I was or what I looked like." He said a real sense of calm had begun to settle over him.

And, with all of these renovations in his mental and emotional states, had also come a physical improvement as well. "My sensitivity to box elders [trees] has gotten noticeably better," he insisted. "My eyes don't run or itch as much as they did a while back." Raymond thinks that in due time, with more overhauling of a badly bruised and mauled ego, his allergy will disappear of its own accord.

Sweating Out His Drug Residues Made Ken's Eczema Disappear. Kenneth was a 26-year-old finishing up his master's degree in business when he was referred to our research center. He took a quarter's worth of classes from us in ethnomedicine. During that period I was covering some of the purification rituals of the Plains Indians, and he asked somewhat laconically one day, "Do you think sweating would help to get rid of this?" while at the same time running his hand over scaly and reddened skin on the side and nape of his neck.

The condition had been with him ever since high school. I suspected it was linked to a number of inoculations he must have received and queried him on this point. His responses confirmed my suspicions. In the 12th grade, he was hospitalized for a week or less to have his appendix removed. Doctors prescribed a host of drugs to curb a hospital-contracted staph infection. Then he went to a small South American country on a two-year mission for his church (Mormon) and had to get a number of immunizations before he left. After this, he returned home and joined the Marine Corps. "At Camp Pendleton," he recalled, "they lined us up in rows without our shirts and marched us between doctors who made pin cushions of both arms." In a word, his system had become overloaded with enough drugs to stock a small pharmacy as it were. No wonder his eczema worsened after each ordeal.

I handed him an article from the October/December 1919 *American Anthropologist* on a typical buffalo sweatlodge ritual. "Maybe there's some things in this you can cull out," I said, adding that the true Native American sweat was an elaborate religious ritual—something to be experienced—and not just a matter of ducking into a fancy sauna for a quick cleansing.

Lack of materials and suitable space prevented him from actually erecting a sweatlodge of his own, but he improvised with a glass-enclosed shower. "Rubbing myself with red clay before climbing in . . . now that was *wild*," he joked. Burning sweet incense in the bathroom with the door closed for at least 20 minutes *prior* to turning on the hot water, didn't seem to pose a problem for him. Nor did drinking several large glasses of cold Mount Olympus spring water during the half-hour he was in there.

After about 10 of these in-home sessions spread over a couple of weeks, he noticed his eczema starting to clear up. A month later, it was 90% gone and he felt terrific!

"Getting the Lead Out" Is More than Just a Figure of Speech. Mercedes was a bright and gregarious young lady of 23½ at the time this chapter was being written. Ever one for small details, she had insisted that I include the ½ when writing up her story.

Always a lover of pets, especially furry felines, she had suddenly developed a terrible reaction to her cat named "Killer." Her violent sneezes, watery eyes, and incessant scratching brought her to my office one day. Even after reminding her that the medical portion of my profession was as *an anthropologist* and not as an licensed physician, she still insisted that I help her in some way.

After ruling out all of the likely dietary, emotional, and environmental considerations that I could think of, I turned my attention to other things within her home. For instance, that cute ceramic coffee mug her folks had brought back with them from Cancun. It was usually what she drank her morning coffee from, she stated. Why? Was there something wrong with it? And that glazed crock-pot she sometimes cooked her favorite bean dishes in . . . how long had she been using that, I wondered aloud. I told her to get a good blood workup from a local chemical toxicologist and get back to me with the results.

Sometime later she returned with the results of this lead-screening test. They showed incredibly high lead levels exceeding 1,000 mcg. in some instances. This was totally unacceptable to the view expressed in the November/December 1986 issue of *Harrowsmith*: "The correct value for blood lead is *zero!*"

The first thing Mercedes did was to have the plumbing in her house checked for lead pipes or lead soldering around any of them that might be copper, and replaced them with plastic ones. Next, she discarded *all* glazed ceramic ware in her possession, opting for inexpensive heavy plastic dinnerware instead.

Then she went on a special diet that I had composed for her, consuming foods high in a water-soluble sulphur amino acid called cysteine. (In the body it's found more often in the form of cysteine instead.)

Cysteine-Containing Foods

Wheat germ	Cabbage
Granola	Brussels sprouts
Oat flakes	Broccoli
Yogurt	Cauliflower
Roast duck*	Baked beef liver (organic if possible)†

*Exceptionally high in cysteine.

†Very, very high in glutathione, a compound synthesized from cysteine, which is *the most important* member of the body's entire toxic waste disposal team.

I also recommended other foods high in vitamin E and selenium, which complement glutathione metabolism very nicely, thereby expediting removal of lead from her system more rapidly. Such foods included raw nuts, certain organ meats, trout and salmon (or other fish), lobster and brown rice.

In about a month on this program, Mercedes's allergic reactions to her cat had just about disappeared. Only an occasional sneeze was all that remained. And new blood-screening tests showed less than 45 mcg. of lead remaining in her body.

Mom's Difficult Diets During Pregnancy Led to Health Difference in Teenage Daughters. Renee and Linda H. are sisters. Renee, the older, is 16 and has only another year of high school before graduating; Linda, 14, just started in the same Salt Lake City high school in September 1990 as a sophomore. Their mother has been a student of mine.

Renee is often lethargic, easily prone to head colds, and can't seem to get rid of an excess buildup of mucus. Linda is spry and lively, seldom sick and hardly ever bothered with phlegm.

The difference between their present states of health isn't so much what they eat but rather what their mother ate when she was pregnant with each of them. Mrs. H. was a heavy milk drinker and ice cream gourmet as well as a frequent hamburger eater during her pregnancy with Renee. But before Linda came along, she had radically changed her dietary life-style, becoming a total vegan (someone who abstains from animal food of any kind, including milk, eggs, cheese, and seafood). The result was a much healthier and allergy-free younger daughter, who was also somewhat slimmer than her slightly round older sister. This shows just how dramatically a mother's diet can affect the health of her unborn child.

◆◆◆◆◆

ASTHMA, BRONCHITIS, AND EMPHYSEMA

Similarities Among Three Kinds of Suffocation

I've combined these three allergy-based diseases for two reasons. First, they're usually brought on by the same sets of conditions, that is, poor nutrition in early life, polluted air, and emotional stress, among other things. Second, the same "bad news" bacteria gang tends to wreck havoc with the immune system but in slightly different ways.

Asthma is a condition characterized by episodes of obstructed bronchi. Some asthmatics suffer due to things they're allergic to in their environment (feathers, fur, molds, dust, pollen, etc.). Others asthmatics are extremely sensitive to certain chemicals in the air, on the job, or in foods and medicines they need. In still others, respiratory infections can trigger asthmatic attacks at any time.

When an asthmatic inhales some pollen, eats a certain food, or otherwise comes in contact with substances to which he or she is allergic, the lungs react very dramatically. Small bronchial airways (the bronchioles) become narrow as muscle fibers tighten in spasm. At the same time, the allergic reaction causes a thickening and congesting of the mucous lining of these bronchioles, narrowing them even further. A third reaction that is common is that the mucus thickens up and plugs some smaller airways.

The effect of these reactions is to cause panting or difficult breathing, which is what the Greek word *asthma* means. During an attack the asthmatic can inhale and suck air into his alveoli, but when he commences to exhale, the tiny airways narrow even more and he has to exert extra pressure to blow the old air out. This means he has to exhale with great force to overcome the airway obstruction. As the air passes irregular narrowings, it often produces a wheezing sound. Then he coughs up phlegm or sputum to clear out the obstructing mucus.

Bronchitis (also called chronic bronchitis) is an even greater irritation of the airways and, as a rule, far more secretion of mucus occurs with fewer cilia to help bring it up. As a result, considerable coughing results. Every cough is a reflex respiratory explosion triggered by the weight of fluid on bronchial branches. The result is a rather "juicy" or productive cough that brings up the sputum. Such coughing and spitting must occur for 3 months out of 12 and for 2 years in a row to qualify as chronic bronchitis.

A hacking "smoker's cough" usually characterizes chronic bronchitis, even if the sufferer isn't a smoker. It comes early in the morning, but sometimes can occur at night, waking a person up. It's often accompanied by wheezing sounds in the chest that can be heard in the quiet of night and in the stillness of bed. The sputum is usually gray or speckled with black. Chronic bronchitis generally follows a bad chest cold or nasty bout of flu.

Emphysema can be easily discerned from the two previous forms of allergy suffocation. The cough isn't the juicy cough of asthma or bronchitis, in which sputum is spit up, but instead more of a dry nonproductive cough. But, as in bronchitis and asthma, the small airways of the lungs—irritated by many different air pollutants—become inflamed and swollen and offer tremendous resistance to exhaled air. This is further complicated by the thick mucus accumulating in the airways, due to the absence of cilia to move it upward. The situation can be additionally complicated by a touch of bronchitis.

The making of emphysema isn't simple. It's a process that results in the steady loss of the lungs' supporting tissues. It occurs silently with the victim who is unaware of the deterioration of his lungs. But it can likewise occur in various isolated sections of an individual's lungs and in different parts at various times. The ultimate destruction is of the lung's gas exchange "machinery," known as the alveolar membrane.

Some doctors believe that as American men become older, they may develop some undetected degree of emphysema. In 1970, Dr. Thomas L. Petty of the University of Colorado in Boulder stated that "perhaps 50% of men over the age of 40 have some degree of emphysema." And Dr. John A. Pierce of St.

Louis wrote that every person fortunate enough to attain 90 years of age "is unlucky enough to get some form of emphysema."

How a Doctor Got His Patient to Breathe Again

This is the true account of what a New England physician did for one of his patients who had started out with bronchial asthma but ended up with the early stages of emphysema as well. This remarkable episode of healing took place over two decades in Boston, Massachusetts. The physician was Dr. Gordon L. Snider, then professor of medicine and head of the Respiratory Disease Section, Department of Medicine, Boston University School of Medicine, and chief of the Pulmonary Disease Section at Boston University Hospital and Chief of the Pulmonary section, V.A. Hospital in Boston.

The patient was Lt. O'M., a veteran cop with the Boston Police Department. The family of the late Lt. O'M. supplied me with the details of Dr. Snider's therapy which had helped their father successfully cope with his respiratory problems for many years. Here are the basic points to that program, which should be of immense help to anyone else suffering from asthma, bronchitis, or emphysema or a combination of some of these.

The first thing Snider did with his patient was to have him stop smoking, period! He also insisted that his patient *not* be around any other smokers, so as not to further irritate his lungs. With what we now know about secondhand smoke, this advice makes quite a bit of sense.

Second, he got O'M. into the habit of *drinking more liquids each day!* This is critical to the success of the entire program. The body simply can't add enough moisture to the air that is breathed or to mucus unless it has some to start with. So O'M. had to be sure he was drinking enough fluids every day. Dr. Snider recommended tap water, fruit juices, hot clear soups, hot tea and coffee, some white wine, and a little nip of warm brandy a couple of times each week.

The third thing Snider had his patient do was to buy for himself a nebulizer, a device that makes water droplets by passing a jet of air over the end of a thin water tube or capillary, much like you'd find in a perfume atomizer. Unlike a home humidifier, a nebulizer produces more minute water droplets which can get beyond the throat and major airways.

But instead of using ordinary water, Dr. Snider had O'M. use salt water. The salt stabilized the droplets physically so that they would not evaporate and could travel deeper into O'M.'s airways. And since it was more like body fluids (which are certainly not pure water), the saline readily mixed with mucus. Also, the saline droplets didn't trigger as much coughing as ordinary water might have. O'M. made his own solution by dissolving 1 tbsp. of ordinary table salt into 1 quart of distilled water. Snider also advised his patient to use *very warm* water, which would feel more comfortable upon the lungs and make for a more effective mist as well.

O'M.'s daughter told me that her father had experimented a little himself with different items to include in with his saline solution. After a little trial and error, he discovered that a few drops of peppermint oil in the warm saltwater actually improved his breathing considerably. A good-quality peppermint oil can be obtained form Pure Herbs of Madison Heights, Michigan (see the appendix for details).

A fourth and very vital routine was actually a combination of two different procedures—posturnal drainage and chest wall percussion or vibration. The basic idea here was to let gravity work in the man's behalf and to move his body around so that specific airways were perpendicular to the floor or at least tilted down, so that the mucus could be pulled toward the larger airways, from which the phlegm could then be coughed up more easily. Snider had O'M. do it twice a day for 20 minutes each time after his mist treatments every morning and just before retiring each evening.

The drainage position was horizontal supine: O'M. lay on his back with a (nonfeather) pillow under his knees so his hips could be slightly elevated. The foot of his bed was raised 20 inches above the floor with bricks. This position drained his airways at the front of his lungs very nicely. On occasion, the patient was made to lay in the horizontal prone position, or face down, again with his feet lifted. A cushion placed under his hips spared his back considerable discomfort. This position allowed him to drain his lower bronchi and the back of his lungs.

Dr. Snider showed O'M.'s wife how to perform percussion or cupping, which assisted in loosening up accumulated mucus in the airways for easier expectoration later on. She clapped the outside of his chest at certain spots with her hands, while he was in one of several postural drainage positions. Her fingers and palms were held so that the hand assumed a sort of cupped configuration to trap a cushion of air. Then the cupped hands were clapped against the chest, much as one might clap the bottom of a bottle to get catsup out. Both hands were used alternately in rapid sequence for several seconds at a time. Later, she switched to a mechanical hand-held vibrator that did the job more effectively.

A fifth and equally important part of Snider's program was to retrain O'M. in proper breathing procedures: inhaling from the *abdomen* instead of the chest and exhaling with *pursed lips* (as when you pucker up to whistle) instead of an open mouth. Snider had successfully taught yoga breathing exercises to hundreds of other respiratory disease patients in Chicago and Milwaukee. This breathing routine is more slow and measured, but definitely better for those suffering from asthma, bronchitis, or emphysema.

The main concern in learning abdominal breathing is what to do with the stomach. O'M. was told to direct his attention away from his chest entirely and to, instead, concentrate solely on the muscles of his abdomen, on protruding it forward as he inhaled and squeezing it tighter as he exhaled. This little ditty helped him, and may help you, remember what to do:

Breath in, belly out,
Breathe out, belly in.

Learning to coordinate movements of his chest and abdomen in breathing, when sitting, standing, and walking was something else O'M. had to do. For instance, while putting his shoes on, he inhaled deeply as he sat upright with shoe in hand, then exhaled slowly as he leaned forward to put his foot in the shoe. When he walked, he was taught to take two steps inhaling and then four steps exhaling. Dr. Snider also taught him to not stand ramrod straight but to bend forward slightly to ease the tension on his abdominal muscles and to relieve the strain on his lower back.

The final part of Snider's remarkable program consisted of putting O'M. on a *gradual but steady* exercise routine, which combined leisurely strolling, pedaling a bicycle, and *slowly* going up and down steps. These daily exercises became an integral part of the overall reconditioning of O'M.'s sick body.

The end result of all this, according to O'M.'s son-in-law and daughter, was that he lived an additional 17 years of quality life with only *minimal* breathing difficulties. And all of this was done with little or no medication or other supplements or remedies. The retired police officer eventually gave up dairy products and eggs once he discovered just how mucus forming they were. And, so, one of Boston's finest became a well man again.

The Role of Diet

Those suffering from asthma, chronic bronchitis, or emphysema may obtain new dietary strategies for moderating their periodic respiratory distress, according to a study involving 9,074 adults aged 30 and older. As part of the Second National Health and Nutrition Exam Survey (NHANES II) conducted between 1976 and 1980, researchers asked volunteers to recall what they had eaten the day before. Scott T. Weiss at the Harvard Medical School in Boston and Joel Schwartz of the Environmental Protection Agency in Washington, D.C., have now analyzed the recalled food choices in light of the respondents' respiratory histories, as determined during NHANES II thorough medical exams and personal interviews.

In the July 1990 *American Journal of Epidemiology*, they reported that diets low in vitamin C, fish, or their zinc-to-copper ratio as well as diets with a high sodium-to-potassium ratio, increased the risk of bronchitis and wheezing, regardless of a person's age, gender, smoking history, or area of residence. Low niacin levels also correlated with a risk of wheezing. The new findings even suggest that "diet may play a role in the susceptibility of certain smokers to the development of chronic bronchitis and emphysema," they say.

Onions also seem to be beneficial. The May/June 1984 issue of *Agents Actions* reported that when guinea pigs were pretreated with a crude onion extract, a protective effect against allergen-induced bronchial obstruction was noticed. The report's two authors speculated that onion could prove very useful in bronchial asthma treatment in humans as well.

◆◆◆◆◆

CHRONIC FATIGUE SYNDROME

Symptoms that Baffle the Mind

In 1974, an Albuquerque, New Mexico, housewife named Nancy K. felt as if she were slowly dying. She was weak, profoundly tired, and plagued by constant bladder infections. Her muscles ached terribly. Her mood shifted unpredictably. Her memory seemed to be failing. "If this is menopause," she remembers thinking, "then this is horrible, even worse than I ever imagined it could be." A hysterectomy followed and then later came extensive psychoanalysis because it was believed that she was "mourning her lost uterus." By 1987, she had been to *212 different doctors* until the last one correctly identified her problem as chronic fatigue syndrome.

In 1984, people in a small resort town on the north shore of Lake Tahoe, Nevada, started experiencing a disease that was hard to define as well as treat. In less than three months, nearly 200 of the 20,000 residents of Incline Village had developed the same symptoms; worse yet, no one was getting any better. Nearly all of the victims were mass-producing antibodies to Epstein-Barr, the herpes virus known to cause infectious mononucleosis. But mono is rare in adults and *epidemics* of adult mono have *never* been heard of. The Atlanta-based Centers for Disease Control finally identified it as chronic fatigue syndrome (CFS).

And the most bizarre of all cases on a somewhat massive scale occurred in Great Britain in 1990. It all started in Bristol with an ordinary house cat named Max. The furry feline ate some cooked beef and promptly succumbed to the ravages of mad cow disease or bovine spongiform encephalopathy (BSE), which until then was largely ignored by the British press. This mysterious malady was turning cows' brains to mush, making the beasts mad, bad, and potentially dangerous to eat. Otherwise normal cows contentedly grazing in pastures would suddenly start staggering and snapping before flopping on the ground to die. Well over 20,000 cows died, and British beef consumption plunged almost 40% in the process. A cover story on CFS in the November 12, 1990 issue of *Newsweek* magazine linked this malady to it.

From these examples we can see that not only can CFS mimic other problems and possibly be transmitted from person to person, but it can also go from one species to another in a very short period of time. *Newsweek* accurately described it as "the disease of the '90s," which now afflicts between 2 and 5 million Americans. And as *The New York Times* piece in September 5, 1990 issue noted, CFS "is also known as 'yuppie flu' because it tends to strike well-educated people in their 30's."

Common symptoms include fevers and lymph-node swelling, night sweats, persistent diarrhea, joint and muscle pain, and rapid weight loss. Say, don't they have a disturbingly similar ring to them? If you're acquainted with AIDS, then you'd be apt to find certain frightening similarities between the two. But this gray plague doesn't kill people—it just turns them into confused and helpless invalids. Many patients suffer mood swings or panic attacks (common in hypoglycemia), and most develop a low-grade dementia of some sort. Sleep disturbances and vision problems are frequent. And though the illness sometimes lifts after a few hellish months, it can linger for years—or recede only to return.

The fact that CFS comes and goes at random, often making sudden appearances, has led some scientists at the University of Miami to suggest that dormant viruses might immediately become activated by another virus. It's believed that something as simple as cold or flu germs can trigger either the Epstein-Barr virus, cytomegalovirus, of HHV-6 virus into quick activity after they've remained dormant for years.

At a special conference sponsored by the Chronic Fatigue Immune Disease Syndrome Association held on November 18, 1990 in Charlotte, South Carolina, Dr. Jay Levy, a professor of medicine and a leading AIDS researcher at the University of California-San Francisco, reported that once such viruses are reactivated, they, in turn, can stimulate immune system cells. These immune defenses start cranking out infection-fighting substances known as cytokines. Typical of such cytokines would be interferon and tumor necrosis factor, which are known to produce symptoms found in CFS patients, he said. While such activation is normal when someone is infected with a cold or flu virus, the reaction usually subsides relatively soon. But in fatigue patients, the activation seems to continue for years, he noted, almost like a leaky faucet of sorts.

In comparing the immune systems of 120 patients with CFS to nearly 80 others who were healthy or had other diseases, Dr. Levy discovered that the CFS group had "chronically elevated levels of one type of white blood cells called CD8 killer T cells. This dysfunction impairment within the immune system leads to an almost immediate drop in energy levels, hence the debilitating fatigue that follows.

Drug-Induced Plagues

A growing body of medical and scientific literature has appeared supporting a rather novel explanation for the appearance of such new and never-before-heard-of maladies like AIDS and CFS—the widespread use of antibiotics in humans and in animal feed. This single factor, say the experts, has laid sufficient groundwork in the last couple of decades for the sudden appearances of the diseases we're now seeing in near epidemic proportions.

According to the July 6, 1990 issue of *Science*, this has been primarily responsible for the *increased* "rise of drug resistance among harmless and harmful bacteria alike." Worse still says the periodical, such antibiotics have induced the harmless bacteria "to serve as a reservoir for resistance genes, which can then be transferred to virulent strains within an individual." These developments spawn a microbial one-two punch of sorts: a highly poisonous and resistant pathogen capable of wrecking unbelievable havoc within the immune system!

The *Newsweek* feature on CFS pointed out an interesting thread common to 87% of those afflicted with this infectious disease: many of them have either had a history of allergies or else have been occasionally allergic to simple things. "We're discovering as we work with more chronic fatigue syndrome patients," one Houston doctor told me recently, "that the majority have had allergies of some sort." It's the opinion of Dr. C. K. Duncan that "allergies serve as a type of precursor [forerunner] to things like this [CFS]." If allergies can be brought under control, he feels, "then a lot of this syndrome would disappear of its own accord." Allergies, he thinks, contribute to the reactivation of certain lethal viruses from their dormant states. We've already discussed the link between antibiotics and allergy formation.

What a Texas Physician Did to Conquer CFS

Dr. Charles Kilroy Duncan is a holistic healer with an independent mind. "I do what I want, when I want, and to whom I want!" he said with an air of authority during my 1986 visit with him on the outskirts of Houston. But one thing that has set C.K. apart from most other doctors (besides his middle name, of course) is the program he's developed over the years to help many of his CFS patients get well again. While some nonsupplemental aspects to it duplicate Dr. Snider's treatment for asthma, bronchitis, and emphysema, some of the most important parts of his therapy are the different herbs and nutrients he insists that his patients take *on a regular daily basis.* "You have to be faithful to the remedial side of my program," he points out, "or else those viruses will just flare up again like one of them oil well fires that hasn't been completely put out yet."

C.K. discovered that certain Oriental herbal compounds, when taken together, worked synergistically to boost the body's output of physical and mental energies. "It came about quite by accident," he said, "when I was attending a medical conference in Seattle, Washington." In between lecture sessions, he visited a downtown Chinese herb shop and discovered the Li Chung Yun formulas. "I brought a few bottles of different formulas," he continued, "and took them back home with me more as souveniers, I suppose, than anything serious in the way of supplementation." Soon, he was having a few of his office staff try them out "for fun" to see if they'd really work. "Imagine my surprise when they reported to met that their stamina seemed increased more after taking these products. That's when I started to investigate them more closely," he finished. The result was that three of the products became an integral part of his recovery program for CFS patients.

In the morning each patient is instructed to take 3 capsules of Li Chung Yun L Formula 18 with 6 fl. oz. of *mineral* water. "I've found that Perrier works the best in assisting these herbs to rejuvenate the liver," he maintains. Sometime before noon, he has patients take the Li Chung Yun Super Compound Formula 3 to help them "shift their gears into overdrive, if necessary" so they can get through the rest of the day. The same amount of these is taken as well, but with *warm* ginseng herbal tea or black or green tea instead.

By midafternoon the body is ready for a good compound that can perk up the immune system, but also keep energy at an optimal level. The Li Chung Yun Pei Pai Li Formula 4 has ingredients like wild cherry bark, horehound herb, and golden-seal root which exert a decided antibiotic influence upon the body, and other herbs like cayenne fruit, ginger and licorice roots, and orange peel that keep vitality high. "It's really got the best of both worlds," Dr. Duncan insists. "You have immune boosters and energy stimulants all in one formula." Patients are advised to take 4 capsules daily *with warm herb tea* of some kind. "I think *what* these formulas are taken with is just as important as how many capsules to swallow at one time," he said.

In the evening and again just before retiring for the night, he recommends that this CFS patients drink a couple of cups of ginseng tea. All these formulas can be readily obtained from most Chinese herb shops and a few selected health food stores. (Albi Imports is a good source; see the appendix for details.)

Dr. Duncan recognizes the importance of certain nutrients crucial for energy production. Energy is stored in the body in the form of glycogen, a compound produced from the carbohydrates we eat and stored in the liver and muscles. When energy is needed, glycogen is converted into glucose, which is then converted (through a complex chain of 10 intermediate steps) into an energy-storage compound called adenosine triphosphate (commonly known as ATP). When ATP splits, it releases the energy needed to move muscles.

"Vitamin B-6 is critical to those recovering from chronic fatigue syndrome," he reminded me. This particular vitamin contains over 50 different enzymes, some of which play a strong role in carbohydrate metabolism to break down glycogen into glucose. Organic beef liver (or dessicated liver tablets from any health food store), canned tunafish, banana, lentils and split peas, broccoli, green snap beans, green peas, and carrots are just some of the foods high in vitamin B-6. Spinach is an additional source of this nutrient. In supplement form about 50 milligrams of vitamin B-6 every *other* day is useful, he says. (Quest Vitamins is a good source for this; see the appendix for details.)

C.K. feels that enzymes are a sorely neglected part of any *good* CFS recovery program. For the uninitiated, enzymes are nothing more than very large proteins that activate certain reactions in the body to form specific substances. All biochemical reactions are essentially enzyme motivated, each by a particular enzyme; and each cell contains many different enzymes. In fact, most chemical reactions in cells would occur too slowly to support life were it not for activation by enzymes.

Two of the very best foods for supplying the body with badly needed enzymes to boost energy levels are *raw* pineapple and papaya. Each contains a unique proteolytic enzyme— bromelain from pineapple and papain from papaya—which can stimulate not only the release of energy from the liver, but can do the same for certain immune system cells as well. A pair of concentrated food supplements developed in Japan by the Wakunaga Pharmaceutical Corp. (makers of the odor-modified garlic called kyolic) are also quite helpful in replenishing those enzymes necessary for strength. Two Kyo-Dophilus capsules taken with 8 fl. oz. of Kyo-Green (1 level tsp. of powder in water) gives the body unbelievable energy (see the appendix for details). Dr. Duncan's program works—just ask his patients who've been helped by it!

◆◆◆◆◆

CONJUNCTIVITIS

Doing Something About "Pink Eye"

Commonly called "pink eye," conjunctivitis has generally been associated with a bad cold or flu. More recently, though, a number of allergens have been provoking many incidents of it in children and adults. An infected or irritated eye is typically bright pink where it ought to be white and produces a yellowish discharge that may cause the eyelids to stick together during sleep.

Such discharge can be removed with cotton balls moistened in a little boric acid solution. (Boric acid powder is available from most drugstores; follow the directions on the container.) The cotton balls should then be discarded after one use. Make a cool compress by soaking a clean wash cloth in a solution of mint/chamomile tea, wring out the excess liquid, and then place it over the closed eyes for relief. To make the tea, boil 1 pint of water, turn off heat, add ½ tsp. of each herb, cover with lid and steep 30 minutes before straining.

Since infectious or allergic conjunctivitis can spread rapidly among family members and friends, the person with it should take exceptional care to avoid touching the eye and should wash the hands thoroughly after any contact with the eye. No one should share that person's wash cloths or towels.

A Remedy for Contact Lens Allergy

One of my students has been wearing contact lenses since he was 13 years old. Not too long ago, his eyes were afflicted by vernal keratoconjunctivitis, a condition of extreme itchiness and sensitivity to light. A stringy, yellowish mucus discharge was prevalent, and beneath each of his upper lids, large pimples appeared.

He tried several antihistamine/decongestant eye medications, but with rather poor results. One day after class, he asked me what alternative remedies there were. I told him how to make an eye lotion out of elder flowers, elecampane root, and eyebright herb.

First, I said, he should boil up a pint of Mt. Olympus spring water and then add ½ tsp. of dried, cut elecampane root, cover with a lid, turn down the heat and simmer for about 4 minutes. Then he should uncover the pot, add ½ tsp. of eyebright herb, cover again and simmer for *only* 1½ minutes. Then uncover a final time, adding the dried elder flowers, put the lid back on and steep for 20 minutes. After straining the contents, he was to put several drops of the *lukewarm* liquid in each eye and leave there for 10 minutes with his head tilted back. Additionally, he took 25,000 I.U. of fish-oil vitamin A and 3,500 mg. of citrus-derived vitamin C. In about two weeks he reported to me that a local ophthalmologist in rechecking his eyes had said that they were now much better than before.

An Eye Formula that Works

Back in the late 1970s early 1980s, I spent some time lecturing, writing, and doing research in the Canadian province of Quebec. During my time there, I accumulated a wealth of medical folklore, some of which eventually went into the creation of a rather interesting herbal formula for vision problems in general.

A couple of years ago, a small Quebec herb company, Les Produits (Elite Products, Inc.), in Beaconsfield (a bedroom suburb of Montreal) bought the formula and marketed it under the name of Iris. It differed from other herbal eye products in one respect: 50% of the ingredients focused primarily on rebuilding the health of the *liver*, of all things! The rest of the herbs in it dealt strictly with improving the vision. I met the owners again in Toronto in late October, 1990 while I was speaking at the Canadian Health Food Association, and they told me of the many successes which people were having with this particular product. (See the appendix for more details.)

◆◆◆◆◆

ECOLOGICAL ILLNESS

Allergic to Life

A new breed of doctors specialize in something loosely termed "clinical ecology." Their patients are those with the ultimate allergies—multiple reactions to just about everything around them. They have become ultrasensitive victims to an increasingly polluted environment.

Such victims experience myriad ills from allergies induced by everything from polyester wear to sipping disodium guanylate in their chowder to no-wax floors, office copiers, perfumes, and even ordinary hamburgers. The symptoms of these silent insults to weakened immune systems are many and varied: nausea, diarrhea, headaches, blurred vision, dizziness, fatigue, confusion, cramps, wobbly knees, asthma, fevers, "brain fag," anxiety, schizophrenia, arthritis, alcoholism, and so forth.

"About 90% of us have some type of sensitivity—to a soap or cleaning agent that may make our eyes water or our skin itch, to some food that could put us to sleep," ecologist Dr. Alfred Johnson, then of the Environmental Health Center in Dallas, Texas, told me back in the fall of 1983. But all of these are "normal allergenic responses" as he put it. However, the bodies of hypersensitive people are unable to cope with the vast array of chemicals in our polluted world. As a result their systems become overloaded and, in time, completely short circuit, Dr. Johnson noted. "Some of my patients," he said, "have to wear special natural fabric gloves to turn the pages of books they wish to read."

A recent issue (October 1990) of *The Times* of London blamed pollution in general for the many environmental allergies people seem to suffer from these days. "Each generation is getting weaker as pollution builds up and wears down the immune system," claims allergy specialist Dr. Jean Monro of Britain's Breakspear Hospital for Allergy and Environmental Medicine. Environmental pollution, failure to breast-feed babies, the addition of chemicals to food and water supplies, and an unwise use of medicines and drugs are cited as contributing factors. Diseases ranging from asthma to cancer, and even child behavioral problems, result. An estimated 17 million people, some 30% of Britain's entire population could be suffering from environmentally induced ailments, many without ever realizing it, the newspaper reported.

Focusing on the Liver-Mind Connection

Michael Tierra, a clinical herbalist from Santa Cruz, California, whom I've known for years, thinks "that the liver should be the central focus of allergy treatments . . . "If the liver is continually overworked in the process of detoxification," he asserts, "then all of its myriad functions become faulty, and various diseases such as allergy will naturally manifest."

Michael takes a truly holistic approach to the problems resulting from ecological illnesses. Besides just recommending tremendous liver herbs like dandelion, burdock and sarsaparilla roots, sweet flag or calamus rhizome, chamomile flowers, and cascara sagrada bark, he also believes that "the mind plays an equally significant role and may often be the root of the problem" with the liver itself. As Dr. Tierra told me a couple of years ago, "Negative feelings, thoughts, and attitudes can produce hormonal reactions harmful to the liver. For instance, John, someone who is easily angered has an adrenalin rush each time he blows up. This constant release of internal toxins further burdens the liver. If the anger persists—especially in the context of overeating and too much fatty, oily food—the liver becomes overtaxed and begins to function improperly, sometimes resulting in allergenic tendencies. . . . If the spirit is sick, the body will not change."

Theron G. Randolph, M.D., of Chicago, a founder of clinical ecology, thinks that the liver-mind connection postulated by Dr. Tierra has medical relevance "in terms of what we're seeing on a daily basis with our own patients." He and others like him scattered around the country testify to a great deal of mental anxiety and emotional uncertainty in the majority of their ultra-sensitive patients.

One south Florida doctor put it quite bluntly: "To hell with liver, I say, and just work on the patient's mind. Once you can get the brain unscrewed and a person's thinking straightened out about how he sees the world or himself in general, then I think you've got a pretty good handle on the rest of that individual's problems." This particular physician, in fact, emphasizes the importance of strong self-esteem with his patients. "I think that respect for self is about 40% of the therapy to ecological health problems," he insists. "Hell, a little pride never hurt anybody. Just look at me . . . I have an ego as big as an elephant, and hell, I've *never* had a *single* allergy in my life!" Well, arrogance may not be for everybody, but a feeling of *strong* self-worth probably makes for an equally strong liver, which Dr. Tierra would obviously agreed with, too.

A Food Treatment for Ecological Poisoning

Within the last several years I've had a chance to personally speak or correspond with some of those rare individuals who've become basically allergic to just about everything in the environment that might irritate the immune system in some way or another. Two of these are Sandy S., a woman in her late thirties, and Jolene O.'s 20-year-old daughter, Janae.

Both women have accurately portrayed themselves as virtual "environmental reactors" to anything synthetic and manmade. Their symptoms are similar, and while their remedial approaches have taken somewhat different paths, yet in at least one thing they have held to a common course—that being a simple food treatment for sick livers, which has enabled them to cope pretty well with their respective ecological illnesses.

Sandy informed me that her tomato-lemon juice concoction "really has been fantastic for doing a detox on my liver." In fact, she said, "I find that I don't react nearly as badly to things like soap, soft water, or bleaches when I follow this cleansing routine on a regular basis than when I neglect it." Young Janae also testified that this food treatment "has been helping me show some improvement with all of my allergies."

In a nutshell, here is what their simple program consists of. *Organic* tomatoes (and they *must be* organically grown, too) are cut up into small pieces and simmered in a waterless cookware stainless steel pot with about half-a-cup of lemon juice and a pinch of cayenne pepper, covered, for approximately 20 minutes. When cool, the mixture is put through a food blender and a 10-fl.-oz. glass drunk before the main meal of the day. Janae also consumes quite a bit of *organic* cooked cabbage as well. And both women have replaced regular conventional lighting with *full-spectrum* lighting fixtures, believing that it helps in some measure, too.

Sandy also spoke highly of the European herb, milk thistle, which has been medically documented to be one of the very best things for environmentally poisoned livers. Nature's Way sells this herb in a product called Thisilyn, available at nearly all health food stores. While these few things can't solve all the problems connected with ecological illness, they can certainly bring some improvements to a very puzzling disease.

◆◆◆◆◆

FOOD ALLERGIES

Symptoms to Look For

My good friend, Lendon Smith, M.D., a retired Oregon pediatrician, prefers to call such allergies "food intolerances" or "food sensitivities," because they more correctly describe the problems involved. Lendon believes that close to 90% of *all* food intolerances in adults began when they were very young, and their moms attempted to feed them solid foods before they were old enough (one year) to handle such things properly. Such a dietary stress imposed during infancy makes most young bodies extremely susceptible to food-modulated allergens.

Lendon believes that the common diagnostic tool of the allergist, namely, skin testing, is virtually worthless. "The patient would do better by testing himself," he argues. Look for common symptoms first, he suggests: headache, postnasal drip ("snorting," "sniffing," "throat clearing," "zonking"), stomachache, diarrhea, tissue edema ("puffy eyes," "fullness in head and chest," "leg aches"), bed wetting, plugged nose, intestinal gas ("a lot of fartin' "), abdominal pain, anal itching, and even insomnia.

Once any of these symptoms have been detected, he says, then try to isolate those particular foods which seem to bring such physical miseries on. After eliminating each offending food from the diet, watch to see whether or not any of these symptoms returns. If they don't, then you know that you have an unusual sensitivity toward that particular staple. And if you want to make doubly sure, just add that food back into your regular diet for a couple of days and see if the same mean cycle repeats itself.

More interesting is the fact that a particular food intolerance will typically "move from one organ to another," Smith states. "I had a patient," he said, "who had a stomach reaction to milk as an infant in the form of colic. Then it moved to his lungs as asthma when he drank the stuff at 18 months of age. From there it relocated in the kidneys and bladder, and he started bed wetting at age 7. Now that he's a grown young man of 21, he gets a skin rash whenever he drinks too much milk."

Also, some symptoms of food intolerance can be quite subtle and require greater detective work to spot. For instance, muscle cramps might be due to low calcium, but a food sensitivity could *also* induce the same spasm. So a person might drink milk in the belief that he needs calcium, but is only exacerbating his problem. Lendon recalls the time he "had a father tell me about his daughter, who couldn't relax and go to sleep at a reasonable bedtime until she stopped drinking milk." Yet the mother kept encouraging their girl to drink a warm glass of milk assuming that it would calm her down. Under normal circumstances, it would do this very thing, but *not* when someone has developed an intolerance to it. Lendon tried to explain to the father that his wife's chronic bronchitis was due to the same exact sensitivity to milk that afflicted their daughter, only that it had moved to a different organ system in the older woman. But he didn't have much success in convincing the man of this fact.

The most common food allergens are cow's milk, corn, wheat, sugar, eggs, yeast, and soy in that approximate order. But just because you abstain from these things *directly* is no guarantee that you won't get them in some other way *indirectly*. For instance, you might avoid straight cow's milk, but never imagine that the creamed soup, cream vegetables, or processed meats you're using are loaded with *powdered* milk! And what about that delicious cob of corn! Why, of course, you'd avoid it if you knew it was causing allergic symptoms. But what about those jams, jellies, peanut butter, cookies, chewing gum, catsup, mayonnaise, luncheon meats, and even soft drinks and beer? Well, *all* of them contain corn syrup as a sweetening agent (not to mention sugar). And most products labeled as "vegetable oil" usually contain corn oil.

Dr. Smith recalled two rather bizarre cases in which two of his patients, who had severe reactions to *anything* with corn in it, couldn't figure out just what was causing their allergic flareups. After weeks and weeks of eliminating *every single thing* in their diets they could think of that contained corn in some form, they finally narrowed the culprits down to two *non*food items: the glue on the back of envelopes and stamps, which one woman in her secretarial job kept licking with her tongue, and a brand of toothpaste used by the other lady regularly to brush her teeth.

So just remember this when it comes to food intolerances: the obvious may not always be as apparent. You may, in fact, have to do some serious investigative work until the *real* offense is found! With food intolerances, nothing ever should be taken for granted or face value, Lendon warns. It is also interesting to note, he says, "that 80% of people with food intolerances have *hypoglycemia* as well!"

Nutritional Therapy a Doctor Recommends

My friend Lendon practiced medicine for almost 40 years. He served as a clinical professor of pediatrics at the University of Oregon Medical School for a number of years and hosted a very popular syndicated health show on the ABC television network. His books have sold in the millions, making him a virtual household name from coast to coast. Thus, many, many people have come to trust what he says.

Occasionally we've had the good pleasure of being on the same panel together at this or that health or medical convention around the country. During such moments, I've quizzed him on what supplements he'd recommend for food intolerances, and here's what he came up with:

- *Vitamin A.* Take an average of 20,000 I.U. daily.
- *Vitamin B-6.* Take around 300 mg. daily.
- *Folic acid* (B-complex group). "Helps with food absorption." About 10 mg. daily is what he prescribes.
- *Niacin* (B-complex group). "Helps to control food intolerance nicely." Between 8–10 *grams* daily, he says.
- *Panthothenic acid* (B-complex group). About 750 mg. daily.
- *Vitamin C.* A daily "maintenance dose" of about 12,000 mg., but can "be increased daily by 1,000 mg. until one's stools are a little loose," he insists. Vitamin C has a *strong antihistamine* action useful in all allergies!
- *Vitamin E.* On this, he gave no specific amounts only to say that it helps "potentiate the A" more. (I suggest *no more* than 400 I.U. daily.)
- *Vitamin D.* Helps with calcium absorption. Get out in the sun more to get your daily dose of D!

- *Calcium.* Again no specific amounts were given by him, but I'd recommend about 1,000 mg. daily.
- *Magnesium.* He gave no firm amounts, but I'd say 400 mg. daily.
- *Selenium.* 50–150 mg. may protect the cell walls against food intolerance, he believes.
- *Zinc, chromium, and manganese.* An all-purpose trace mineral tablet [containing these] is good to take, he thinks.

Quest Vitamins of Vancouver, Canada probably has the best single vitamins and minerals anywhere in the industry. They're also available in the United States as well. And a good trace mineral compound called Aqua-Vite may be obtained from Great American Natural Products of St. Petersburg, Florida. (See the appendix for more details.)

Diet Programs for Reducing Food Allergens

My colleague Lendon has several sure solutions for eliminating most of the symptoms common to food intolerances. One of the most basic is a four-day fast, taking nothing but distilled water, routinely performed every month or six weeks. Usually a weekend or a long holiday period is best because not so much physical energy is required. Obviously, those afflicted with diabetes or hypoglycemia will need to modify this diet somewhat with mild foods to keep their energy levels up.

If a water-only diet is not for you, Lendon recommends the following simple program which should eliminate the most common allergens.

Breakfast: Small cube steak or cooked oatmeal, 1 small banana, 1 medium apple, 5 pineapple rings, or 1 cup of prunes.

Lunch: Tender veal, 1 cup of either almonds or walnuts, half a cup of *organically grown* raisins (other kinds are heavily saturated with DDT and can actually aggravate existing symptoms).

Supper: Fresh- or saltwater fish (steamed or baked) or roast lamb, cooked brown rice or sweet potato, carrots and *organic* red leafy lettuce (not iceberg).

Dr. Smith points out that with his water fast, many food-sensitive people will encounter headaches, fatigue, and other withdrawal symptoms on the second and third day, but by the fourth start noticing definite improvements in how they feel. If an offending item isn't eaten for three months, it can be eaten again every four to five days without side effects. On his modified diet, several days must pass before enough of the allergens are gone for the person to start feeling better.

On an elimination diet to get rid of food allergens, the produce listed on the next page, preferably organic, is permitted.

One final point that Lendon has stressed to thousands of his patients throughout the years, "If you leave white sugar and sugary foods alone, most of your allergies will *completely disappear* of their own accord!"

How a Rotation Diet Saved One Scientist's Life

Ms. Elaine C. is an immunologist, who studies the progress of certain diseases. During a recent medical conference we both attended, she shared the following true story with me and gave her consent for me to use it here.

In 1976, Ms. C. was doing some histocompatibility studies on T cells at the National Institutes of Health in Bethesda, Maryland. The work required her lab to kill, shave, and remove the lymph glands of several guinea pigs each day. "There was fur everywhere," she recalled, "each and every day. We became rather cavalier about the whole thing; we'd dig the fur out of our noses and just go right back to work. Sometimes we'd joke with each other about who might have the biggest fur ball in their gut."

But then she began to take things more seriously when she noticed she was short of breath after bicycling to work a couple of mornings. "I was blue in the face from lack of sufficient oxygen. I would have to sit at my desk in order to catch my breath," she said. Barely 30 years old, she imagined the worst and believed she had coronary heart disease. Only after the attacks began occurring more frequently, even when she hadn't

VEGETABLES	FRUITS
Asparagus	Apples
Cauliflower	Berries (different kinds)
Brussels sprouts	Citrus
Cabbage	Figs
Radish	Dates
Celery	Melons (different
Beets	kinds)
Cucumber	Plums
Avocado	Nectarines
Kale	Peaches
Kohl-rabi	Pears
Okra	Cherries
Carrot	Cranberries
Parsnip	Bananas
Yam	Grapes
Sweet potato	Raisins
Green pepper	Apricots
Broccoli	Persimmons
Beans (string, lima)	
Squash (different kinds)	
Greens (beet, mustard, spinach, turnip, collards)	
Bean sprouts	

been out exercising, did she finally go see a physician. "He ran a series of tests and informed me that I had what appeared to be asthma," she explained. "He put me on different medications for this, but none of them helped. The symptoms just got worse. So I decided to start wearing a full-face mask, complete with air filters, to keep that fur out of my system. It seemed to help a little in the beginning, but my shortness of breath soon returned even *after* I had left our laboratory at the end of every day."

A friend referred her to a local doctor specializing in ecological medicine and food intolerances. A lengthy questionnaire that she had to fill out soon told the physician what he needed to know. "He basically said that my hamburgers, french fries, milk shakes, doughnuts, colas, and soft drinks had to go," she replied. "In other words, the guinea pig fur was merely a surface irritant for a more deeply rooted allergy, namely, my inability to handle junk food."

Elaine was put on a special rotation diet, in which she could group together members of the same food family. These foods were consumed on the same day, since they were chemically similar. For instance, asparagus, garlic, leeks, and onions belong to the same family, so she was able to eat any of them in the same day. However, the program was flexible enough to allow members of the same food family to be eaten on different days, just so long as there were two days intervening. For instance, she could have grapefruit on Monday, and then eat oranges on Thursday.

Now each rotation diet is different and needs to be built around those "safe" foods that only *your* body chemistry can tolerate. Ms. C.'s diet was established for her own physiological needs, but probably isn't very useful for someone else. She had to stay away from all of her problem foods for at least four months. She told me that "In less than five weeks time, my breathing returned to normal and I've had no further problems since."

In the event someone had severe multiple food intolerances, there might be only enough safe foods to eat one per meal, but that person could eat as much of that food as he or she desired. After a while the person might try adding more foods, one at a time, to his or her own rotation diet. Then if there were a reaction, the food should be eliminated again for several months.

Spices Help Reduce Food Intolerances

Over the years in my visits with hundreds of different folk healers from numerous cultures, I've discovered that spices contain valuable healing properties often overlooked by the medical profession. One of their virtues is their ability to *diminish* food intolerances. And they seem to do it quite nicely in the process.

Some friends of mine from Tempe, Arizona, Rick and Vicki W., have a couple of boys who were afflicted with celiac disease when they were just youngsters. Their parents took them to every specialist they could think of, but to no avail. Nothing really seemed to work except to feed their sons gluten-*free* bread and cereal.

One time when I was in the Phoenix area to lecture at a medical conference, I dropped by for a short visit. They asked what natural substances were available to help with this malady. I recommended the powdered spice cardamom, and suggested the following recipe:

To a pot of cooked oatmeal that would yield four average servings, add a level teaspoonful of cardamom about 2 minutes before it is ready to take from the stove. My friends tried this and discovered to their delight that their boys could easily eat this cereal without encountering the usual smelly diarrhea and abdominal swelling typical of this food intolerance. They also put cardamom into the oatmeal cookies with good results.

A more recent and very bizarre case came to my attention in October 1990. A white, middle-class, female, age 45, who stands 5-foot 1-inch in stockings and weighs just 116 lb. wrote me two lengthy letters from her home in Fresh Meadows, New York. A portion of R.A.'s first letter to me dated October 6 read as follows:

> I neglected to say that about the age of 26, I developed a severe reaction to *heavy* electronic fields. When I walked under high power tension lines, near *color* T.V.s, I would feel my whole metabolism speeding up, feel electric shocks on my nerves, get dizzy and tense and the next day break out in acne. It felt as if my body was in some way picking up the electromagnetic field.
>
> ... At 33 my symptoms began to change. The colitis improved somewhat, but I came down with severe *clinical* depression (some say this can happen when meditating too much) and horrible nervousness, also severe migraine.
>
> ... I finally went to an allergist who gave me a R.A.S.T. Test and found me incredibly [sic] allergic to *most all*

foods. What's more, when I went near electrical equipment, the allergies were greatly exacerbated. . . .

So what do I eat, you must be asking. By trial and error I found I could eat *parsley*, which seems to calm me, dill, parsnips and turnips and asparagus. And when I feel a little better I have a hamburger, maybe with a little rosemary or time [sic] on it. I find that some cooking spices help me not to be so allergic to foods.

Another interesting point is that when I go to a saltwater bay area and stay for the day, my allergic symptoms diminish and I can eat much more foods to which I am usually allergic to at home. One allergist said that being around saltwater areas helps many allergic patients. I can actually feel my body calming down there. There is also an essence of saltwater being sold in Europe which *calms* tense people upon inhaling it.

To help overcome your own food sensitivities, learn to season your meals with sea salt, anise seed, basil, bay, caraway seed, cardamom, celery seed, chervil, cinnamon, cloves, coriander, cumin, dill, fennel seed, fenugreek seed, garlic, ginger, mace, marjoram, mustard, nutmeg, onion, oregano, paprika, parsley, pepper (black, red, white), rosemary, sage, savory, sesame seed (decorticated), tarragon, thyme, and turmeric.

In "How I Came Clean," journalist David Steinman reported his own experience in the June 1990 issue of *California* magazine. Discovering that he had astronomical levels of DDT in his bloodstream, he radically changed the way he ate. Central to this one man's diet back from the brink were certain key spices, which helped to flush toxic residues from his body for good.

◆◆◆◆◆

HAY FEVER

How I Control My Own Hay Fever

For the first five years of my life, I grew up on a farm in Sandy, Utah. You wouldn't know it now, but then it was covered with hundreds of peach trees and stream-fed pastures for our grazing cows. During this time, I drank *a lot* of *raw* milk without any apparent problems.

It was only when my parents sold their land and moved into the city, where I started drinking *pasteurized* milk, that my allergy problems began. The symptoms common to hay fever gradually worsened in my late teens and twenties. During most of my thirties, we lived on a small farm in the central Utah community of Manti, where we kept a nice herd of Nubian and Toggenberg goats. I had access to all the *raw* milk our nannies could produce.

I soon discovered that my summertime sneezing, runny nose, and itchy red eyes, from the alfalfa hay we harvested, was beginning to subside for the first time in years. Within a year, *all* of my hay fever symptoms had entirely disappeared. In 1981, we sold our property and bought a very large cattle ranch in the remote wilderness of southern Utah, near Bryce Canyon, but our temporary home is in Salt Lake City.

For the past decade, I've had to return to using regular pasteurized cow's milk in my morning and late evening cereals. But I've noticed that as long as I limit my intake to these amounts (almost two 8-fl.-oz. glasses daily) and don't drink any extra milk, my hay fever symptoms are held in check pretty well. However, if I commit several dietary indiscretions for a few days in a row and consume more than I should, then my allergy acts up again.

The Onion Treatment for Hay Fever and Asthma

By the end of 1990, some 30 million Americans suffered from hay fever reported the National Center for Health Statistics. This and other common allergic conditions account for almost 9% of all visits to the doctor. But if more sufferers knew about onions, then maybe they wouldn't have to see an physician so often.

Robert S., age 68, of Newbury Park, California, happened to be attending the 1990 Cancer Control Society Convention at the Pasadena Hilton when I spoke. He came up and reintroduced himself; he had heard me speak some nine years before this.

Now Bob is an accomplished singer and has worked as a tenor, but he has periodically suffered from chest congestion and belabored breathing, attributed in part to borderline hay fever-asthma.

When we first met, I told him about the value of onion therapy, and just happened to have two reports to this effect with me from *Agents Actions* (May/June 1984) and the *European Journal of Pharmacology* (vol. 107, 1985, pp. 17–24). Impressed with the evidence before him, he asked how one went about taking this spice.

My reply was to make a simple tea by brewing just one slice of chopped onion in 1 quart of distilled water, and then drinking *only ½ cups* every 4 hours or whenever symptoms appeared to be at their worst. When we met again he reported that he was singing his heart out again without much difficulty, but now had encountered a new and very different kind of problem. "Because of my breath, my audience now prefers sitting farther away than they did before," he moaned.

◆◆◆◆◆

LYME DISEASE

News-Making Disease Misread as an Allergy

During much of 1989 and 1990, a new kind of disease with horrible side effects made headlines in newspapers and scientific journals and on radio and television broadcasts all over the country. It's called Lyme disease, named appropriately enough for the small Connecticut town where it was first identified in 1977. It's this country's most frequently diagnosed tickborne illness, and it occurs on all continents save for Antarctica.

A pinhead-sized specimen of deer tick of the genus *Ixodes* that is virtually invisible in its immature, nymph form, is the cause of Lyme disease. Symptoms of the disease seem to cover a baffling range. A bull's-eye rash, so called because it's often found darker at its edges and sometimes feels hard at its center, usually appears between two days and five weeks after a bite. Later, the victim may experience muscle pains, dizziness, shortness of breath, clogged sinuses, and heart irregularities severe enough in some instances to require a temporary pacemaker.

According to a feature story in the May/June 1989 issue of *Hippocrates* health magazine, Lyme disease has been repeatedly misdiagnosed by hundreds of physicians all around the country.

Since many of the initial symptoms mimic an allergy of some kind, doctors usually misinterpret it as just that and nothing else. But as the disease rapidly spreads through nearly all fifty states (except Alaska, Arizona, Hawaii, Montana, Nebraska, New Mexico, and Wyoming), and 10,000 new cases turn up each year, epidemiologists at the Centers for Disease Control in Atlanta are taking it much more seriously. This is especially true because of the *secondary* symptoms which usually show up months later: rheumatoid arthritis in knees and other joints, insomnia, extreme mood swings, dementia, and so forth. These later reactions sometimes resemble other disorders, such as hypoglycemia, Alzheimer's disease, or even multiple sclerosis. In 1988 a persons chances of contracting Lyme disease were roughly 1 in 30,000; in 1989 1 in 23,000; and in 1990 1 in 17,000.

How to Avoid Ticks

Nancy Sturhan of Humptulips, Washington, worked for some time as a forester in the state of Louisiana. In a short letter contributed to the April 29, 1989 issue of *Science News*, she reported that the best way she'd found to avoid tick bites was by fastening a cat flea-and-tick collar around each ankle just outside her workboot. With the legs of her jeans covering the flea collars, she had created a tick death chamber on each leg. She still found ticks on both legs, but they were never attached, were dead, and never made it past her knees. She employed this method routinely for a year with perfect results.

What to Do If You Are Bitten by a Tick

Should you be unlucky enough to get bitten by a tick, there is a correct procedure for removing the little bugger. Grab the tick as close to your skin as possible, using tweezers or fingers covered with rubber gloves or a paper towel. Pull upward steadily, without squeezing the body, until the anthropod detaches. Keep in mind that you're attempting to prevent contact with its bodily fluids, so don't handle the tick or crush it between your nails once it's loose. Flush it down a toilet or bury it in the ground somewhere. If the mouthparts remain in your skin, try to remove them the same way you would a splinter. Then disinfect the bite and wash your hands. One doctor suggests Betadine for this; I recommend your own urine if ammonia isn't handy. Hydrogen peroxide isn't strong enough to do the job.

Cleansing Ritual to Reduce Symptoms

A letter dated July 14, 1990, came from my friends, Loyal and Ethel. Ethel brought up the subject of Lyme disease. "Loyal has had and removed many ticks in the past himself, big ones and itty bitty ones." But, she observed, he *never once* got sick with *any* kind of fever, nor came down with symptoms common to Lyme disease. "Loyal went hiking with a friend of ours some time back," she continued. "Both had ticks on them when they got back. Loyal and Charles removed them. But while Loyal never got sick, Charles did. Came down with joint pains, memory loss. Felt terrible."

The reasons why one got sick and the other didn't depended on two things. One, Loyal is basically a vegetarian in that he eats *no* red meat. Second, and more important, he always goes on a 24- or 36-hour cleansing routine in which he flushes his system out with nothing but mineral water and lemon juice. He may sometimes drink a cup or two of burdock root tea, and maybe take up to 10,000 mg. of vitamin C, but he usually just sticks with the water-and-citrus fast instead.

"Loyal has been doing this for many years," she added, "and never once has got sick that I know of." To make the tonic, just add 1 level Tbsp. of lemon or lime juice to a pint of Evian or Perrier spring water and drink about 3 to 4 pints daily. To make the tea, just add 2 Tbsp. of coarse, dried roots to 1 quart of boiling water, cover and simmer for 5 minutes, then steep for ½ hour. Drink 3 cups daily.

PNEUMONIA

Elizabeth Taylor's Presumed "Allergy"

According to press reports (*USA Today*, November 20, 1990, and *People* magazine, December 10, 1990), it all started with those very slight conditions so typical of a normal spring allergy: sore throat, runny nose, and itchy eyes. At least that's what the first doctor thought when actress Elizabeth Taylor went to see him. From there her problem was diagnosed by several other physicians as sinusitis and just a bad case of influenza. Then a low-grade fever set in to complicate matters further.

So the lady who rode a horse to fame 46 years ago in *National Velvet* decided to check herself and her long medical history into the Daniel Freeman Marina Hospital in Los Angeles. But the bacteria that is known to mimic other types of respiratory infections or allergies had already taken command of Taylor's body in the form of a rare type of viral pneumonia.

Once the doctors realized what she really had, they transferred her to St. John's Hospital in Santa Monica in April 1990. She remained there in intensive care for almost three months.

This is what makes pneumonia in *any* form such an insidious disease. It can masquerade as several different ailments within a short period of time. It can fool even the smartest doctors. And as it nearly proved to be in Taylor's case, once the virus finally decides to throw off these disguises and make its presence known, the consequences can be fatal *if prompt medical attention* isn't sought right away.

A Medical Recovery Program That Works

Due to rising health costs, more people are opting for self-care these days instead of always relying upon the medical profession to do their treating for them. However, there are some diseases best left in the hands of skilled physicians, and pneumonia happens to be one of these.

However, in addition to the life-saving techniques offered in hospitals for viral pneumonia, there are also some health food supplements that can be taken to boost the body's own immune defenses. Goldenseal root and kyolic garlic have demonstrated antibiotic value in cases like this. Two capsules of powdered goldenseal and 2 capsules of the liquid kyolic garlic should be taken every 4 hours where pneumonia persists. And every 6 hours up to 100,000 I.U. of vitamin A (usually 4 25,000 I.U. fish oil capsules) and 25,000 mg. of vitamin C (25 1,000 mg. tablets crushed or 2 Tbsp. of powder stirred into 8 fl. oz. of water) should be taken as well. These are easily obtainable in health food stores. (See the appendix for more information.)

A cup of *hot* herbal tea on an empty stomach every few hours is very helpful as well. To make the tea, bring 1 quart of water to a boil and add 1 level tsp. of wild cherry bark. Cover, reduce heat, and simmer 5 minutes. Uncover and add ½ tsp. each of horehound herb and coltsfoot leaves. Stir, cover, turn off heat, and steep 45 minutes. Strain, sweeten with a little dark honey, and drink often during course of illness.

In addition, there are some other things that can be done to help overcome something as difficult as pneumonia. For example, Taylor's successful comeback from her second near-death experience with this disease (the first was in 1961 during the filming of *Cleopatra*) was also due to a strict life-style program she was put on by her physicians. Cover stories in both *USA Today* (November 20, 1990) and *People* magazine (December 10, 1990) reported some of its highlights.

First, she can never smoke again, or be around others who do, because the contact smoke alone from just one person would be the equivalent of one pack of cigarettes to her scarred lungs. Passive smoke is just as deadly for recovered pneumonia victims as smoking itself.

Taylor was also encouraged to take frequent walks by the ocean, as the misty salt air helps to strengthen the respiratory system. Without this breathing therapy occasionally, doctors think that the smog, for which L.A. is unfortunately renowned, could do severe harm to her lungs.

Second, Taylor's diet had to undergo some radical changes. No more alcohol, period! doctors ordered. And dairy products, including eggs, had to go too. While in the hospital, she lost 30 pounds due to vegetarian-style meals with an occasional helping of meat. And, oh yes, there was one thing more: very little deep-fried or fried food.

Next her formerly hectic pace underwent radical transformation. Doctors told her to s-l-o-w down or she'd be dead in no time at all. Her entire body needed about a year's time for recuperation, so plenty of lounging around and doing practically nothing that was stressful was their chief prescription. According to neighbors, Ms. Taylor rises early, watches some television, takes in a movie, goes for a leisurely drive, enjoys picnic outings, and spends a great deal of time with her live animals. The pet therapy, close friends insist, has helped her the most in overcoming whatever boredom or depression might go with sudden life-style changes like this.

And though she still travels a great deal, she has, at last, learned how to relax. This, above anything else, probably accounts for her most dramatic turnaround in health, physicians say. For, if the body isn't given plenty of time in which to rebuild itself from something as devastating as pneumonia, then all other efforts are merely Band-Aid approaches to a temporary comeback at best.

◆◆◆◆◆

SINUSITIS, SKIN RASH, AND SORE THROAT

A European Grandmother's Remedies

In late November and early December, in between some important health conventions I had to speak at, the Anthropological Research Center here in Salt Lake City, Utah, sponsored an "Herb Information" educational series. These classes were conducted by me and members of my staff.

One of those who attended all the lectures was a 77-year-old German grandmother by the name of Gerda Olds. For pretty much all of her life, she has been actively involved in the health care-giving process in some way. During the course of the series, she contributed many valuable, tried-and-true remedies for this or that ailment. She kindly permitted the use of both her name and some of her wonderful folk cures for this chapter.

Herbal Tea for Sinusitis. Gerda employs the following herbs for reducing temporary inflammation of the nasal cavities. She boils up a pint of water in a closed pot with a tight-fitting lid. Then turns the heat off, uncovers it, and adds ½ tsp. each of the following: sage leaves, yarrow herb, *powdered* white oak bark, and coarsely shredded (*not* powdered) slippery elm inner bark. The mixture is stirred a couple of times, the lid is replaced and the contents permitted to steep for ½ hour.

To use as an inhalant, she says, just uncover and hold the face a couple of inches above the pot with a bath towel or baby blanket thrown over the top of the head and back of the neck to hold vapors in better. Inhale *through the nose* for about 5 minutes. The tea may also be strained and taken internally in 1 cup amounts several times daily on an empty stomach.

Mrs. Old's Skin Rash Remedy. Mrs. Olds prefers a two-part approach to any type of surface rash. First wash the afflicted area with an herbal solution. This can be either a tea or, preferably, a fluid extract. The herbs best suited for his are bay leaves, thyme herb, and chaparral stems and leaves.

Make a tea out of them according to the instructions previously given. But let them simmer for a few minutes on low heat before removing and steeping. The mixture should steep for up to 10 hours to be effective. The liquid is strained and used to wash the skin gently. The best way to do this, she says, is to soak some cotton balls in the tea and then squeeze the liquid on to the skin, letting it run over the area needed. Then allow it to dry of its own accord without wiping it.

Next combine some *powdered* chickweed herb (½ tsp.) and comfrey root and leaves (1 tsp.) in a container. In a separate container, blend together some fluid extract of lobelia or Indian tobacco (½ tsp.) with wheat germ oil (1 tsp.) and a little honey (¼ tsp.) Then mix the dry ingredients in with the wet ones and combine thoroughly. A little practice may be needed to get the proportions exact enough so that a smooth paste with the even consistency of cooked Cream 'o Wheat cereal is the result.

Then apply this paste to the afflicted surface and cover with a single, *loose* dressing of gauze. Keep it this way overnight, if possible. She claims it really helps to clear up bad rashes of any type.

Gargling Your Way to Relief Gerda says she has a sure way of getting ride of sore throats. Bring a pint of any commercial *seltzer* or carbonated water to a boil. Reduce the heat to a lower setting and add 1 tsp. each of coarsely cut rosemary, sage, and thyme. Then add a tablespoon of coarsely chopped or shredded pomegranate fruit rind and seeds. Cover and simmer 5 minutes. Remove from the heat and steep an hour. Strain and rewarm each time you wish to gargle with ½ cup. When rewarmed be sure to add ¼ tsp. of honey to improve the flavor somewhat. Gargle periodically with this solution throughout the course of the day. It really helps to clear up any type of sore throat, she insists.

All the things that Gerda recommends may be found at most health food stores or nutrition centers. (See the appendix for anything not easily obtainable.)

Summary

1. Allergies can be provoked by shyness, fear, and stress as well as by environmental factors.
2. Many allergies have their foundations in antibiotics accumulated early in life from ingested foods, immunizations, and the like.
3. "Bad news" bacteria also invade physiological systems a lot easier when heavy metal toxins are present.
4. These tricky bacteria develop tough resistance to modern drugs and chemicals and can survive for long periods of time.
5. Allergies can even start in the prenatal stage of life due to the poor diets of many expectant mothers.
6. Self-confidence can help diminish allergic reactions.
7. Sweating out chemical toxins is one way of improving the the immune system.
8. Lead poisoning occurs in the most unlikely places; look for it in ceramic ware, soldering around water pipes, and so on.
9. Asthma, bronchitis, and emphysema share some similarities.
10. Corrective measures for the aforementioned diseases include stop smoking, drink lots of fluids, use a mist machine filled with saltwater solution often, recline the body in different tilted positions, massage chest, inhale and exhale properly, and practice moderate exercises routinely.
11. Onions may be good for asthma.

12. Chronic fatigue syndrome is a baffling malady that mimics a host of other problems.

13. New epidemics of this kind may be partly induced by the overuse of many chemical drugs used for innoculations and other medical reasons.

14. Modern diseases that are allergy-related may be helped by Oriental herbs, vitamins, and enzymes sometimes.

15. Herbs and boric acid solution clear up conjunctivitis.

16. Those suffering from ecological illnesses are essentially allergic to the environment itself or at least many things therein.

17. The state of the mind and condition of the liver reflects how well or badly one can handle environmental pollutions.

18. Environmental suffering may be eased with tomato and lemon juices.

19. Food allergies begin during infancy and continue on well into adulthood, with symptoms that can mimic other problems.

20. Food allergies can shift focus and direction several times in the course of one's life.

21. Most of those with food allergies also suffer from hypoglycemia.

22. A strong vitamin-mineral program is necessary to alleviate food intolerances.

23. Either a short-term weekend fast on fluids or a simple elimination diet will help allergic reactions to certain foods gradually subside.

24. Get all forms of sugar out of the diet and most allergies will disappear by themselves.

25. Practice food rotation to clear up your allergies.

26. Spices seem to reduce food intolerances.

27. The drinking of pasteurized over raw milk can aggravate hay fever.

28. Onions have therapeutic value for hay fever and asthma.

29. Lyme disease is often misdiagnosed.

30. Vegetarians run lower risks of contracting Lyme disease from infected ticks than do meat-eaters.

31. Pneumonia is one of those serious ailments that requires prompt medical attention, regardless of the holistic measures used.

32. Smoke-free air, walking by the ocean, no alcohol or junk food, and learning to relax help in recovery from pneumonia.

33. Common herbs can relieve sinusitis, rash, and sore throat.

7

Winning the War Against the Epidemics of the 1990s

AN ERA OF PLAGUES

A PASTOR at the huge Phoenix First Assembly [of God] in Arizona, warned his 6,500-member congregation members sometime ago in a typical hell fire-and-damnation sermon that "this nation has entered an era of plagues . . . far worse than what Egypt experienced in the days of Moses." He cited Revelation 9:20 and 11:6 as scriptural proof of this.

This book isn't the place to debate the correctness of his remarks, but it's certainly interesting to consider that this century began with the great influenza epidemic of 1918, which claimed 25 million lives, and now just before the twentieth century ends we find ourselves facing the prospect of another, more insidious plague in the form of AIDS.

Concurrent with AIDS, there have been dramatic upswings in other major diseases, some of which had been all but forgotten by many of this modern generation. Just one example: The *Toronto Star* for Monday, April 22, 1991, reported that probably we are going to have cholera in all of the countries of Latin America.

Then, too, acts of hostility and aggression have soared of late due to economic stress, drug abuse, unemployment, and the threat of war. Such anger-induced violence is now considered a major *health* threat to society by the medical profession. So the epidemics examined in this chapter are as follows:

AIDS	Cancer
Anger	Hepatitis
Bubonic Plague	Tuberculosis

254

◆◆◆◆◆

ACQUIRED IMMUNE DEFICIENCY SYNDROME

AIDS Strikes in USA Every 14 Minutes

The numbers just keep getting worse, it seems. According to Dr. James Curran, head of AIDS programs at the Center for Disease Control in Atlanta, "AIDS strikes someone in the USA every 14 minutes!" That was reported in the June 14, 1988 issue of *USA Today*. That figure had *dropped* by 2 minutes by the end of 1990, according to Dr. Curran. "Better figure one American every 12 minutes gets the virus now," he said when I spoke to him recently by phone.

Monthly statistics keep appearing that make things look grimmer all the time. The June 25, 1990 issue of *Newsweek* quoted the World Health Organization as saying that almost 1 million people worldwide developed AIDS in 1990 and up to *10 million* have contracted the virus that causes it. By the end of this decade about *30 million* will have become infected with it.

And America has the lion's share of victims. For all of 1984, fewer than 4,500 actual cases had been reported. By the end of 1990, 3,400 cases of AIDS were reported *every month* in this country. The Thursday, August 30, 1990 edition of *The New York Times* reported that almost *half* of all autopsies routinely done by the New York City Medical Examiner's office reveal AIDS infection to some degree.

Separate polls published at different times in *USA Today* found that the American public fears AIDS more than any other single disease, including cancer and heart attacks. The May 12, 1987 issue of the paper noted that of 1,304 adults polled, close to 50% fear this disease more than any other. And the June 16, 1988 issue reported that, among those interviewed, 43% listed the "spread of AIDS" as the top national concern over other issues such as crime (33%), drug abuse (32%), inflation (28%), and homelessness (25%).

The *Journal of the American Medical Association* for September 11, 1987 phrased the situation best when it noted that "socially, politically, and economically, AIDS is an ever-worsening disaster!"

How AIDS Devastates the Immune System

A decade ago, epidemic diseases were considered a thing of the past. Not any more, though, for the human immunodeficiency virus (or HIV) known to cause AIDS changed that thinking for good.

HIV has no life of its own. Unlike a bacterium, it doesn't absorb nutrients, generate waste, or reproduce by dividing. It's just a protein capsule containing two short strands of genetic material (RNA) and a few enzymes. It happens to use human cells to perpetutate itself. After infecting someone, HIV may spend 10 years or more quietly snuggled away within various tissues and organs like an unsuspecting mouse in your basement or attic somewhere. But when fully activated, it turns certain immune cells into virus factories, which produce a flurry of new virus capsules. Soon after cells become infected and the immune system inevitably tumbles like a house of playing cards.

The immune system is an elaborate, internal defense network that includes different types of blood cells. Among these immune cells, the ones that identify an intruder and authorize an immediate attack on it are called T4 lymphocytes or "helper T cells." Every T4 cell has appendages called CD4 receptors, through which it exchanges information with other immune cells. And it is through these CD4 receptors that HIV attacks. The outer shell of the HIV capsule (known as the envelope) is equipped with an appendage called gp120. This distinctive protein molecule happens to fit the CD4 receptor rather nicely, much like an electric plug fits into a wall socket. When the two molecules dock, the contents of the viral capsule—the RNA and the enzymes—flow freely into the cell's interior.

Once inside, HIV becomes a permanent feature of the cell. First, an enzyme called reverse transcriptase uses information encoded in the RNA to manufacture a double strand of DNA—a piece of software that can direct the cell to manufacture more virus. This DNA, known as the provirus, then integrates itself into the host cell's chromosomes. It represents just a tiny segment of the cell's genetic code. Once activated, however, it's the only segment that counts.

The trouble begins when the provirus starts directing enzymes in the host cell to produce new strands of viral RNA.

These rogue pieces of RNA serve as a blueprint, from which other enzymes start churning out the raw material for new virus capsules. These raw materials (long protein molecules) get chopped into shorter pieces by an enzyme called protease. Those pieces then clip together to form new HIV particles, which burst from the surface of the host cell and float off to infect others. The host cell is killed in the process.

According to a report in *Newsweek*, June 25, 1990, one reason HIV poses such a challenge is that the infection itself isn't even *theoretically* curable: modern biologists, for all their technological ingenuity, are far from knowing just how to purge unwanted DNA sequences from human chromosomes. There is little if any likelihood of AIDS ever becoming a chronic but manageable condition, much like diabetes or hypertension.

A Master of Disguises

The AIDS virus, unlike the leopard, not only can change its spots but dots—quite often and very fast, as a matter of fact. Researchers have known for some time that the virus genome differs from one infected person to the next. In other words, no two people have the same exact virus. Scientists have now learned that it can even show dramatic variation within a single individual. Moreover, HIV may be spinning off many different variants because it's inherently prone to making mistakes as it keeps reproducing itself.

The AIDS virus is one of the most elusive ever known. Very recent research has discovered that HIV can reside inside of people for up to nine years without ever triggering production of the antibodies that doctors have heretofore relied upon as their chief evidence of AIDS infection.

During the first weekend in June 1988, Dr. Monte S. Meltzer of Walter Reed Army Institute of Research in Washington, D.C., reported some of his own findings about HIV's sneaky ways at an AIDS workshop in New York City sponsored by the Cancer Research Institute. His investigative work revealed that HIV prefers to hide away in macrophages, a type of immune system scavenger cell found in tissue, in semen and vaginal fluid, in blood throughout the body, and in the brain. When in the blood, these cells are usually called monocytes.

The Army finding is based on a study of three gay men who had had repeated sexual intercourse without condoms with people known to be virus carriers. All three were healthy and all three had tested negative in widely used tests for AIDS virus antibodies. In addition the researchers had failed to find signs of HIV in the mens' T4 cells, where it often hangs out in its active state. But when Dr. Meltzer and his colleagues looked for the AIDS virus in the mens' macrophages, they found a lot of it quietly stashed away. They followed these men for up to a year and found that not one of them had developed any of the customary antibodies. New studies by several other groups indicate that everyone who has AIDS antibodies also has the virus in their macrophages. The virus can live and grow in macrophages without ever killing these helpful immune cells, even when the macrophages are filled almost to the bursting point with HIV.

Hence, normal methods of AIDS detection that depend upon the presence of antibodies may be worthless.

External Ways of Detecting AIDS

In an epidemic just waiting to happen, like AIDS, certain external observations are sometimes more useful in determining if a person is carrying HIV than some sophisticated, technological methods of diagnoses are.

For one thing, the mouth *never* lies. Look for any kind of oral lesion, but especially a white one on the tongue or mouth floor often characterized by rough projections that look like hairs. It isn't found anywhere else in the body. Along with hairy leukoplakia, there is usually oral yeast infection and herpes simplex as well. If all three are present in some form, that individual probably has AIDS.

Other, more obvious, signs are sudden loss of weight, extreme fatigue, skin blotches that won't clear up, fetid or "dragon" breath, periodic diarrhea, occasional insomnia, dark circles under the eyes, and inability to digest food properly marked by consistent and recurrent intestinal gas. There are other external signs, but these are some of the more prominent ones to look for.

AIDS can be treated with natural remedies and certain

kinds of food. These measures *won't cure* a person of HIV, but they will, at least, help hold the virus in check.

How Two Men Controlled AIDS

To those who've been unfortunate enough to have contracted HIV, there is a ray of hope on an otherwise dark horizon: AIDS can be controlled with extensive dietary modifications. The following two examples serve as proof of this. The first account is excerpted from the *Journal of Orthomolecular Medicine* (Vol. 5, 1990, pp. 25–31) and used with the permission of the editors. The second case study is based on several personal interviews I had with L.N. of Van Nuys, California.

The pseudonym of Calaph Timmerson was used by the author of the article, "A Few Simple Techniques for Staying Alive: Home Remedies for the A.I.D.S. Holocaust." He has had AIDS since 1985. Doctors all but gave him up for dead; however, he rallied back much to their astonishment. "The amazing thing is that I look and feel completely healthy and appear to be increasingly healthy and energetic every day," he wrote. "Four years ago, I looked like grim death. . . . Since then, I gained ten pounds. . . . Frequently, people are complimenting me on how well I look—the same people who thought I was dying a few years ago. They tell me, in confidential tones, that a few years ago, they thought I had AIDS, but since my condition always seems to be improving, they know it couldn't be AIDS."

What's his secret? Why spices, of course. "About every two days, I eat very spicy food from one of many countries that use hot spices, such as Mexico, Brazil, Burma, China (Szechuan/Hunan), Thailand, and Korea. Each cuisine is based upon the local spices, which are different, and seem to affect different microorganisms in different ways. The most dramatic effect is from the Korean spicy pickled cabbage called *kim-chi*, which has a lot of red cayenne pepper.

"At least once per week I have a kim-chi stew called kim-chi jige, which is liquid fire. I eat this together with a large amount of beef, fruit, and vegetables. I try to vary the menu and the types of spices, including several that are not notoriously hot. Milder spices, such as Thai lemon grass and holy basil, are dramatically effective in eliminating gas and the bloated feeling. In Mexican restaurants I always finish the bowl of hot sauce, using the curved tacos that are shaped like a spoon. Eating *guacamole* together with the hot sauce seems to make the *salsa picante* easier and more pleasant to finish, and makes it "stick to the ribs" more.

"Every few days I eat some kind of spicy food. Among the different spicy or pungent foods I eat are hot Chinese mustard, a Japanese green mustard called *wasabe*, ordinary mustard, garlic, ginger, and horseradish. . . . I have spoken with several other long-term survivors who have very low T4 levels, *but* who appear to be in robust health, and who are energetic, working full time, and putting on weight. I have discovered, to my surprise, that most of the long-term survivors I know are also eating spicy food, and particularly the Korean *kim-chi*, at least once per week. They don't think of spicy food as any kind of therapy—they just happen to like it. A friend of mine who is still working full time as a computer analyst, even though his T4 [cell] counts is around 10, says that, at this point, he can only eat spicy food, because bland food makes him nauseous and full of gas."

He concludes his observations on spices by saying that the reason they seem to work so well in checking HIV is because of their ability to "inhibit or kill various microbes, but which are safe for human ingestion." His final testimonial states: "Since I have started conscientiously eating spicy food, I have been consistently much more alert and able to work than I have been at any other time during the past ten years."

In the case of L.N., also of Van Nuys, California, a variety of things seemed to have worked for him. In May 1983 he was diagnosed as having Kaposi sarcoma, the skin cancer usually associated with AIDS. A year's worth of conventional medical treatments left him more ill from the side effects. So he turned to natural alternatives with convincing results. Almost eight years later, at the close of 1990, he had managed the nearly impossible: becoming one of just a select handful of this nation's only known long-term survivors of AIDS.

When I first interviewed him at an "AIDS Therapies" workshop in Anaheim, California, on April 8, 1988, sponsored by the Natural Foods Expo, he was rather muscular and had a stocky build. His weight was a solid 165 lb. for a height of 5 feet 9 inches. He radiated a picture of near-perfect health to all outward appearances at least.

His dietary program then consisted of whole grains and fresh fruit for breakfast. Along with fresh carrot juice, he took a number of nutritional supplements, including kyolic garlic, vitamins A, C, and E, zinc, germanium, and homemade egg-lecithin formulation. He worked out every day on weights at a local health club.

I questioned him closely for the particulars to this very useful regimen. His favorite fruits tended to be oranges, apples, bananas, cantaloupes, and other melons. Occasionally he would make himself some poached eggs on whole wheat toast, but other than this, he avoided dairy products.

Lunch was "never a big meal of mine," he admitted. He stayed mostly with more fresh fruits and lots of cooked brown rice. "I found this gave me the energy I needed while working out in the gym," he said.

Dinner was usually his biggest meal. He would rotate different kinds of fresh- or saltwater fish (poached) with skinless chicken (barbecued, broiled, or baked). Vegetables like broccoli, cauliflower, and brussels sprouts were always lightly steamed. Fresh salads would almost always include raw spinach and Romaine lettuce, along with cherry tomatoes, slice of raw onion and cucumber, slices of cooked beets, and some chopped fresh mushrooms.

Of his different supplements, these few stood out: kyolic garlic (3 capsules at night), Pines' wheatgrass (3 tablets), liquid vitamin A (1 drop of 10,000 I.U. in juice), Wholesale Nutrition's vitamin C (8–10 grams daily), and Alta Health Products' fluid extract of pau d'arco (18 drops in juice each day). Most of these products can be obtained in health food stores across the country. If you can't find some of them, consult the appendix for further information.

L.N.'s conversation with me a couple of years ago was considerably animated and sprinkled with a lot of enthusiasm "I go to the gym regularly to stimulate my physical immune system," he said. "The key to my workouts, though, is to stimulate, not suppress, my immune capabilities. I find that constant exercise stimulates everything in me—the physical, mental, spiritual, and emotional bases. They're all extremely important to me."

Two other foods that L.N. believes were critical to his recovery are onions—"I eat lots of them . . . never can get enough of them"—and citrus fruit—"I take lemon juice in cold water as a potent blood cleanser . . . dynamic stuff!" He reminded me, though, "Don't have your readers leave their doctors. They have decent ideas, too. It's important to have a combination of both Eastern and Western philosophy."

A little over 2½ years after this, I interviewed him again. This time things were a little different. Louie no longer exercised as religously. Nor was he bubbling over with the same levels of energy and enthusiasm. He was much quieter, spoke in softer tones of voice, and not for very long at that. His weight had dropped to 135 lb., which was still in line with his height, however.

He said 1990 had been his roughest year yet, and he hoped the following year would be better. He explained that those like himself who've been able to put their AIDS into remission for so long, eventually become susceptible to what he termed "opportunistic infections." In his case, a combination of MAI or mycobacterium avium intracellulare (a malabsorption problem with the intestinal tract similar to giardia) and PCP or pneumocystis carinii (a lung infection), had plagued him for most of the year.

"I found myself losing weight like crazy," he said. "I couldn't keep any food down to speak of. Kept vomiting stuff up. And I've been continually bothered with frequent bouts of diarrhea. My muscles ache a lot and I get many cramps in my stomach. I'm always fatigued, no matter how much I try to eat."

To remedy this situation, he switched to a much different kind of diet. While still retaining some of the natural and organic foods to which his body had grown accustomed, he started consuming things that were densely packed in calories. "Items I'd never otherwise touch have become my mainstays of late," he reluctantly admitted. "Once I wouldn't have touched any dairy products at all, but just tonight I had two tuna melts with lots of cheese and butter on the bread. A couple of days ago I ate a Winchell's doughnut. And when I was over to my mom's for dinner recently, I had two big helpings of pumpkin pie with whipping cream on it. I also indulge myself in peanut butter sandwiches, a dish of ice cream now and then, and anything else I can lay my hands on that is calorie-rich."

The result of all this has been a slight resurgence in his energy levels, a modest weight gain of 3 lb., a temporary halt in his diarrhea, and an end to his regurgitation problem. "I've discovered with AIDS that you have to change your diet according to how your symptoms change," he concluded. However, his supplement program remains virtually unchanged from what it was before.

◆◆◆◆◆

ANGER

Hostility Can Ruin More than Your Day

A recent wealth of scientific data suggests that chronic anger is so damaging to the body that it ranks with, or even exceeds, cigarette smoking, obesity, and a high-fat diet as a powerful risk factor for early death. "Our studies indicate that hostile, suspicious anger is right up there with any other health hazard we know about," said Dr. Redford Williams, a researcher in behavioral medicine at the Duke University Medical Center, in Durham, North Carolina.

In results presented at a recent meeting of the American Heart Association, held in November 1990, Dr. Williams reported that people who scored high on a hostility scale as teenagers were much more likely than their more cheerful peers to have elevated cholesterol levels as adults, suggesting a strong link between unremitting anger and heart disease.

In a second recent study, Dr. Mara Julius, an epidemiologist at the University of Michigan, Ann Arbor, analyzed the effects of chronic anger on women over the age of 18. She found that women who had answered initial test questions with obvious signs of long-term, suppressed anger were three times more likely to have died than were those who did not harbor such hostile feelings.

To rank as a chronically hostile person, one need not be pathologically maladapted and living on the edge of society. Indeed, said Dr. Williams, many of the world's mistrustful cynics don't even realize that they have a problem. In fact, "they may even be rather proud of being hard-nosed and tough-minded," he finished.

Dr. Julius discovered in her research that women are far more likely to be at risk when suppressing their anger than men are. She thinks maybe the extra burden of guilt they carry within themselves concerning their anger may be one reason for this.

But scientists claim that the effect of anger on the body is "very profound," regardless of whether it's stifled or expressed via a tantrum. They know that hostile people have a more reactive sympathetic nervous system than do others. Their bodies tend to produce abnormally high levels of stress hormones like adrenaline and noradrenaline whenever they feel that somebody is picking on them. Those hormones can stimulate a wide spectrum of effects, raising blood pressure, quickening the heart beat, and dilating the pupils.

However, many angry people also have an underactive parasympathetic nervous system that fails to produce the common hormone acetylcholine, which normally turns off the harsh effects of adrenaline. Over time, too much adrenaline and too little acetylcholine can lead to a host of health problems. The arteries grow stiffer from constantly elevated blood pressure and the heart weakens from being overexerted. Stress hormones have been shown to damage the liver and kidney and to release too much fat from fat stores, which could explain why those who are hostile as teenagers have high cholesterol levels as adults.

Anger Injures Immunity

Two excellent books explain in some detail the effects of anger upon the immune system. Norman Cousins's *Head First: The Biology of Hope* (1989) mentions that for six different emotional states, namely, anger, fear, surprise, disgust, sadness, and happiness, there were separate effects upon the heart, immune system, and body temperature. Anger, for instance, was characterized by a high heart rate, a sudden plunge in killer cells (necessary to fight major infections like cancer), and an increase in body temperature. Happiness, on the other hand, led to low rises in heart and body temperature, and a very stabilized output of killer cells (as it should be anyway). Additional research at

Yale University Department of Psychology demonstrated that anger during exercise raised human heart rates an average of 33 beats per minute—more than double the increase during neutral (or normal) exercise and sometimes flattened white blood cell counts.

The second book, *Perfect Health* by Deepak Chopra, M.D., takes an Ayurvedic look at anger's deadly effects upon the human system. He likens anger to a fast-moving car, which suddenly brakes for no reason at all. The inevitable skid marks from burned rubber on the asphalt is equivalent to about what happens biologically within the body. The nerves are frayed, their protective myelin sheathing material is chemically "worn down," by an overabundance of adrenaline and similarly produced substances. And the whole immune system is, literally, "whipped" into a frenzy for no reason at all. Too many infection-fighting cells are made, and these, in turn, can hurt the body later on by turning against it in the form of autoimmune diseases.

Anger: A Lethal Disease

The level of personal anger and frustration in the United States is at an all-time high. So notes the December 17, 1990 issue of *Newsweek* magazine. It may be seen in the spiraling rise in homicides and spousal and child abuse of late. So bad have these become that now homicides and similar acts of anger are routinely reported *not* by the federal crime center but instead by the government Centers for Disease Control (CDC) in Atlanta, Georgia.

The reason for this is evidently clear, said John Chancellor of the NBC "Nightly News," *Thursday evening*, December 13, 1990. "Hostility is now considered to be an *epidemic* disease affecting the health of our whole society." That is why the CDC now has the job of keeping such statistics, he explained in his editorial commentary.

How to Get Rid of Anger

A close friend of mine, Larry H., had a serious temper as he grew up. In his teenage years, he pointed a loaded pistol at his younger brother's head and threatened to pull the trigger (he didn't). Another time he was picked up by Provo, Utah, police officers while in the act of carrying a loaded rifle over to someone else's house. When stopped and asked what he was doing, he replied very coolly that he was intending to kill a high school buddy of his, because "the kid stole my date away from me." When the Vietnam war was on, he received a 4-Y classification because of his hair-trigger temper.

Today, he is a respected social scientist and religious leader in his own community. He has counseled hundreds of men, women, and young people about the deadly consequences of anger. Just what, you may ask, prompted this turnaround?

Several things come to mind. One, he got himself into several steady relationships with people who could truly understand him and fulfill his needs of being loved and wanted. Two, he was placed in different positions of leadership, which demanded a cool head and level thinking. To have done otherwise would have jeopardized his opportunities for success. Third, he plunged himself into social services, working with the *emotionally* handicapped like himself, but concentrating his energies mostly with suicidally prone youth. Four, he availed himself of physically-demanding sports whenever he felt his temper about to rise. Boxing and, later on, karate helped him to find healthy outlets through which to challenge some of his pent-up rage. Five, he became a firm disciple of communication and openly talked about his occasional feelings of hostility with his close friends and relatives. He sought and got their advice and understanding, so he was never really alone with his anger. Six, he began developing in his late thirties a pattern of living that was more conducive to peace than anything else. His hobbies and pasttimes became less aggressive and more congenial. Finally, he started to develop a spiritual respect for other life forms around him, and ended up with an inner desire to never want to knowingly hurt another creature of God's, be it man or beast, as long as he lived.

Another neighbor, Ethel W., had a history of domestic violence since the age of 19. The physical and verbal abuse her kids received was legendary in the area in which we lived and in the church (Mormon meetinghouse) nearly everyone attended. Her outbursts also affected her social relationships.

Interestingly, this highly unpleasant side to her took shape at about the same time she went to a dentist to have several cavities filled. Before this, she had been one of the sweetest, most endearing girls anyone could have had the pleasure of knowing. During her first decade of marriage, it seemed that every trip to the dentist for a filling, resulted in a more explosive personality later on.

Someone told her about the hidden dangers in these amalgam fillings. At first, she didn't take this information seriously, but one day she almost strangled her fourth child, an 11-month-old baby, because he was crying excessively and for no apparent reason. It was then she realized she needed help, and badly!

A local Salt Lake City dental surgeon agreed to replace everyone of her silver-mercury fillings with gold. It was an expensive procedure that occupied the better part of 13 weeks and cost almost $10,000. But within just a few weeks, her inclination to fly off the handle at the most trivial things had disappeared. Now, on those rare occasions when she becomes angry, it's a normally controlled reaction without the urge for violence.

A segment of the popular television news program "Sixty Minutes," which aired on CBS December 16, 1990, dealt with this very thing. A leading allergist, who specializes in studying the awful reactions that thousands of people seem to have to amalgam fillings, told Morley Safer that "a significant number" of his violent-prone patients watched their hostilities almost "disappear overnight" when they had their old amalgam fillings replaced with something safer like enamel or gold.

◆◆◆◆◆

BUBONIC PLAGUE

Is the "Black Death" Coming Back?

As if rising unemployment, a burgeoning national debt, and the soaring rate of AIDS isn't enough to make even the most optimistic of us somewhat gloomy, now there comes the very real possibility that bubonic plague may be lurking just around the corner.

Evidence for this comes from two sources, one religious

and the other scientific. The holy scriptures of Protestants, Catholics, Jews, Muslims, and Mormons all point to awful and terrible diseases reminiscent of the Black Death in medieval times, which seem to hang over us like the proverbial sword of Damocles just waiting to fall at the slightest move. And recent reports on "The Bubonic Plague" (*Scientific American*, February and July 1988) and on "Fleas, The Lethal Leapers" (*National Geographic*, May 1988), which carry it, suggest an ominous comeback of this disease.

Forget about the decade-long outbreaks all over New Mexico, which eventually spilled over into neighboring Utah, Arizona, and Colorado. Forget about that fellow, Dr. Allan Barnes with the Centers for Disease Control, who warned us in 1978, "It could take only a spark to get the country on an epidemic course [of Black Death]." Forget the *hundreds* of recently reported bubonic cases in the dry scrublands behind the coast of northeast Brazil around Joao Pessoa in 1987. And don't even pay much mind to what former Health and Human Services Secretary Otis R. Bowen said in 1987 about " 'Black Death' dwarfing the current AIDS epidemic" in the coming decade (1990s).

But think instead of rats, and *lots* of them at that! Without giving you nightmares, there are a couple of things you should know about these city-bred rodents. First, they're virtually indestructible. According to the October 1979 *Chicagoland Monthly* article on "Super Rats," "when subjected to nuclear radiation from postwar atomic bomb tests in the Pacific, *rats thrived!*" Second, third, and fourth, noted the January 1980 *Ciba-Geigy Journal* on "Rats," rodents are "devilishly, deadly clever and cunning" to say the least.

Worst of all, though, declared both publications is that these *tens of millions* of rodents found in all major metropolitan areas of this country are absolutely *filthy*. Many of them, in fact, are potential "walking disease factories," quite capable of causing all manners of sickness, *including* the bubonic plague. And as poverty flourishes in our inner cities and the standards of living keep dropping, we will soon come to find that these endless multitudes of rodents will repeat history again, as their four-legged ancestors did between 1346 and 1352 A.D. when 25 million people died in Europe alone!

Plague Prevention: "Four Thieves Vinegar"

A remedy from the Dark Ages is reputed to be about the most effective way to treat plague symptoms, which include fever, prostration, delirium, and swelling of the lymph glands, especially in the armpit or groin. Such hard swellings are called buboes, sometimes accompanied by black blotches.

In medieval Europe, those who consumed garlic or made liberal use of a specific garlic vinegar never contracted the plague. A few, who used either form of garlic in large quantities early on in their sickness, managed somehow to survive, though barely.

The city of Toulouse, France, was struck by the bubonic plague in 1630. At that time, a band of four thieves went throughout the city, entering infected houses and helping themselves to whatever they wanted from the dead and dying. Yet, despite such enormous risks, they *never* got sick! In time the local authorities captured them and put them on trial. Upon being sentenced to death, they pleaded for mercy. In exchange for their secret remedy against the Black Death, the judge granted them clemency.

In their subsequent deposition, they revealed their methods of preparing it. This document lay buried in the archives of Toulouse for several centuries, until recently rediscovered by a famous French herbalist, Maurice Mességué. He gave the details of it in his book, *C'est la Nature Qui à Raison*, published in France some years ago.

The thieves first made a vinegar out of some cheap wine by drinking a few swigs each and then expectorating their mouthfuls *back into* the container with the rest of the wine. This solution was then covered and set in a warm place for sometime until it had entirely gone sour. Today, you can just purchase a quart of apple cider or wine vinegar.

Next they collected the *fresh* herbs—sage leaves, savory herb, thyme herb, rosemary leaves, lavender flowers and leaves, peppermint leaves, bergamot (Oswego tea or bee balm) leaves and flowers, and some eucalyptus leaves—coarsely chopped them up, and added equal parts to the amount of vinegar they had. If you cannot get fresh herbs, then their essential oils may be substituted, but, remember, when using the expressed oils of any herb that they are extremely potent, a few drops goes a long way! So, for instance, oils of peppermint and eucalyptus can be substituted, but only about 6–8 *drops* of each should be added to 1 quart of cider or wine vinegar.

The vinegar mixture was allowed to set for a week or so, being stirred a few times every day. After this the thieves rubbed the liquid over their entire bodies. Since these aromatic herbs are strong germicides, it's easy to see how well protected they were while ransacking the houses and bodies of the sick and dying. In modern times, this "Four Thieves Vinegar" has some application in cases of contagious diseases like influenza or even the common cold, for example. Judiciously rubbing *small* amounts of this on the hands, around the mouth, beneath the nostrils, and on the cheeks should help to reduce your susceptibility to these diseases. Of course, caution needs to be used in putting it around the eyes or if you are allergic to any of these particular herbs.

CANCER

The Four Major Cancers

There are many different types of cancer. Some are fairly common like leukemia (cancer of the blood), while others, such as mucoepidermoid carcinoma (tumor of the salivary gland ducts), rarely occur. Because of space limitations, only the four leading cancers in this country will be covered here. The dietary and remedial information offered applies to all of them and is solely intended as nutritional support, not as a substitute for regular medical or alternative treatments of choice. The four leading cancers are lung, colo-rectal, breast, and prostate.

Is Cancer an Epidemic?

In some of my public speaking appearances recently, I've frequently been asked the question, "Is cancer considered an epidemic?" That often depends on whom you ask, is my usual response. Most physicians *downplay* the ominous statistics, even though the number of cases is increasing by leaps and bounds every year. Recent evidence suggests that, at least for one type of cancer, it has reached epidemic proportions.

A Harvard Medical School oncologist has looked at cancer in women in her book, *Dr. Susan Love's Breast Book* (Reading, Massachusetts: Addison-Wesley, 1990). In 1960, 1 in every 20 American women developed breast cancer in her lifetime; now it's 1 in 10. Over 155,000 women in the United States will be diagnosed with breast cancer this year. And over 25% of them will die as a result of it. With statistics like that, argues Dr. Love, "it's an epidemic for sure, and it's going to get worst before it gets better!"

Herbs That Help Fight Cancer

I've worked with hundreds of herbs over the last several decades of my life, and have interviewed some 135 different folk healers from all over the world. I've studied their ways and compiled some highly interesting facts in the course of my global research.

1. Cultures that have high-fiber diets (*un*polished rice, whole wheat bread, *un*peeled root vegetables) don't get colo-rectal cancer.

2. Women in cultures that consume a lot of onions and garlic have substantially lower rates of breast cancer.

3. In cultures that tend to have more spicy cuisines (Indian, Thai, Indonesian, Mexican, Chinese), there is far less incidence of prostate and colo-rectal cancers than in other cultures with blander diets.

4. In those parts of the world (some Indonesian islands, the Philippines, Granada, and the West Indies) where the air is heavily scented with certain aromatic spices (cinnamon and nutmeg), there is virtually no lung cancer.

In addition, I've discovered several important herbs used here in America that are quite potent against the four major cancers in general. Each of them works best in a different form.

Chaparral *(Larrea divaricata).* An octogenarian named Ernest Farr, residing in Mesa, Arizona, came down with malignant melanoma in the late 1970s. Physicians at the University of Utah Medical Center in Salt Lake City, where he went for observation and a biopsy, said there was very little they could do. So he went back home and started drinking chaparral tea every day. He added 2 Tbsp. of dried chaparral to 1 quart of boiling water, covered, and simmered it on low heat for about 10 minutes. Then he removed the pot from the burner and let it steep for an additional *10–12 hours!* He strained what he needed and drank three cups daily in between meals. His melanoma soon disappeared, much to the amazement of the same doctors who checked him over again a year later. His story was reported as an "anonymous" case study in the *Rocky Mountain Medical Journal* (November 1970) and *Cancer Chemotherapy Reports* (April 1969). Chaparral is available at most health food stores (see the appendix).

Goldenseal *(Hydrastis canadensis).* Solomon Yoder of the Amish community in Sarasota, Florida, developed stomach cancer about four years ago. Declining surgery but accepting limited chemotherapy, he soon discovered that didn't help either. So he began experimenting with different herbs and found that *powdered* goldenseal root worked the best of all. He took 3 capsules every morning before breakfast for the first week, and then increased it to 4 capsules a couple of weeks later. A third medical exam several months later showed his intestinal tumor to be in remission. He also added to his daily regimen several other herbal combinations containing goldenseal. He took 3 capsules of Old Amish Resist-All and 3 capsules of Old Amish Formula 83 late in the morning or early afternoon. (See the appendix for more information on Old Amish Products.) Goldenseal powder by itself, however, can be obtained from most health food stores or nutrition centers, and empty gelatin capsules can be purchased from most drugstores. Note: People with hypoglycemia should use this herb with caution, since it lowers blood sugar levels.

Pau D'Arco *(Tabebuia* **species***).* In 1960 in the Brazilian suburb of Americana near Sao Paulo, an elderly gentleman was operated on for prostate cancer. But further examination showed that the tumor had severely metastasized. Doctors, therefore, gave him about a month to 40 days to live. Shortly after their dreadful prognosis, he went to see his dentist to get a cavity filled. The dentist, Dr. Dei Santi, noticed how gloomy his patient was and, upon learning about the supposedly incurable cancer, he recommended that the old fellow start drinking some pau d'arco or lapacho. The man made the tea by putting approximately half-a-cup of the dried bark into a coffee pot filled two-thirds with boiling water, and letting the brew perk for 15 minutes or so. Later, he would drink 4 cups of the *lukewarm* tea every day on an empty stomach. After 15 days, his excruciating pain left. After 30 days, he was able to move around quite well. He survived another seven years in pretty good health. This and other proven cases were reported in a feature-length article in the highly respected Brazilian periodical, *O Cruzeiro* (March 18, 1967). The best and purest source for this hard-to-find herb is Alta Health Products of Pasadena, California, where it can be purchased in tea, fluid extract, capsule, and powder forms, but I suggest that the liquids be used for maximum effectiveness. (See the appendix for details.)

Red Beets *(Beta vulgaris).* D.G., a Hungarian woman of 30, was admitted to the district hospital in Csoma, Hungary, on March 10, 1957. She had been sick for three months and lost considerable weight. Her temperature soared to 38.5°C. Dr. Alexander Ferenczi, her attending physician and renowned for his famous cancer cures with beets, detected nodules as large as prune pits in both breasts and under her armpits. The test excision disclosed an adenocarcinoma. She was subsequently treated with beet liquid (made by reconstituting dehydrated red beet juice), blood transfusion, iron tablets, and injections of neoperheparine. Two weeks later her tumor nodules decreased in size and by March 26 no further traces of them could be detected in her breasts. And the lymphatic nodules in both armpits had also reduced to about one-fourth of their original size. The patient was discharged at the end of the month and sent home. This and numerous other remarkable cures effected by Dr. Ferenczi's amazing beet root therapy appeared in a lengthy medical article in the July 1986 issue of *International Clinical Nutrition Review*. Quality organic beet root powder in bulk can be purchased from Pines' International of Lawrence, Kansas (see the appendix). Just add 1 level tsp. of beet powder to an 8-oz. glass of water or juice and drink every morning for preventive measures. Or as a nutritional supplement to existing forms of cancer already receiving proper medical treatment, this amount should be tripled; in other words, drink three glasses a day instead of just one.

Garlic *(Allium sativum)*. Benjamin Lau, M.D., Ph.D., is a respected professor of medical microbiology and immunology in the Department of Microbiology at California's Loma Linda School of Medicine. Both as a practicing physician and as a researcher, he has discovered garlic's incredible anticancer properties. With his kind permission, I've excerpted a few things from his recent book, *Garlic for Health.*

> For the past ten years, my associates and I have studied cancer biology and immunology. Ten years ago we reported that cancer cells secrete substances that repel cancer-fighting cells, particularly those we call phagocytes. As a result our research has centered on ways to enhance phagocyte activity through various immune stimulants referred to as "biological response modifier." We've experimented both with live bacterial vaccine and killed bacterial vaccine; both strengthen the body's control against cancer.... We've also centered our research efforts on the role of nutrition in cancer development and prevention.... During the past several years, I have collaborated with several urologists in the study of bladder cancer.... We have used both live and killed bacterial vaccines and have included garlic extract in our testing. Test results published in the *Journal of Urology* show that treatment with a liquid garlic extract (kyolic from Wakunaga Pharmaceutical) produced the lowest incidence of bladder cancer.... What happens? Garlic apparently stimulates the body's immune system, particularly enhancing the macrophages and lymphocytes, which destroy cancer cells.... We are understandably excited to see that a natural substance can have such impact on cancer prevention! Several energetic physicians and researchers are now working with me, using modern analytic tools to fully explore the effects of each component of garlic. So far, our evidence shows that garlic can help inhibit tumor growth—but we also have experimental data showing that garlic can enhance the body's own immune system,

You don't need a prescription for kyolic garlic, which is readily available in nearly all health food stores or nutrition centers nationwide. Holistic-minded medical doctors, whom I know that treat cancer, recommend that their patients take up to 10 liquid-filled capsules daily. Otherwise, for general maintenance purposes and to prevent getting cancer, they suggest between 2 and 3 capsules daily with meals. (*Garlic for Health* and another book, *Garlic in Nutrition & Medicine* by Robert I-San Lin, Ph.D., are *free* for the asking. Just send $3.00 to cover postage to Anthropological Research Center, P.O. Box 11471, Salt Lake City, Utah 84147. They are intended solely for educational purposes.)

Chlorophyll. Linda Y., a 33-year-old Chinese American from Los Angeles, shared a recent experience with me that she hoped would benefit some of my readers. It happened this way: I was doing a two-hour early-morning nationwide talk show in late December 1990 on The InfoTainment Radio Network. The show was "The Billy Goodman Happening," and Linda was one of many callers who phoned in either with questions or with personal health success stories of some kind. She told us that about eight months earlier, a pigmented mole on her right thigh started giving her some problems, so she consulted several skin specialists. They referred her to a prominent oncologist at UCLA Medical Center. He pronounced it as a rare form of melanocarcinoma, which he thought was treatable with combined chemotherapy and radiation. Upon learning of the drastic side effects of both, however, she decided to take her chances with more natural things instead. Someone told her about bakuryokuso from Japan, which she started taking faithfully. She reported that her melanocarcinoma began subsiding within seven weeks of taking the bakuryokuso. For the benefit of the rest of us, who didn't know what in the heck this stuff was, I asked what it was. "Oh, it's plain green barley juice powder," she chimed in with enthusiasm. And told us how much she took each day: "One teaspoonful in a glass of juice or plain water with every meal." Green barley juice and wheatgrass juice is very popular in the East. One product very popular throughout Japan and now just recently introduced into America and Canada is Kyo-Green. It consists of organically grown young barley and wheat grass, with kelp seaweed, unpolished (brown) rice, and Bulgarian chlorella (a mineral-rich algae). (See under Wakunaga in the appendix.) Better still, I encourage you to invest in a good juicer and make your own green drink consisting of spinach leaves, Romaine lettuce, parsley, endive, and celery. Blend one-third green juice with one-third carrot juice and one-third pineapple juice for a truely flavorful and zesty drink!

Tijuana Cancer Clinic's "Recovery Diet"

Of all the Mexican cancer clinics that I've visited over the years, the one formerly called Agua Caliente Valparaiso, but now known as the East/West Wellness Center, has impressed me the most. Owned and operated by a distinguished Korean doctor from Seoul with a long and laudable record of healing success to his credit, this Tijuana facility resembles more a luxurious health resort than a cancer clinic. Dr. Henry Yun has specialized in a nutritional approach toward cancer by focusing on those foods that will help to rebuild the body so it can fight back against this dread disease.

In early September 1990, I visited Dr. Yun and spent time with him, his dietitians, and kitchen staff. I also observed as well as interviewed specific cancer patients, both Asian and Caucasian, during my short stay there. I came away with a profound respect for a man who has used *nutritional* chemotherapy, essentially food, as his chief weapon against cancer. Every other healing modality that his center uses to help people get well again revolves around food. "Food is the *centerpiece* of everything good we accomplish here," he reminded me.

Here is a typical two-week meal plan. By following such a diet, you may be able to reduce your own risk of incurring cancer or else better manage any existing conditions. For more precise details, contact Dr. Yun at his East/West Wellness Center in Tijuana. (See the appendix for details.)

A Cancer Treatment Diet

Breakfast

Sunday—Rice/millet cereal with almonds, honey, goat's milk.

Monday—Poached egg on bed of spinach; fresh papaya.

Tuesday—Cooked oatmeat with honey; goat's milk; grapefruit.

Wednesday—Wheatina cereal with apple juice; honey; goat's milk.

Thursday—Seven grain cereal with honey and goat's milk (includes corn, rice, rye, oats, barley, buckwheat, millet).

Friday—Cooked rye cereal with sliced banana, goat's milk.

Saturday—Buckwheat/buttermilk pancakes with blueberry syrup, and fresh papaya.

(Seven-grain toast and chamomile tea served with every breakfast.)

Lunch

(Lunch is always the main meal of the day at the East/West Wellness Center or Agua Caliente Valparaiso in Tijuana, Mexico.)

Sunday—Baked potato, tossed green salad (includes cherry tomato, red onion, fresh basil, watercress, etc.) with apple cider vinegar and olive oil dressing on the side.

Monday—Rotini pasta (made from spinach, beets, carrots, whole wheat flour) salad with the following ingredients included: broccoflowers (genetic cross between broccoli and cauliflower), green pepper, sliced garlic, parmesan cheese, lemon juice, olive oil, basil, red onion. Served with soy bread and garlic on top. Also soup of the day can vary. May be either angel hair (made out of garlic and parsley), soba (Japanese noodle soup made with buckwheat flour) or something else. (Monday is *always* pasta day.)

Tuesday—"Festival of vegetables" plate, which includes carrots, broccoli, cauliflower, brussels sprouts, red bell pepper, and green beans. All lightly steamed and served with sesame seed–amino acid–olive oil dressing. Steamed brown rice served on the side as well.

Wednesday—Corn patties (made with corn, green onions, whole wheat flower and Parmesan cheese). They are baked, *never* fried or grilled. Served with green salad, consisting of Romaine and butter lettuce, red onions, fresh cooked beets, and water cress. Covered with an avocado dressing.

Thursday—Stuffed bell peppers filled with mixture of cooked millet, rice, and almonds. Served with a vegetable salad on the side, consisting of sliced beets, red onion, and cucumber.

Friday—Fish of the day is poached or baked. (Type served rotates every week between sea bass, salmon, sole, halibut or mahi-mahi.) Served with steamed brown rice, steamed medley of vegetables (brussels sprouts, snow peas and carrots), and steamed red Pontiac potatoes.

Saturday—Miso (seaweed) soup (fixed different ways). Also steam-fried vegetable mixture consisting of snow peas, green and red and bokchoy and napa cabbages, carrots, green peppers, bean sprouts, oyster and shiitake mushrooms, and celery. Served with steamed brown rice and some cooked soba noodles with green onions on the side.

(Chamomile tea is served with every lunch.)

Dinner

All evening meals are much lighter than lunch. Typical dinners include some type of soup, whole-grain breads, muffins, cookies or cakes (sweetened with honey), generous helpings of fresh fruits (melons, peaches, pears, apples, apricots, grapes or whatever else happens to be in season then). Plenty of Hungarian or German chamomile tea is the available beverage.

The varieties of soup include the following: garlic, onion, lentil, cabbage, spinach, barley, garbanzo, vegetable, seaweed, soba, and miso. A particular favorite of both Oriental as well as Hispanic and Caucasian patients is an incredibly delicious 15-bean soup. It consists of the following legumes: Great Northern, pinto, lima, black-eye, garbanzo, small white, green split pea, baby lima, pear barley, kidney, white kidney, cranberry bean, pink, small red, black, yellow split pea, and navy.

The clinic's two chefs, Oscar Flores and Eva Moreno, make all of their own breads, muffins, cookies, and cakes with almond nut milk or goat's milk and canola oil or flaxseed oil. Their bakery items include banana bread, blueberry muffins, pineapple-upside down bread, raspberry muffins, pineapple bread, almond bread, oatmeal cookies, carob cookies, raisin and oatmeal cookies, orange bread, ginger-apple cookies or bread, apple strudel, almond Danish, poppyseed muffins, and coffee cake. They only use whole wheat flour, *never* bleached white flour, which Dr. Yun believes is detrimental to one's health.

If none of these bakery delectables is available for the evening meal, then a generous helping of fresh fruit is served. When I was there at the beginning of September 1990, the patients feasted on ripe mango slices.

Often a very tempting fruit salad is served at night. Ingredients for it will include finger bananas from the Yucatan, nectarines and miniature oranges from Acapulco, mangos from Mazatlan, papaya from Mexico City, and apples, pears, prunes, raisins, and almonds from wherever. A cottage cheese-yogurt mixture is then blended in to give everything else a more solid base.

Interestingly enough, melons are the only fruit served *alone*. Dr. Yun discovered that they digest a lot easier by themselves than when combined with other fruits.

How the Mind Can Help the Body Fight Cancer

Max Lerner is an unusually lucky fellow. In January 1981, just a month before he turned 78, his long-time internist friend came back with some very bad news following a barium enema and the customary abdominal scan. "You have a problem . . . well, actually *two* of them to be quite frank! You have large-cell lymphoma, always a very difficult cancer to deal with. And yours is advanced." They had also detected a tumor on his prostate gland.

Lerner soon discovered the truth of the old adage that "when it rains, it pours." While doctors attempted to treat him for both cancers, he sustained a severe heart attack in the hospital. His attending physicians and nurses finally resolved to "patch the guy up best we can and get him outta' here" so he could go home to die.

But as Lerner outlined in his best-seller, *Wrestling with the Angel,* (New York: Norton, 1990) and in an interview with me, he wasn't about to pull up stakes just yet. Through all these horrible ordeals he came to grasp the true significance of health as a working equilibrium of the systems of the body—a kind of functioning balance. Illness is the breaking of that equilibrium, throwing each of us into chaos. But recovery is the achieving of a *new* type of equilibrium or something different where you don't return to the old status quo.

Lerner found that healing is simply the restoration of order to our physical, mental, and emotional beings. He discovered rituals or set periods for sleeping and waking, for work and play, for meditation, and so forth. While reading a King James Bible placed in his room by the Gideons, he happened onto the opening verses of the third chapter of Ecclesiastes. There in front of him, in plain English, he said, "Were the very answers I'd been looking for. To everything there is a season, and a time to every purpose under the heaven. A time to be born, and a time to die. . . . A time to kill, and a time to heal; a time to break down, and a time to build up; a time to weep, and a time to laugh . . . I figured," he said, "that my time for healing, building up, and laughing had come."

He began striving for more orderly patterns of daily living than had heretofore been the case. "I adopted a *will therapy* or an active struggle against my illness. I decided to fight the essentially passive role assigned to me by the medical profession. I would no longer be just another 'good patient' complacently accepting whatever they told me or gave me to merely suit their own convenient schedules. Instead, I began using my God-given intelligence and experience to help restore my equilibrium.

"I became a very difficult patient for them to handle. Our sense of values clashed often. I remembered what Thomas Hobbes once said—that 'when two men ride one horse, one of them must ride up front.' So I decided that I must hold the reins in my own doctor-patient relationship. I began seeking for greater *autonomy* to what *I* wanted and not so much to what they imagined I needed. For once in my life, *I started to take charge of my OWN body* for a change. And boy! did it ever feel good, I tell you," he continued.

Lerner started to pursue a variety of adjunct therapies, from regular exercise to visualization techniques, in which he imagined the triumph of his immune system cells in battle over the cancer cells. And whenever he could, he wrote—from ambitious book outlines to his daily personal journal. He attended parties, even in his weaker moments. He learned to laugh again, to dance, to enjoy life to its fullest as much as his own strength would permit him to. "I was fully determined to preserve my core selfhood," he said.

In the most problematic phases of his sickness, he would constantly jot down in his diary: "I *must* live! I *must* live! For there is *so* much yet to do, to see, to enjoy! So, I *have* to live!" He doesn't remember just when this resolve turned into the possibility that he *could* live. But a turning point in his conditions came sometime in 1982 when his physician informed him that his white cell count was finally swinging upward again.

"I now felt the elation of the upward arc of healing," he says. "I stopped losing weight, and ate well without forcing myself to. My new-found energy took me outdoors in walks and gathering firewood. This helped my digestion and made me sleep better without nightmares of dying. My concentration improved, my imagery grew more confident, the memory losses were minimized. My web of relations became closer and stronger."

It wasn't too long before Lerner's "I can live" became reality: "I *shall* live!" At the close of 1990, this spry, old gentleman was getting ready to celebrate his 89th birthday with all of the exhuberance and enthusiasm of a 16-year-old kid. It's been over a decade now since both cancers went into *total* remission and his body bounced back from the effects of his near-death heart attack. To Max Lerner, the seeds of death *and life* are in each one of us. And what we do with them inevitably determines just how long we will last in the face of the bleakest and most despairing adversities imaginable!

◆◆◆◆◆

HEPATITIS

Knowing Your Disease Alphabet

Hepatitis is one of those illnesses with its own series of alphabet letters. A few years ago the two main forms of viruses that caused hepatitis were categorized as A and B. Now other viruses causing this difficult disease have been identified, earning it other letters, C, D, and E. Incidents of hepatitis E, which causes acute diarrhea, are rarely encountered in the United States, since the virus is usually contracted from sewage-containing water. D is found only in the presence of B—researchers do not yet know why.

However, hepatitis C is the one we should be most concerned about right now since it accounts for almost 40% of the estimated 800,000 cases of hepatitis in the United States each year and is responsible for most of those that go on to produce long-term complications. A recent medical study suggests that at least 20% of people with chronic hepatitis C will go on to develop scarring of the liver known as cirrhosis. Finally, hepatitis C is being implicated more and more in the alarming rise of liver cancers these days. Although the death toll from hepatitis C isn't precisely known, the virus is believed to account for most of the annual 25,000 deaths from chronic liver disease in America, notes the October 1990 issue of the *Harvard Medical School Health Letter*.

A Canadian Doctor's Program for Treating Liver Problems

A Canadian Naturopathic doctor, Rolf Edwards, has about the best program for treating hepatitis that I know of. He has put together an herbal program for his hepatitis cases that *works!* "Hepatitis is not your everyday garden-variety type of disease," he reminded me at a recent Canadian Health Food Association convention in Toronto. "Your arsenal of weapons must include things that deliver therapeutic action to the liver, besides just high hopes and expectations to your patient's psyche."

First, he removes the following foods from the diets of his hepatitis patients: legumes (beans or split peas), highly seasoned or fried/deep-fried foods, cabbage dishes, and raw fruit. All of them produce great irritation to the liver and result in terrible physical discomforts.

Second, Rolf has found that "by shopping around some" a person can put together a nice group of products to take from several different companies. "No one manufacturer or single line of products has all the solutions for something as nasty as hepatitis," he insists. The following products form the foundation of his therapy:

Li Chung Yun Formulas 15 & 18. Both herbal combinations were developed by top Oriental healers specifically for the Asiatic people. They are very popular items found in many American and Canadian Chinese herb shops. Dr. Edwards likes Formula 15 because it helps his patients to digest their food better and relieves some of the physical pressure brought on by a deteriorated liver. It includes the Chinese herb pai shu (atractylus), kan ts'ao (licorice root), tang sen (codonopsitis), baishao (peony root), fu ling (poria cocos), ch'en p'i (citrus rind), kanchiang (ginger root), and papaya extract. His patients are instructed to take 2 capsules twice daily with meals. The "L" formula (#18) contains these liver-rejuvenating herbs: dandelion root, black radish, ho-shou-wu, barberry root, bupleurum, pai-shao, golden seal and ginger roots, and capsicum. Dr. Edwards says about 5 capsules a day in between meals is essential for hepatitis cases, less than this (only two) is sufficient for noninfected livers.

Rocky Mountain Multi Minerals. Rolf prescribes 3 tablets daily with meals for any patients suffering from liver disorders (including hepatitis, of course).

Heaven Grade Korean Red Ginseng Extract. Rolf insists that this is one of the most concentrated ginseng root extracts he's ever seen on the market. It contains no water or alcohol. He has his patients put 1 to 2 measuring spoonfuls in a cup of very warm water, then stir the contents thoroughly before *sipping*.

All of these products can be obtained from a Vancouver, B.C., company, Albi Imports. The firm also has an outlet in Washington State to accommodate their American customers. (See the appendix for details.)

Dr. Edwards also finds that wormwood is very useful for liver conditions, including hepatitis. If it's available in your area from a specialty food and beverage store, try to get some wormwood wine. He prefers the Italian varieties like Cinzano and Martini. Amazingly enough, *small* wineglassfuls each day will *not* further injure the livers of alcoholics, but actually help them to a certain extent. A good wormwood fluid extract works just as well if the wine can't be procured. About 15 drops three times daily in 6 fl. oz. of water is suggested. (See Pure Herbs in the appendix for a good source of wormwood fluid extract.) Hot wormwood tea, taken an hour after a meal, is also helpful, but should not be taken for too long (less than a month).

This Canadian naturopathic physician is aware of the recent scientific data to have emerged from Germany regarding the wonderful effects of milk or marian thistle (*Silybum marianum*) upon the liver. If anything can reverse hepatitis besides the Li Chung Yun formulas, he claims, "then surely these would be the ones." He likes the Thisilyn product put out by Nature's Way the best—"I find it works better than some of the other brands." (Thisilyn is available at most health food stores. See the appendix for more details.)

To Edwards's fine supplement program, I'd like to add several things of my own, which experience has shown to be very good for rebuilding injured livers. An 8-fl.-oz. glass of tomato juice or low-sodium V-8 juice with a squirt of lemon juice in it, every afternoon for lunch or evening for dinner, really gives that organ a badly needed boost of energy. (See *The Tohoku Journal of Experimental Medicine*, Vol. 27, 1952, pp. 343–348, for several reports on fresh tomato juice therapy for liver disturbances.) Also cooked artichoke and its juice plays a significant role in revitalizing worn-out livers.

Most of the standard treatments previously used for liver problems have proven ineffective or at least not up to what had been expected of them. These include lipotropic compounds, amino acids, hydrolyzed liver extract, and vitamin B-complex. However, some things like vitamin C (20,000 mg.) and vitamin A (50,000 I.U.) are helpful, when used with the rest of Dr. Edwards's therapy.

◆◆◆◆◆

TUBERCULOSIS

Resurgence of an Old Public Health Menace

The July 15, 1990 *The New York Times* front page carried this ominous headline: "Tuberculosis Germ Resurges as Peril to Public Health." Because of rising tides of AIDS, homelessness, and drug/alcohol abuse, tuberculosis (TB) is reemerging as a public health threat in the United States, especially in the inner cities. During the 1960s and 1970s, when the number of TB cases steadily decreased, and public health officials predicted its near elimination by the turn of the century. But for most of this decade new cases have been rising 5% each year.

Experts say the revival of TB is mainly linked to the AIDS epidemic, largely because people infected with AIDS virus are unusually susceptible to this disease, and, like anyone with active TB, these patients can spread the disease to others. The tuberculosis resurgence is by far the worst in the inner cities, where infection with the AIDS virus overlaps with other conditions associated with a high risk for TB: homelessness, malnutrition, drug use, alcoholism, crowded living conditions, and immigration from underdeveloped countries where TB rates are high. Some of these conditions weaken the immune system; others increase the risk of being exposed to the germ.

Tuberculosis is a chronic wasting disease caused by the mycobacterium tuberculosis, which can be spread through the air, with repeated exposures, particularly in poorly ventilated spaces. While many people carry the germ, the disease can be spread only by the very small number who have active TB, characterized by vigorous coughing and large pockets of the germ in the lung.

Herbal Treatments for Tuberculosis

Tuberculosis is still endemic to many countries of the Pacific Rim (nations situated around the edges of the Pacific Ocean). In my travels to many of them, I've discovered a number of reliable herbal remedies, which can help to delay the progress of or outrightly cure the disease altogether. The following list comes from my initial work with folk healers and doctors in Taiwan, Korea, Thailand, Hong Kong, Burma, Singapore, Malaysia, and Indonesia.

Acorns (Quercus species). Used to reduce TB nodules in Korea and Manchuria (part of mainland China). Remove shells by hand. Cover with water and boil until nearly cooked, then discard liquid. Cover again with fresh water and add 2 tsp. of powdered charcoal to help remove strong tannic acid taste. Boil and discard water again. Cover with water third time and boil again. Strain and drink 1 cup warm several times each day in between meals.

Asparagus. If using fresh asparagus, be sure to break off the woody portions before cooking. But whether using fresh or frozen, cover with almost *double* the amount of water needed; then cook them until they nearly fall to pieces. The idea here is to *over*cook rather than undercook in order to get enough liquid to drink. Strain and drink 1 cup of the warm juice every few hours as needed.

Cinnamon. Small cut pieces of this bark can be purchased in any grocery store or local supermarket. Boil a tablespoonful of bark pieces in 1 pint of water for 5 minutes; then reduce heat to simmer for 25 additional minutes. Strain and drink 1 cup lukewarm as needed.

Coltsfoot Leaves. To 1 pint of boiling water, add 1 tsp. leaves. Stir, cover and steep away from heat 30 minutes. Strain and drink 1 cup warm as needed.

Dandelion Flowers. Pick a handful of fresh dandelion blossoms from an *un*sprayed lawn, pasture, or meadow. Rinse under cold water in wire strain or metal sieve to clean. Immerse in boiling water, cover, and let steep 1 hour; strain and drink 2 cups while still hot.

Dang Quei. A homeopathic physician in Taipei, Taiwan (Dr. Hsu), informed me in 1986 while I was visiting his country that he used the root of Angelica sinensis in powdered form to help cure some of his patients suffering from tuberculosis. He gave them 12 small pills the size of buckshot twice daily for up to three months with good results. An equivalent amount of quality dang quei root from the Orient may be taken as 4 capsules each day of the brand Quan Yin, available by mail order from Albi Imports. (See the appendix for more details.)

Gotu Kola (Hydrocotyle asiatica/Centella asiatica). This is a common weed found throughout much of Malaysia, Indonesia, and the Philippines. Try to cultivate the stuff in a well tended garden and it will die on you. But just throw a handful of seeds in a dirt driveway or pathway which receives a lot of abuse and neglect and watch it grow like crazy! Hot tea is the best way to take this herb for bleeding lungs. Follow directions under coltsfoot leaves for making the tea. Can be ordered from Albi

Imports if local health food stores don't carry it. (See the appendix.)

Hibiscus Rose/Rose of China (an ornamental). Usually available from local nurseries. Quite safe for internal use so long as it hasn't been sprayed for bugs. One handful of the flowers and half a handful of the leaves in a quart of boiling water and steeped for 30 minutes with the pot covered makes a helpful and healing drink for distressed lungs. A cup of the warm tea is suggested 3 times daily.

Marjoram/Oregano (common culinary spice). In parts of Indo-China, it's common for TB sufferers to take a pinch (about ⅛ tsp.) of the powder and mix it into 1 cup of plain hot water before drinking.

Mistletoe. In parts of Burma and Malaysia, folk healers make a broth for the lungs by cooking some of the leaves and twigs with a piece of pork for up to an hour. A chop or other cut of pork will suffice, along with 1 large Tbsp. of the dried twigs and leaves in 1¼ quarts of water, boiled down to ¾ quart and taken while still warm. Very, very good for TB in children and the elderly. The pork seems to neutralize any negative effects that the mistletoe may have.

Prickly Ash (Zanthoxylum americanum). Difficult to find in the crude form for tea making. But a liquid tincture or extract is satisfactory enough. Some of the Chinese homeopathic doctors I met in Singapore a while back used this herb extensively on their TB patients. Between 15 and 20 drops of the fluid extract should be taken sublingually (beneath the tongue) twice daily in between meals. (Pure Herbs of Madison Heights, Michigan, carries the fluid extract; see the appendix.)

Violet and Pansy. Both are common garden flowers and very pretty to look at. They are often used by European and Chinese herbalists for lung disorders of all kinds, including tuberculosis and pneumonia. Not only are the flowers used, but also the roots of the plants as well. The roots require several minutes of simmering on low heat, before adding the flowers. But *don't boil* the flowers or you'll lose their value. Cover and steep contents an hour. Strain and drink a cup while still warm.

Woundwort/All-heal/Prunella. This is a widespread weed in China, Taiwan, Japan and Korea. Use the dried stalk, leaves and flowering spikes. Make a tea as you might for mistletoe, but omit the pork. Drink a cup warm to soothe inflamed and infected lungs.

Summary

1. Because of promiscuous and riotous life-styles, substance abuse, poverty, and other social ills, some diseases of an epidemic scale are health realities of the nineties.

2. The AIDS virus is an elusive, ever-changing microbe masquerading under a number of different disguises.

3. Some external detection for the AIDS virus is better than the biochemical kind.

4. Spicey foods seem to help retard the AIDS virus.

5. Long-term survivors of AIDS must cope with a different set of illnesses known as "opportunistic infections"; hence, their programs must be constantly revised and updated to match the particular ailments bothering them.

6. Anger can damage the body just as much as smoking, a high-fat diet, chronic alcoholism, or obesity can.

7. Social solutions help allay chronic anger, as well as replacing the amalgam fillings in one's teeth sometimes.

8. A vinegar made with aromatic herbs affords protection against the bubonic plague.

9. Antibiotic herbs and nourishing foods are the best prevention/treatment program for lung, colo-rectal, breast, and prostate cancers.

10. Oriental and Western herbs and nutritional supplements help to combat hepatitis and tuberculosis.

⚜ 8 ⚜

"Power Eating" With Recipes to Fight Infection

I AM INDEBTED to Chef Paul Buck, formerly of Hampstead, England, for helping me formulate the recipes here. At one time he worked for the British Broadcasting Corporation (the BBC) and cooked for top recording artists like the Beatles, the Rolling Stones, and Elton John, who "were all into health food themselves." Here is where he learned healthier cooking practices. Paul was executive chef for the Mount Irvine Bay Hotel in Tobago, West Indies, for a while—"a true island paradise," he recalls with a warm smile. Since then, he has been the main chef in some of the South's classiest restaurants, working in Florida, Georgia, and the Carolinas.

The following recipes are guidelines. Paul and I have intended them to be working models of what good meals ought to be for successful recuperation from illnesses. Individual foods that may complement a particular condition are included with some of these recipes. The recipes here are intended for the following problems, but are not limited to them.

AIDS and cancer	Fever
Allergies	Ecological illness
Asthma and bronchitis	Gastroenteritis
Candidiasis	Infection (general)
Chickenpox, measles, mumps	Sexually transmissible diseases
	Sore throat
Chronic fatigue syndrome	Systemic lupus erythematosus
Common cold, influenza	Tonsillitis
Constipation	Tuberculosis

289

AIDS AND CANCER

Item: "Protease inhibitors in beans and grains prevent radiation-induced carcinogenesis and enhance tissue resistance to invasion by tumor cells." (*Journal of The National Cancer Institute*, December 1984)

Whole Black Beans

Ingredients:

8 oz. whole black beans	2 pints water
2½–3 tsp. sea salt	12 finely cut cloves of garlic
1 oz. finely cut ginger root	½ oz. clarified butter (ghee)
4 dried red chilies	

Method:

1. Remove the grit from the beans and wash them 3–4 times.
2. Boil the water and add salt, beans, garlic, ginger, red chilies, and butter.
3. Cover with a lid. When it comes to a boil, reduce the heat and simmer 3–4 minutes. Serves two to four.

Item: "Dr. Saxon Graham and others reported: "We found decreased risks in cancers of the colon and rectum associated with *frequent* ingestion of vegetables, and *especially* cabbage, brussels sprouts, and broccoli. (*Journal of the National Cancer Institute*, September 1978).

Braised Red Cabbage

Ingredients:

¾ lb. red cabbage	2 oz. butter
¼ pint apple cider vinegar	4 oz. cooking apples
½ oz. brown sugar (or 1 tsp. honey)	pinch of kelp (seaweed)

Method:

1. Quarter, trim, and shred cabbage.

2. Wash well and drain; then season with *coarse* kelp.

3. *Place* in a well-buttered ovenproof casserole pan. *Do not* use aluminum or iron.

4. Add vinegar and cover with a buttered piece of paper and the lid.

5. Bake in a moderate oven for approximately 1 ½ hours.

6. Add the peeled, cored apples diced into ½" pieces. Recover the lid and continue cooking until tender, about 2 hours total. If a little dry use stock to moisten. Serves three.

Brussels Sprouts

Ingredients:

    Brussel sprouts
    Chestnuts
    Butter

Methods:

Cook sprouts until a little firm. Drain well and mix with equal amounts of chestnuts that have been peeled and cooked in stock. Butter nicely and serve.

Broccoli Salad

Ingredients:

broccoli flowerets	smidgen of brown sugar
2 tsp. tarragon vinegar	4 tsp. olive oil
sea salt and kelp to taste	1 tsp. tomato puree

Method:

1. Soak broccoli in cold water 30 minutes. Then break broccoli into flowerets. Tie flowerets loosely in a piece of muslin and cook in boiling water for 10 minutes. Drain and chill.

2. Make a dressing of the tarragon vinegar, salt, kelp, sugar, and olive oil. Mix well and add tomato puree.

3. Put flowerets in salad bowl and toss gently. If enough broccoli is used, this should serve four.

Complementary Foods: Carrots, radishes, green and red onions, garlic, cauliflower, mustard greens, spinach, Oriental mushrooms (shiitake), kale, and kohlrabi all have chemopreventive and chemotherapeutic value for treating AIDS and cancer nutritionally. And clinical work done by Japanese scientists indicate that *fresh* figs help to reduce tumors as much as 50%, said *Agricultural & Biological Chemistry* (July 1978) and *Cancer Treatment Reports* (January 1980).

◆◆◆◆◆

ALLERGIES

ITEM: Over the past six years, several research teams have shown that tannic acid can chemically alter house dust, pollen, and dust-mite antigens so that they no longer elicit allergic reactions. (*Science News*, Vol. 138; p. 109).

Refreshing Teas & Soups

Oriental teas (black, green, and mixed combinations) contain large amounts of tannins. The *Encyclopedia of Common Natural Ingredients Used in Food, Drugs & Cosmetics* (New York: John Wiley & Sons, 1980) reports that this can be as much as 27%. Green tea generally ranks a little higher in tannic acid than does black tea, but not by much. Use these teas not only as tangy beverages but also as potential *stock* bases for a number of vegetarian consommés.

The following varieties of black and green teas will help to alleviate many types of allergies. And may be successfully used without much worry about worsening any existing allergies, except in the rarest instances. They can be ordered in bulk from Frontier Herbs or Great American Natural Products (see the appendix).

Assam. A flowering orange pekoe with a robust, rich, malty taste and a cloudy, amber color from the Assam Province in Northeast India.

Ceylon. An intense, flowery aroma and flavor characterize this imported tea from Sri Lanka.

Darjeeling. Another flowery orange pekoe with a full-bodied, delicate flavor and a dark amber color from India.

Earl Grey. A hearty and aromatic black tea that's been sprayed with French bergamot oil. Recommended for different soup bases. Works well with fish, particularly salmon.

English Breakfast. A fine quality tea from Taiwan, characterized with a rich, mellow, Chinese flavor and fragrant aroma. This black tea is a combination of Assam flowery orange pekoe and Ceylon broken orange pekoe. Also very good to use in consommés. Use with Navy beans.

Formosa Black. An inexpensive standard grade that may be combined with cinnamon bark or cloves or orange peel. When mixed with any of the foregoing spices, goes great with small peeled pumpkin or sweet potato chunks.

Gunpowder Green. Has a round, bold character, is a little pungent and bitter. Brews up to a yellow-green color. Works surprisingly well in leek or onion soups. Tangy vegetables like radishes and endive complement it, too.

Irish Breakfast. Will tempt the palates of even the most discriminating tea drinkers. This combination of Assam flowery orange pekoe and Ceylon orange pekoe goes well with delicate flowers (rose petals, marigolds, tulips) and slightly tangy greens like spinach or watercress. The broth base should be boiling hot before such ingredients are added. Then remove from heat, cover, and steep 10 minutes before serving.

Jasmine. A sweet-smelling tea made by adding scented white jasmine flowers during the final firing of Pouchong tea. Makes a remarkable base for certain "fruit" soups, for example, finely diced *fresh*, ripened, peeled peaches or pears.

Keemun Congou. Similar to English Breakfast, but of much higher quality. Dark amber in color, it's considered China's finest black tea. Good with most legumes.

Kukicha Twig. Considered to be the lowest grade of tea. But for those wanting something without tannic acid or caffeine and nutritionally good (high in calcium), then this is the one. Preferred among macrobiotic diet enthusiasts. Needs to be simmered 15 minutes on low heat to bring out the mellow flavor, though. See what this can do for chickpeas, slit peas, and lentils!

Lapsang Souchong. This Taiwan black tea has a strong, distinctive, smoky flavor to it. If you don't object to pork, throw in a ham hock bone along with some diced turnips. One-quarter teaspoons of low-sodium Worcestershire, soy, and Tabasco sauces may also be added *provided* one isn't allergic to any of them.

Long Jing. A black tea from the province of Hanchow, noted for its light, fresh flavor and smooth scented aroma. Also good for certain "fruit" soups, especially when soaking pieces of *homemade* dried fruit in it for a while.

Oolong. An exquisite tea famous for its delicate, subtle, fruity taste and light color. Try soaking organic (*un*sprayed) raisins in some of this hot brew.

Yunnan. A flowery orange pekoe black tea from China.

◆◆◆◆

Two Tea Recipes

Method I:

1. Boil fresh water until it's bubbling fiercely.

2. Rinse your teapot with boiling water, then drain it, keeping it warm.

3. Use a clean, dry spoon to remove the bulk leaves from the container. (Use about 1 tsp. of tea per cup, plus 1 for the pot). Put the tea in your teapot.

4. Quickly transfer the boiling water to the pot, pouring directly over the leaves. Cover and steep for 3 to 5 minutes. If desired, small quantities of fresh or canned *goat's* milk can be added, but avoid too much as it will spoil the aroma and flavor.

Method II:

1. Large mesh tea infusers are excellent for making big jars of tea for icing.

2. Simply fill the ball with loose tea and place in a clean gallon jar full of cool water.

3. Place in the sun until steeped to desired strength.

4. Then strain and add ice cubes formed from *distilled* or pure *spring* water.

◆◆◆◆◆

A Pumpkin Tea Soup

This recipe serves as a working model for making other soups.

Ingredients:

2 lb. pumpkin, peeled and chopped into 2" chunks

4 cups of spicy Formosa black tea

½ lb. sweet potato, chopped

1 scallion, crushed (if allergic, then omit)*

1 clove garlic (if allergic, then omit)*

1 sprig fresh thyme or 1 tsp. dried herb

2 Tbsp. barley miso or sea salt to taste

*Dill may be substituted for scallion or garlic if allergic to them.

Method:

1. In a medium-sized saucepan, add pumpkin to 2 cups tea. Cook until the pumpkin is soft enough to crush or purée.

2. While pumpkin is cooking, in a separate saucepan add the sweet potato to 2 cups of tea and cook until it's soft but not mushy.

3. Drain tea purée the sweet potato or mash it with a fork, and add it to the pumpkin with the scallion/garlic and thyme or dill and thyme.

4. Add more tea if the mixture is too thick.

5. Add sea salt, if not using miso.

6. Cook for 10 minutes.

7. Take out ¼ cup of the soup and dissolve miso in it.

8. Return to pot and heat for 3 more minutes (don't boil).
Serves four.

◆◆◆◆◆

Legume Tea Soup

Ingredients:

1 cup red peas, dried broad beans, or adkuki beans

1 cup goat's milk

1 cup English Breakfast or Keemun Congou or Lapsang Souchong Tea

3 sprigs fresh thyme or 3 tsp. dried or some dill

4 whole allspice berries

1 peppercorn

coarsely granulated kelp for flavor

Method:

1. Wash beans or peas and add to pot. Add milk and tea.

2. Cook the legumes until they're soft but not mushy.

3. When cooked, add spices and kelp.

4. Simmer until soft, adding more tea if necessary.
Serves four.

◆◆◆◆◆

ASTHMA & BRONCHITIS

ITEM: "Caffeine [can] result in bronchodilation in asthmatic children. . . . Caffeine . . . can produce significant improvement . . . in adult asthmatics." (*American Review of Respiratory Disease*, Vol. 135, 1987, pp. 173–75)

ITEM: "One or more components of crude onion extract appear to have a protective effect against allergen-induced bronchial obstruction in the guinea pig and may prove useful in bronchial asthma treatment in humans." (*Agents Actions*, Vol 14, May-June 1984, pp. 626–629)

Both black and green tea contain about 5% caffein. Use some Gunpowder Green Tea with onions for a soup base.

◆◆◆◆

Breathe Easier soup

Ingredients:

    3 cups of Gunpowder Green Tea
    1 onion, finely minced (or ¼ cup onion flakes)
    1 carrot, diced (or ¼ cup dried or frozen diced carrots)
    2 tablespoons of yerba maté tea leaves
    ½ teaspoons of coarse kelp, basil, oregano and parsley flakes.

Method:

Cook all the ingredients together on medium heat, until carrots are done. Discard yerba maté leaves and serve hot. Serves four.

◆◆◆◆◆

CANDIDIASIS

ITEM: "The consumption of vegetables from the mustard family as a means of enhancing the immune system's ability to resist recurrent candidal infections, has been advocated by one therapist." (*New Zealand Medical Journal*, 98 (780): 450, 1985)

The mustard family is quite large and includes all those vegetables belonging to the genus Brassica, as follows:

Black, brown, or grocer's mustard (B. nigra)

White mustard, charlock, or salad mustard (B. or Sinapis alba)

Field mustard (B. campestris)

Chinese or Indian mustard (B. juncea)

Tansy mustard (Sisymbrium incisa, S. pinnata)

Hedge mustard (S. officinale)

Common green cabbage (B. oleracea)

Red or purple cabbage (B. oleracea rubra)

Broccoli (B. oleracea italica)

Kale and collards (B. oleracea acephala)

Kohlrabi (B. oleracea)

Cauliflower (B. oleracea botrytis)

Brussels sprout (B. oleracea gemmifera)

There is also a close relative of the mustards called rocket that grows wild in southern Europe and cultivated as a salad vegetable throughout the British Isles and France. It has a very distinctive spicy falvor, but digests better if consumed with lettuce or purslane.

About half of the foregoing list of items are readily obtainable from any supermarket or green grocer. Some of the varieties of mustard leaves make great salads. Shredded cabbage along with just a few other simple ingredients makes a quick and easy cole slaw. In the South they have different ways of fixing *cooked* "mixed greens" or plain "collards 'n greens." Usually a little lemon or lime juice perks them up a little more.

◆◆◆◆

Whole Cauliflower

Ingredients (for steaming):

1 medium cauliflower	½ oz. ginger
6 cloves garlic	¾ tsp. sea salt
2 green chilies	½ tsp. garam masala
½ tsp. cayenne pepper	1 tsp. lemon juice

Ingredients (for masala paste):

3–4 oz. ghee (Indian clarified butter): Melt 2 lb. butter until it reaches slow, rolling boil. Remove from heat and skim off foam with spoon. Return to heat and repeat this procedure twice more, removing as much of the foam as possible and discarding it. Allow pan to cool 2 minutes and then remove thin film that forms. Let the butter cool and then, while still liquid, pour through a fine-meshed tea strainer, but stop pouring when the heavier solids at bottom of pan move to strainer. Collect ghee in glass jar, cool completely, and cover. Entire process takes less than half an hour. Two pounds of butter yields 1 lb. ghee. Can be stored without refrigeration for 6 months. (I'm grateful to a colleague, Michael Tierra, for these instructions on how to prepare ghee.)

5 crushed garlic cloves	an inch piece of cinnamon
½ oz. coriander seeds	6 cloves
	8 peppercorns
4 oz. tomatoes	4 green cardamoms (if
½ oz. dry shredded coconut	available) (otherwise use 2 tsp. powdered
½ tsp. white cumin seeds	cardamom)
	½ oz. almonds
4 tsp. plain yogurt	¾ tsp. sea salt
4 oz. onions	pinch of nutmeg
½ oz. ginger	½ tsp. garam masala

Method (for steaming cauliflower):

1. Wash and dry cauliflower.
2. Grind garlic, ginger, and green chilies.
3. Add salt, cayenne pepper, and garam masala.
4. Mix lemon juice with ground paste.
5. Put as much paste as possible between flowerets.
6. Place cauliflower with stems down in heatproof dish that can hold it in vertical position.
7. Transfer to trivet (three-legged tripod) in pressure cooker; add ¼ pint water and steam for 3 minutes at 10 lb. pressure. In the absence of a pressure cooker, place in a degchi, add ½ pint of water, and steam 20 minutes or until half-cooked.

Method (for masala paste):

1. Heat the ghee and fry thinly sliced onions and garlic.
2. Grind ginger, coriander seeds, cloves, peppercorns, cinnamon, cardamoms, almonds, and cumin seeds. Then add the shredded coconut. (In some instances, powdered spices may need to be substituted where the fresh spices can't be obtained.)
3. Add the ground masala, salt, and nutmeg to the frying onions and continue cooking with small amounts of yogurt until it's completely utilized.
4. Last add the pulp of 4 oz. tomatoes.

5. Cover the top of the cauliflower with half the masala paste.

6. Coat with ghee and bake in moderate oven (350° F.) for 15 minutes or until the masala is browned and the cauliflower evenly cooked.

7. Remove from oven, pour the remaining masala around it, and bake 5 minutes. Serve, sprinkled with chopped coriander leaves or parsley, green chilies, and garam masala. Serves two to three.

Stuffed Cabbage Rolls

Ingredients:

24 small or 12 large cabbage leaves

2 oz. onions

1 oz. ginger

2 tsp. sea salt

½ tsp. garam masala

8–12 oz. tomato puree

6 cloves garlic

6 green chilies

12 oz. lean mutton or Indian cream cheese

¾ tsp. cayenne pepper

1 tsp. flour

4 oz. ghee

little lime juice

¼ tsp. white pepper

Method:

1. Wash cabbage, carefully separate leaves, and simmer in boiled salted water until they are half-cooked.

2. Remove from water and drain.

3. Mince the raw meat or the panir (cream cheese).

4. Heat some ghee and fry lightly the finely chopped onions, 6 chopped garlic cloves, ½ oz. ginger, and 3 chilies.

5. Add minced meat or panir, sea salt, cayenne, and garam masala. Cook until tender. Remove from heat, cool, and divide into 12 equal parts.

6. Remove hard stems from cabbage leaves and spread them on a table. (If leaves are small place two of them with their edges overlapping on each other.)

7. Put one part of the minced meat mixture on one edge of each leaf; roll and turn the sides gently in.

8. Sprinkle over them a little fresh lime juice, salt, white and red pepper; then roll in dry flour and brown in hot butter or ghee.

9. Remove from ghee and lightly brown in hot butter or ghee remaining onions, ginger, and green chilies.

10. Add the rolls along with 2 tsp. water. Cook covered until tender. When nearly done add the tomato puree and cook uncovered for 10 minutes. Add salt and pepper to taste. Serve hot. Serves four to six.

◆◆◆◆◆◆

CHICKENPOX, MEASLES, AND MUMPS

ITEM: "Of no small importance is the ability of peppermint to inhibit and kill many kinds of micro organisms. . . . A few of these bugs need special mention: . . . Herpes simplex, the source of cold sores [and chickenpox]; mumps virus . . . . [Daniel B. Mowry, *The Scientific Validation of Herbal Medicine* (Lehi, UT: Cormorant Books, 1986), p. 75]."

ITEM: "Hundreds of case histories . . . have come to us, through the carefully controlled clinical research of the American eclectic physicians. . . During the height of their activity, literally hundreds of cases were reported, in which echinacea was used to prevent and treat an incredible variety of infectious diseases: . . . measles . . . mumps, rubella . . . [Daniel B. Mowry, *Next Generation Herbal Medicine* (Lehi, UT: Cormorant Books, 1988), p. 57]."

Cooling Tea

This tea reduces the fever present in these childhood ailments. The child should be given this simple tea in ½ cup amounts several times during the day on an empty stomach, and preferably when slightly cool, but *not* cold either.

Ingredients:

4 Tbsp. cut fresh (or 3 Tbsp. dried) peppermint leaves*
1 pint distilled or spring water
¼ tsp. real vanilla flavor
pinch of cardamom
¼ tsp. dark honey or blackstrap molasses
15 drops fluid extract echinacea herb*

Method:

1. Bring water to rapid boil in pot that *isn't* aluminum.

*2. Add mint leaves and stir. (Oil of peppermint may be substituted if the leaves aren't readily available. But only add between 6 and 8 drops at the most, since it's quite strong.)

3. Then remove from the heat and add vanilla, cardamom powder, and honey or molasses. Stir again and cover with lid to steep about 25 minutes.

4. About halfway through steeping time, add the echinacea fluid extract. (See Pure Herbs in the appendix to obtain this.)

5. Strain and give ½ cup of *slightly* cooled tea to child every few hours on an empty stomach.

◆◆◆◆◆

CHRONIC FATIGUE SYNDROME

ITEM: "The stamina building [and] antistress . . . principle of *Cicer arietinum* [Bengal gram chickpea] has been isolated and identified for the first time to be pangamic acid (D-glucono-dimethylaminoacetic acid). . . . Seeds soaked overnight in water and the sprouted grain are both considered to be extremely nourishing and constitute a regular item of diet for athletes and professional wrestlers in India. . . . Bengal gram [chickpea] is used as a food for horses which gives them an untiring stamina . . . (*Journal of Ethnopharmacology*, Vol.7, 1983, p. 239)."

ITEM: "There are 117.07 milligrams of pangamic acid in 100 grams of Bengal gram (chickpea] (*Indian Drugs*, February 1983, p. 187)."

Chickpea and Vegetable Stew

Ingredients (for cooking chickpeas):

> 2 cups dried chickpeas
> 6 cups water
> ½ tsp. salt (optional)

Method (for cooking chickpeas):

    1. Wash chickpeas and pick out any stones. Soak for 8 hours in cold water or bring beans and water to boil, cook for 2 minutes, turn off heat, and soak for 2 hours.

    2. After beans swell, add enough water to cover; cook in a pressure cooker for 50 minutes or else simmer on the stove for 1½ to 2 hours.

    3. Add the salt 10 minutes before the chickpeas have finished cooking. Pour off excess water before serving. (If desired, reserve the water for making soup.) Serves four by itself or use in stew recipe below.

Ingredients (for cooking millet):

2 cups raw millet grain	pinch of salt
3 cups boiling water	pinch of powdered
3 tsp. butter or sunflower seed or olive oil	cardamom

Method (for cooking millet):

    1. Bring water to boil; then add butter or oil.

    2. Next, sprinkle in the millet a little at a time. Stir briefly and partially cover. Reduce heat to lowest setting possible.

    3. Cook the millet for 15–20 minutes *only*. Overcooking tends to make it mushy. Stir with a fork halfway through cooking and again at the end. This time, it's desirable that the trapped steam escape; otherwise it will keep cooking the millet even after it's removed from direct heat. So fluff it with a fork *a lot* after it's cooked and leave it uncovered. This is the best deterrent to avoid mushiness.

    4. Add the salt and cardamom *after* it's cooked.

Ingredients (for chickpea-vegetable stew):

>   2 cups cooked chickpea
>   4 cups cooked millet
>   2 Tbsp. olive oil
>   2 Tbsp. butter
>   1 cup of chopped white onion
>   1 tsp. salt
>   1 lb. fresh mushrooms, chopped
>   3 Tbsp. fresh lemon juice
>   1 lb. bunch fresh broccoli, chopped
>   ½ cup (packed) currants
>   kelp to taste
>   cayenne pepper to taste
>   ½ tsp. mild paprika
>   1½ cups chopped, toasted cashews

Method (for chickpea-vegetable stew):

1. Cook onion in combined olive oil and butter, with salt, in large, heavy skillet. Keep heat medium-low, and cook for 5 minutes or until onion begins to get tender.

2. Add mushrooms, lemon juice, and broccoli. Cover, and cook over medium-low heat until the broccoli is bright green and barely tender (8–10 minutes for this).

3. Add cooked drained chickpeas and all remaining ingredients, and simmer, covered for another 6 minutes. Serve over millet.

Serves four. Arrange stew in center of a platter, with millet around its edges.

◆◆◆◆◆

COMMON COLD AND INFLUENZA

ITEM: "The present note reports evidence of an inhibiting influence of an aqueous garlic extract on the infectious process developing in mice inoculated with influenza virus A/PR8/34 (H1N1). . . . Garlic extract suppressed rate of lung infection of mice with experimental influenza." (*Revue Roumaine De Medecine-Virologie/Romanian Review of Medicine & Virology*, Vol. 34, 1983, pp. 11—17).

◆◆◆◆◆

West Indian Fish Garlic Soup

Ingredients:

2 lb. assorted fresh fish

½ gal. water

1 cup white wine

1 bay leaf

1 large onion, peeled and sliced

½ cup sliced celery

½ cup chopped raw carrots

2 large raw potatoes, peeled and chopped

¼ tsp. powdered turmeric

2 cloves garlic, finely minced

1 tsp. liquid kyolic garlic (see Wakunaga in the appendix)

1 tsp. coarse granulated kelp

pinch of cayenned pepper

pinch of powdered thyme

pinch of rosemary

Method:

1. Clean and cut up fish—rock cod, bass, or whatever is available. Put fish, head, and tail in a large pot and cover with water. Bring to a rolling boil.

2. Add white wine and bay leaf.

3. Let simmer until fish falls apart, about 1½ hours.

4. Discard bones, fins, heads, and so on.

5. Sauté onions and celery in butter until golden brown. Pour sautéed vegetables into stock, rinsing pan with some of the stock, and add it back into the pot for extra flavor and color.

6. Next add carrots, potatoes, seasonings, and liquid kyolic garlic as well as minced raw garlic.

7. Simmer for another hour or until vegetables are mushy.

8. Remove soup from stove and force everything through a food mill or a large-hole food colander, or blend the entire soup with the vegetables and the fish in a blender, adding a little at a time.

9. Return to pot and bring to another boil. Correct seasonings if necessary.

10. This soup should have consistency of cream soup, but without the benefit of milk or cream or flour or grease. Serves four to five.

◆◆◆◆◆◆

CONSTIPATION

ITEM: "Twenty-five of forty-eight volunteers maintained a daily intake of potatoes approximately to 1 kg. for a minimum of 10 weeks to a maximum of 20 weeks. The average consumption was 0.86 kg., i.e. about 2 lbs., containing an estimated 4.26 grams crude fibre. . . . There was a significant decrease in intestinal transit times and in colo-rectal pressures, and significant increase in stool wieghts." (*Irish Journal of Medical Science*, September, 1977, p. 285).

ITEM: "Concentrations [of minerals] are generally at their highest in raw unpeeled potato and at their lowest in potato peeled before cooking." (*Acta Agriculturae Scandinavica*, Vol. 22, Suppl., 1980, p. 159).

◆◆◆◆◆

Potato, Tomato, and Onion Curry

Ingredients:

1 lb. small potatoes	2–3 oz. ghee (see recipe on p. 298 for preparation)
1 lb. tomatoes	
2 tsp. coarsely granulated kelp	8 oz. small whole onions
	½ tsp. garam masala
pinch of cayenne pepper	3 green chilies
½ tsp. turmeric	1 oz. finely cut ginger root
	½ tsp. honey

Method:

1. Heat the ghee. Skin onions and keeping them whole cook on medium heat for 30 minutes.

2. Then add small whole potatoes or roughly cut large ones, kelp, cayenne pepper, and turmeric and cook on low heat. (Add no liquid but cover the pot with lid, and when potatoes are nearly cooked, add wedges of tomatoes, sliced green chilies, ginger, and honey.

3. Turn heat to highest setting and continue cooking. The potatoes and tomatoes, though cooked, should remain firm. Serve sprinkled with garam masala (available from any specialty food store carrying Indian foods) and chopped fresh parsley. Serves three to four.

◆◆◆◆◆◆

FEVER

ITEM: "Cold is not only antipyretic [anti-fever], but may be applied . . . as a sedative and anodyne [pain-relieving agent]. . . . it may be even used as a local anaesthetic." [J.V. Shoemaker, *A Practical Treatise on Materia Medica & Therapeutics*, 7th rev. ed., (Philadelphia: F.A. Davis, 1908), pp. 1117–1118].

◆◆◆◆

Beverage Body Coolers

Ingredients:

1 cup fresh raspberries	1–2 tsp. pure maple syrup
¾ cup white grape juice	½ cup yogurt or goat's milk (optional)

Method:

1. Blend the chilled berries with the sweetening, and strain.

2. Add the chilled juice and serve in a frosted glass or cup (chilled in the freezer) or with crushed ice if desired. The amount of berries and juice may be altered to suit personal taste. Add extra berries for a redder, richer taste or more juice to lighten the flavor.

Ingredients:

1 cup fresh or frozen blackberries or ripe, dark pitted cherries

¾ cup purple grape juice

1–2 tsp. dark honey or maple syrup

Method:

Prepare in same way as the foregoing recipe.

Ingredients:

> 1 liter spring/distilled water   3–5 Tbsp. maple syrup
> juice of 3 lemons

Method:

1. Mix liquid sweetening into 1 cup of very hot water until it dissolves.

2. Add lemon juice, ice cubes, and cold water until the mixture equals 1 liter. If ice isn't available, use water only and chill before serving. Stir and serve.

Ingredients:

> 1 cup blueberries   1 stick cinnamon
> 1 cup berries of your   1 tsp. grated lemon rind
> choice   ¼ cup lemon juice
> 1½ cups water   1 tsp. powdered slippery
> 2 Tbsp. quick-cooking   elm
> tapioca
> ¼ cup honey

Method:

1. Combine all ingredients in a saucepan. Bring mixture to a boil over medium heat and simmer for 5–7 minutes, stirring frequently.

2. Remove from heat, transfer to chilled pitcher, and refrigerate until liquid is *cool*, but not necessarily cold. This is an excellent drink for children or adults who are recuperating from illness.

◆◆◆◆◆◆

ECOLOGICAL ILLNESS

ITEM: "Allergies may be the missing link in modern medicine, the explanation for what is unexplained. . . . Allergic reactions can resemble the symptoms of almost any disease. Allergy is modern medicine's 'great mimicker.' Allergic reactions can trigger a range of symptoms not traditionally associated with allergies. They can affect how people feel, act, and even think. Allergies can account for countless physical problems. . . . Allergic symptoms are not just limited to physical ills. They can also affect the mind. . . . The can increase a person's susceptibility to [infection] by overloading the body's immune system. Allergies can also cause fluctuations in symptoms associated with other diseases. . . . Although pollens, molds, and dust can cause such dramatic symptoms, allergic people are more likely to react to. . . . other substances: the foods they eat. . . . The foods could be junk foods . . . but they don't have to be. They could be wholesome, nutritious foods because allergies don't discriminate between good and bad foods. . . . Allergens . . . could include what people eat most often. . . ." (*Let's Live*, March 1988, pp. 28–36)

Ecological illness, as defined elsewhere in this book, can be having an allergic reaction to just about anything in the environment, or, put more specifically, to being "allergic to life" in general! But there are ways to cope with this. The most important are "avoidance of selected foods for a minimum of 3 to 6 months [which] can effectively decrease the antibody titers of I_gG and their subclasses [of allergy antigens]," noted the November 1987 issue of *Annals of Allergy*.

Briefly put, it's not so much what you eat but what you must *avoid* consuming to minimize allergic symptoms of ecological illness. Hence, meal recipes should *not* include any of the following items: dairy products, eggs, white/brown sugar, wheat flour (brown or white), baking yeast, chocolate, and so forth. Also, other staples like shellfish, celery, peaches, nectarines, grapes, lettuce, and just about all store-bought meat should be discontinued. In their place, substitute organic chicken, fish, and some types of organic produce.

Learn to revise old recipes and substitute other things in place of items you've been familiar with using for a long time. The following bread recipe is an example of this.

◆◆◆◆◆

Wheatfree Rye Bread

Ingredients I:

1 cup rye flour	½ cup soy flour
1½ cups rice flour	2 Tbsps. aluminum-free baking powder

Method I:

1. Mix the dry ingredients together thoroughly.

Ingredients II:

1 Tbsp. olive oil	1 Tbsp. honey
1 Tbsp. blackstrap molasses	1 tsp. sea salt

Method II:

1. Mix with flour mixture until well combined; then scrape the thick batter into a well-oiled loaf pan (8½ inches x 4½ inches).

2. Make a dome out of aluminum foil and cover the pan with it, but leaving sufficient room for the bread to rise in.

3. Bake about 70 minutes, covered, in an oven preheated to 350°F.

4. Cool on a rack, out of the pan. Makes 24 slices.

When making soups or stews, try using spices in place of table salt and black pepper. Those with ecological illnesses report that seasoning their food with dill herb, thyme, basil, rosemary, and sage keeps their allergic reactions to a minimum. But use them *fresh*, if possible, since most store-bought spices have been fumigated with ethylene oxide to kill insects. Also the use of several other spices like cardamon, for instance, can reduce intolerances to wheat and milk. Use this powdered spice in cooked cereal, in puddings made from goat milk, and in other dishes that call for whole wheat or milk.

Also the manner in which food is cooked sometimes can positively or negatively affect someone suffering form ecological problems. Foods that are steamed, baked, or boiled generally yield the least harmful reactions, while foods that are pan fried, deep-fat dried, barbecued, charbroiled, or microwaved tend to produce the most unpleasant physical and biochemical results.

And, by the way, the type of beverages consumed has a lot to do with how well an ecological illness can be managed. *Any* colas, soft drinks, canned/bottled fruit juices, beer, wine, and hard liquor are obviously taboo. Also forbidden are chlorinated/fluoridated water, tea, and coffee. Most beneficial and *least* reactionary are some fresh fruit juices (kiwis and limes), a few organic vegetable juices (especially carrot), and bottled mineral/spring water. Also the use of baking soda (¼ tsp. in 8 fl. oz.) acidifies the body to minimize reactions.

◆◆◆◆◆

GASTROENTERITIS

ITEM: "Certain spices are proven to be the best remedy for gastroenteritis, as a rule." [John Heinerman. *The Complete Book of Spices* (New Canaan, CT: Keets Publishing, Co., 1983)].

◆◆◆◆

Anti-Inflammatory Tea

Ingredients:

½ tsp. caraway seed	pinches of ginger and
½ tsp. fennel seed	cardamom
½ tsp. dried mint leaves	several drops of pure vanilla
	½ tsp. chamomile flowers

Method:

1. Bring 3 cups of water to a boil.

2. Add caraway and fennel seeds, cover, and simmer on low heat for 5 minutes.

3. Uncover and add mint and chamomile. Stir, cover, and remove from heat and steep 25 minutes.

4. About 15 minutes into steeping, while still quite warm, uncover and add powdered ginger and cardamom and vanilla extract. Stir, recover, and continue steeping.

5. Strain and drink a cup *lukewarm*.

◆◆◆◆◆

INFECTION

ITEM: "Garlic was on the verge of being accepted as a valid antibiotic before the development of synthetic antibiotics in the late 1940s . . . [Filmmaker Les Blank]: In Peru I ate one or two cloves a day chopped in fresh orange juice. I didn't get any of the intestinal parasites others did." [Sheldon Greenberg and Elizabeth L. Ortiz, *The Spice of Life* (New York: The Amaryllis Press, 1983), p. 142].

◆◆◆◆◆

Onion and Garlic Soup

Ingredients:

> ¼ cup butter
>
> 6 large onions, peeled and finely chopped
>
> 4–6 large cloves garlic, peeled and minced
>
> 1 tsp. whole-wheat flour
>
> 2 cups dry white wine (Chablis)
>
> sea salt and coarse kelp, to taste
>
> ½ tsp. crumbled thyme
>
> 4 cups chicken stock
>
> 4 large eggs
>
> 1 cup Gruyère or Emmenthaler cheese, grated
>
> ½ cup whipping cream

Method:

1. Heat the butter in a heavy flameproof casserole.

2. Add the onions and garlic and sauté until the onions are a light, golden brown.

3. Stir in the flour and sauté for 2 minutes longer.

4. Then add the wine, sea salt, kelp, and thyme and simmer, uncovered, over a low heat for half-an-hour, stirring from time to time.

5. Next add the chicken stock, bring back to the boiling point, cover and cook in a preheated moderate oven, 350°F. for 2 hours.

6. Serve the soup in four small ovenproof soup bowls. Beat the eggs separately and add one to each serving, stirring it into the soup to mix well. Sprinkle with the Gruyére or Emmenthaler cheese and cook in the oven for 10 minutes longer.

7. Add 2 Tbsp. whipping cream to each serving. Serve immediately. Makes four servings.

NOTE: If desired, the eggs and whipped cream may be omitted; just use the cheese and return to the oven briefly.

◆◆◆◆◆

SEXUALLY TRANSMISSIBLE DISEASES

ITEM: "A deficiency of vitamin A can result in a . . . decreased resistance to infection." [V. E. Tyler et al., *Pharmacognosy* (Philadelphia: Lea & Febiger, 1988), p. 288)].

ITEM: "Carotenoids are a class of more than 500 yellow-to-red hued pigments, chemically related to vitamin A. Though found predominantly in green and yellow vegetables, they also color tomatoes, carrots, egg yolks, algae and even [fish] oil. Now, Japanese scientists working with cultured human cancer cells report . . . that . . . some of these nontoxic pigments fight cancers [and sexually transmissible diseases] by effectively putting malignant [and infective] cells to sleep and suppressing the expression of a gene that might otherwise foster tumor growth [or viral infection]." (*Science News*, Vol. 136, November 4, 1989, p. 294.)

◆◆◆◆

Baked Carrots

Ingredients:

8 carrots, washed and cut into strips	2 Tbsp. oil
½ cup chopped onion	2 Tbsp. lemon juice
	½ tsp. cinnamon
½ cup raisins	¼ tsp. cloves
1 apple, cored and cut into cubes	½ cup Granola
2 Tbsp. honey	

Method:

1. Place all ingredients in a shallow casserole, cover tightly, and bake at 375° F. for 45 minutes. Serves six.

◆◆◆◆◆

Vitamin A Delight

Ingredients:

½ cup olive oil	2 cloves of garlic
1 onion, sliced thin	1 bay leaf
1 cup plum tomatoes	6 sprigs of parsley
½ green bell pepper, chopped	½ tsp. dried chervil
½ cup chopped celery	1 lb. green beans, cooked until tender and drained
¼ cup water	¼ cup grated Swiss cheese
½ tsp. basil	
¼ cup marjoram	

Method:

1. In a skillet heat the oil, add the onion, and cook until golden brown.

2. Next add the tomatoes, green pepper, celery, water, basil, and marjoram.

3. Tie the garlic, bay leaf, parsley, and chervil in a small cheesecloth bag and add to the vegetables.

4. Simmer, uncovered, about 25 minutes. Then add the beans and continue simmering until they are hot.

5. Remove the spice bag and serve at once topped with cheese. Serves six.

◆◆◆◆◆

Squash Soup

Ingredients:

¼ cup virgin olive oil	1 lb. rutabagas, peeled and diced
4 medium onions, chopped	2 lb. Pontiac potatoes, peeled and cubed
2 tsps. thyme leaves	
½ tsp. ground nutmeg	

16 cups peeled, cubed	3½ quarts fish stock (made
banana, Hubbard, acorn	from boiling fish heads,
or Golden Acorn squash,	bones, and fish scraps
or pumpkin (7 lb.)	together)

Methods:

1. Heat oil in a 10-quart pan over medium-high heat. Add onions, thyme, and nutmeg and cook, stirring frequently, until onions are soft (about 15 minutes).

2. Next add rutabagas, potatoes, and squash; cook, stirring occasionally, until vegetables become tender (about 25 minutes).

3. Then pour in fish broth and bring to a boil over high heat; reduce heat, cover, and simmer until squash mashes easily (about 1¼ hours).

4. Cream vegetables and broth, a little bit at a time, in a blender or food processor until smooth. If made ahead, let cool; then cover and refrigerate until next day. Serves ten.

◆◆◆◆◆◆

SORE THROAT AND TONSILLITIS

ITEM: "[Hot] wine and capsicum [are useful] as gargle in some sore and malignant sore throats." [Samuel O. L. Potter, M.D. *Materia Medica, Pharmacy, and Therapeutics* (Philadelphia: P. Blakiston's Son & Co., 1906), p. 815]

Winter Greens and Potato Drink (I)

Ingredients:

1 lb. frozen mixed greens (mustard, collards, kale, escarole)

2 medium Pontiac (red) potatoes, unpeeled, scrubbed, quartered and thinly sliced

1 Tbsp. virgin olive oil

2 small dried chili peppers, seeds removed, torn into pieces

1 cup white wine

pinch of cayenne pepper powder

2 medium fresh tomatoes, chopped, or 1 16-oz. can, drained and chopped

2 cloves garlic, minced

1 tsp. whole peppercorns

half a lemon, unpeeled, quartered

Method:

1. Remove any leaves from greens that are yellow or wilted and remove any tough, fibrous stems. Chop the leaves, rinse them well, and set aside.

2. Cook potatoes in boiling, salted water until tender, for 10 minutes. Remove with a slotted spoon.

3. Next add the greens to the hot potato water and boil them for 7 minutes; then remove and drain them well.

4. Now put 1 dried chili pepper, 1 garlic clove, the peppercorns, and the lemon into the hot potato-chlorophyll broth and cook for another 10 minutes.

5. Remove them and discard. Finally, add the wine and pinch of cayenne pepper powder, cover, and simmer for 5 minutes.

6. Drink ½ cup of this while *warm,* gargling good with each mouthful taken before swallowing.

◆◆◆◆◆

Winter Greens and Potatoes (II)

Method:

1. Warm the olive oil over a medium heat in a wide, nonstick skillet and add the other chili pepper. When the oil is hot, add the potatoes, stir to coat them sufficiently, and cook for just 1 minute.

2. Next add the cooked greens, tomatoes, and other minced garlic clove. Continue cooking for another 7 minutes, breaking up the potatoes with a wooden spoon. Sprinkle with a touch of powdered cayenne to season. Serves four.

◆◆◆◆◆

SYSTEMIC LUPUS ERYTHEMATOSUS

ITEM: "Marine lipids [fish oils] might have a therapeutic effect on the glomerulonephritis of human systemic lupus erythematosus." (*Prostaglandis*, Vol. 30, July 1985, pp. 51–75).

◆◆◆◆◆

Grouper/Red Snapper Francaise

Chef Paul Buck notes: "This is a nice light recipe for the 'fried fish lover' as the egg acts as a gossimer skin. The fish does not absorb the grease like normal fried fish. You may top this fish with any of your favorite sauces or use my own sauce provencal."

Ingredients:

> 2 lb. grouper or snapper fillet (boneless/skinless)
> seasoned flour
> 3 beaten eggs
> lemon/lime wedges
> 8 oz. margarine

Method:

1. Dredge fillets of fish in seasoned flour, then in beaten egg.

2. Make sure the margarine is hot before adding. Fry until golden brown on both sides. Serve with lemon or lime wedges. Serves 2 to 3.

Sauce Provencal

Ingredients:

> 1½ lb. vine-ripened tomatoes
> (blanched/peeled/seeded)
> 4 oz. onions or shallots
> ½ clove garlic
> 1 sprig thyme
> 4 oz. white wine
> 1 bay leaf
> 2–3 oz. virgin olive oil
> salt and pepper to taste

Method:

1. Sauté onions and garlic together until tender but do not brown.
2. Add the diced tomatoes, thyme, bay leaf, white wine, and salt/pepper to taste.
3. Simmer until tender (about 25 minutes).
4. Top any cooked fish off with this sauce.

Cold Fish Salad

Ingredients:

4 peeled tomatoes sliced	1 hard boiled egg
4 boiled potatoes sliced	¼ pint apple cider vinegar
2 oz. celery cut julienne (french-fry) style	4 Romaine lettuce leaves
1 oz. blanched (in hot water) onion ring	1 small can salmon meat

Method:

1. Mix tomatoes, potatoes, celery, onion rings, and salmon.
2. Blend all of the above with apple cider vinegar marinade.
3. Dress on bed of Romaine lettuce.
4. Sprinkle with chopped or julienne of egg.

Garlic-Fish Cooking Oil

The reader should be cautioned that this cooking oil works better with seafoods and any vegetables that you don't mind imparting a strong fish flavor to; otherwise its use is somewhat limited with many other kinds of foods due to its marine taste. However, for giving lupus victims some theraupeutic relief due to its fish oil content, it's very good.

Ingredients:

1 pint virgin olive oil
2 cloves garlic

½ lb. of some type of *raw* oily fish
(mehaden, salmon, tuna, shark), coarsely chopped
2 sprigs of each fresh thyme, rosemary, and sage

Method:

1. Peel and thinly slice garlic.
2. Add to the oil with raw fish pieces and herbs.
3. Store in closed quart fruit jar in refrigerator for two weeks, shaking each day for 2 minutes. Strain and put into another jar, discarding fish and herbs. Use in salads and for cooking/baking purposes. One teaspoonful daily of this oil can also be taken as a useful food supplement, too.

One food which lupus victims should avoid is alfalfa sprouts, believe it or not. The nonprotein amino acid L-canavanine, a structural analog of L-arginine is found in high concentrations in alfalfa sprouts. When alfalfa sprouts were fed to mice genetically predisposed to autoimmune disease, it severely aggravated lupuslike autoimmune phenomena, according to the July 1985 issue of the *Canadian Journal of Physiology and Pharmacology.*

◆◆◆◆◆

TUBERCULOSIS

ITEM: "Restricted protein intake makes the body more susceptible to tuberculosis. Grafe reported that in Germany during the famine period following World War II, the incidence of infectious diseases increased only slightly but a particular increase in tuberculosis was observed." (*Deutsche Medezin Wochenschrift*, Vol. 75, p. 441).

The following recipes constitute a complete meal for tuberculosis victims. This dinner is not only high in protein and carbohydrates, but also contains a variety of culinary spices noted for both their flavor as well as antibiotic strength. This particular meal was especially planned with the medical adage in mind—"Food is your best medicine"—and a national best-seller of the same title by the late Henry G. Bieler, M.D. (New York: Random House, 1966).

◆◆◆◆◆

Rack of Lamb Dijon

Ingredients:

2 racks of lamb (french trimmed by the butcher)

1 tsp. dried rosemary

Dijon mustard

10 oz. fresh bread crumbs

1 tsp. chopped parsley

1 tsp. finely chopped garlic

2 oz. melted margarine

¼ tsp. thyme

mint jelly

Method:

1. Use enough Dijon mustard to coat the meat side of the lamb racks.

2. Mix together margarine, thyme, rosemary, garlic, parsley, and breadcrumbs. Then pack mixture on top of Dijon-covered lamb and roast in oven at 375°F. for about 25 minutes (or until medium rare). To serve just slice down between bone to have individual chops. Serves four.

◆◆◆◆◆

Fried Potato Curry

Ingredients:

1½ lb. potatoes

4 oz. grated onions

10 cloves garlic

½ tsp. turmeric powder

1 tsp. white cumin seeds

1 Tbsp. coriander seeds

12 peppercorns

½ oz. almonds

2 tsp. salt

½ pint yogurt

½ tsp. garam masala

1 lb. ghee

½ oz. fresh ginger root

1 tsp. cayenne pepper

1 tsp. poppy seeds

6 cloves

2 brown cardamoms

½ oz. dessicated coconut

5 green cardamoms

pinches of nutmeg and mace to taste

¼ pint water

1 tsp. chopped fresh coriander leaves or parsley sprigs

2 finely cut green chilies

Method:

1. Select potatoes that are the size of walnuts. Peel and prick all over with a fork and soak in 1¼ pints ice water and 1 tsp. salt for 30 minutes. Dry them with clean cloth.

2. Heat 1 lb. ghee and fry the potatoes on medium heat until brown. While potatoes are frying, roast coriander seeds on a hot griddle and sift the skins. Likewise roast the poppy seeds, coconut, cumin seeds, cloves, peppercorns, brown cardamoms, the mace, and nutmeg. Grind these along with ginger, garlic and a little water until a fine paste is formed. Note: In the event that green or brown cardamoms, fresh coriander, and fresh ginger root aren't readily available, then the powdered forms may be substituted. In this case, one would use 1 tsp. ginger powder, 1 tsp. coriander, and 2 tsp. cardamom. They would be added at the end with the other ground ingredients into a little water to form a suitable paste.

3. Heat 4 oz. ghee and brown the grated onions. Remove pan from heat, add cayenne pepper, turmeric, crushed green cardamoms, salt and ground paste to the browned onions. Then cook on slow heat. Note: See Candidiasis, Whole Cauliflower recipe, for instructions on making ghee.

4. Beat ½ pint yogurt lightly and add a little of it at a time to the mixture until half of it is used up. Add the fried potatoes and cook for another 5 minutes. Then add the remaining yogurt and ½ pint of hot water. Keep it in the oven or cook on slow heat for 20 minutes longer. Serves three.

◆◆◆◆◆

Once a Year Salad

Ingredients:

4 large vine-ripened tomatoes
(blanched in hot water, peeled)

1 large or 2 small vidalia
(sweet) onions

2 cloves garlic

½ pint virgin olive oil

½ pint red wine vinegar

1 tsp. fresh chopped basil

coarsely granulated kelp (a seaweed) to taste

Method:

1. Thickly slice tomatoes and layer with thinly sliced onions.

2. Combine olive oil, vinegar, crushed garlic, chopped basil, and kelp together. Mix well and pour over salad.

3. Then marinate in refrigerator for 4 hours. If desired, add quartered radishes, green bell pepper rings (and the chopped inner seed core of the pepper), and finely snipped fresh watercress.

◆◆◆◆◆

Appendix:
A Guide to
Companies and Their
Products

Albi Imports Ltd.
7188 Curragh Ave.
Burnaby, B.C.
Canada V5J 4V9

Albi Imports Ltd.
19029 36th Ave. West
Unit B
Linnwood, WA 98036

Heavenly Grade Korean Ginseng (extract, powder, tea)
Li Chung Yun Siberian Ginseng (capsules and liquid extract)
Jing Sam Jung Herbal Tonic
Li Chung Yun Kan-Ts'ao Chinese Licorice Root
Quan Yin Dang Quei
Li Chung Yun Foo-Ti-Teng
Rocky Mountain Multi-Minerals and Vitamin C
Li Chung Yun Gotu Kola
Li Chung Yun Herbal Laxative 1
Li Chung Yun L.B.C. (lower bowel capsules) 2
Li Chung Yun Super Compound 3 (energy)
Li Chung Yun Pei Pa li Capsules 4 (colds)
Li Chung Yun Nirvana 5 (stress)
Li Chung Yun Sum Yuen Li Capsules 6 (heart)
Li Chung Yun A & R Capsules 7 (arthritis)
Li Chung Yun K & B Capsules 8 (kidney and bladder)

Li Chung Yun Shigatze 8 (obesity)
Li Chung Yun Tau-Fa Yuen Capsules 11 (hair)
Li Chung Yun Natural Herb Fiber 12
Li Chung Yun Astragalus 14 (immunity)
Li Chung Yun Po-Chai Capsules 15 (digestion)
Li Chung Yun Hy-Po Capsules 16 (hypoglycemia)
Li Chung Yun "L" 18 (liver)
Li Chung Yun Antler Horn 19 (male tonic)
Quan Yin "For Ladies Only" Formulas I and II
Quan Yin Herbal Energy Formulas: Tiger (men) and Tigress
   (women)
Li Chung Yun Ginkgo Biloba Capsules
Li Chung Yun Super Rei Shi (medicinal mushrooms)
Li Chung Yun Dragon Balm (aching back and sore muscles)

These are some of the most popular herbal formulas in the Orient and may be found in most Chinese herb shops in North America or ordered directly from the exclusive importer of them.

Anthropological Research Center
John Heinerman, Director
P. O. Box 11471
Salt Lake City, UT 84147
1-(801)-521-8824

Garlic for Health by Benjamin Lau, M.D.
Garlic in Nutrition & Medicine by Robert I-San Lin, Ph.D.

To receive copies of the two garlic books free, send 25 30-cent stamps or $7.50 to cover postage,

"Foods and Supplements for Healthier Living"
A two-hour video cassette by Dr. Heinerman; $39.95

"Herbal First Aid," "Herbs for Health Problems," and "Spices as Food & Medicine"
A lecture series of three audio tapes (5½ hours) by Dr. Heinerman; $29.95

Bronson Pharmaceuticals Co.
4526 Rinetti Lane
La Cañada, CA 91011

Arth-Relief Cream

Custom-Made Formulas
P.O. Box 1623
Salt Lake City, UT 84110-1623

Actractylodes tea
Dandelion and Chicory Coffee Substitute
Stevia (an herbal sweetener)
Rex's Wheat Germ Oil
Flaxseed
Sarsaparilla
Slippery elm
Herbal Arthritus Preparation
White Willow
Chaparral
Yarrow
Ayurvedic Anti-Smoking Extract
Assorted Spices

East/West Wellness Center
Agua Calente Val Paraiso
KM 13.5 Sta. Fely
Del Tren Tijuana Tegate Sta Fe & Ave.
Ferrocarril Baja, Calif. (Mexico)
011-526-682-5409/2722

East/West Wellness Center
2036 Dairy Mart Road, Suite 128-122
San Ysidro, CA 92173
1-(800)-233-1360

Frontier Cooperative Herbs,
P.O. Box 299,
Norway, IA 52318

Many varieties of black and green teas

Great American Natural Products, Inc.
4121 16th Street North
St. Petersburg, FL 33703
1-(800)-323-4372

AquaVite Vitamin-Mineral Supplement
Super Herbal C
Watercress powder
Pantothenic acid
PABA cream
Selenium
Super Energy
Buffered C
Natural Calm
Mag/Calm
Garlic oil
Allereze
Sinese
Black and Green Teas

Nature's Way Products, Inc.
10 Mountain Springs
Springville, UT 84663

Cold Care
Allerex
Broncrin
Thisilyn

Old Amish Herbs
4141 Irish St. North
St. Petersburg, FL 33703

FarmLax
Resist-All

Pines, Inc.
P.O. Box 1107
Lawrence, KS 66044
1-(800)-642-PINE

Bulk cereal grasses
Beet Powder

Pure Herbs, Ltd.
32101 Townley
Madison Heights, MI 48071
(313)-585-6922
Specializes in herbal fluid Extracts

Irish moss
Dulse
Valerian
Wild lettuce
Rosemary
Chamomile
Indian tobacco
Goldenseal
Chaparral
Echinacea
St. Johnswort
Prickly ash
Peppermint oil
Herbal adjustment

Quest Vitamins USA, Inc.
1163 Chess Dr., Suite F
Foster City, CA 94404
(415)-349-1233

Nutri-Health Data Computer Software
Electro-C Powder
Vitamin A
Vitamin B-complex
Powdered mineral supplement
Vitamins D and E

Wakunaga of America Co., Ltd.
23501 Madero
Mission Viejo, CA 92691
California 1-(800)-544-5800
Nationwide 1-(800)-421-2998

Kyolic odorless garlic
Kyo-Dophilus
Kyo-Green
Goldenseal root

Index of Specific Diseases

General Index

A

Acne, remedy for, 146
Acorns, and tuberculosis, 285
Acupuncture, quitting smoking, 113
Addison's disease, 38–40
  and cholesterol, 39–40
  preventive care, 38–39
  symptoms of, 38
Adenoids, swollen, remedy for, 146–47
AIDS, 17, 255–67
  dietary control of, 259–63
  external signs of, 258–59
  and immune system, 256–57
  increase in spread of, 255
  power diet recipes, 290–92
  virus in, 257–59
Alanine, sleep induction, 135
Alcoholism, 80–86
  good nutrition against, 81–86
  and immune system, 80–81
  nutritional supplements for, 83–84
Alkalinizing diet, quitting smoking, 140–41
Allergies
  allergy-inducing bacteria, 209–11
  and chronic fatigue syndrome, 225–26
  and chronic ulcerative colitis, 44
  elimination of, case examples, 212–16
  nature of, 208–12
  and rheumatoid arthritis, 66
  and shyness, 208–9
  teas/soups for alleviation of, 294–96
  See also specific types of allergies

Amphetamines, 90–91
  natural alternatives to, 91
  psychosis induced by, 91
Angel dust, 103–4
Angelica root, and rheumatoid arthritis, 68
Anger
  effects of, 263–64, 265
  getting rid of, 265–67
  and immune system, 264–65
Ankylosing spondylitis, 40–43
  areas affected by, 40
  and positive attitude, 41–42
  symptoms of, 40
  Vitamin C, 42–43
Anxiety attacks, 86–90
  epidemic stress syndrome, 87–90
Appendicitis, cure for attack of, 149–50
Asparagus, and tuberculosis, 286
Asthma
  characteristics of, 217–18
  soup for, 297
Atherosclerosis
  dietary control of, 184–86
  and ginger, 192–93
  and onions, 195–97
  viral link to, 180–83
Atherosclerosis, 176–86
  in young people, 177–78
Atractylodes tea, and colds, 7
Autoimmune diseases
  Addison's disease, 38–40
  ankylosing spondylitis, 40–43
  celiac disease, 43–44
  chronic ulcerative colitis, 44–46
  Crohn's disease, 46–48
  diabetes mellitus, 48–55
  Graves's disease, 55–57